THE TROUBLE WITH
DOCTORS

The Trouble with Doctors

ISBN: 979-8-9883724-0-0 (paperback)
         979-8-9883724-1-7 (ebook)

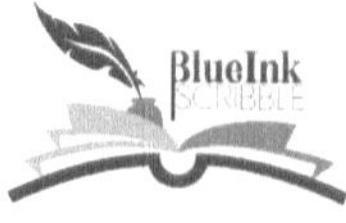

Printed in the United States of America

THE TROUBLE WITH
DOCTORS

FRAUD AND DECEIT IN MEDICINE

DR JOHN "JOCK" ANDERSON
AND HELEN WEINEL

First, do no harm.

Primum non nocere. Above all, do no harm!

Thomas Inman, later attributed to Hippocrates.

TABLE OF CONTENTS

PREFACE

Physicians or surgeons use their experience, wisdom, knowledge, and intuition to bring about the best outcomes for the patients under their care. It can be a delicate balancing act in which they must consider the possible hurt that an intervention might cause as well as its potential benefits.

Is it better to do something or to do nothing at all?

A quick Google search of the words "First do no harm" or "Do no harm" produces a blog post written by Robert H. Shmerling, MD, senior faculty editor, Harvard Health, on June 22, 2020, for Harvard Health Publishing at Harvard Medical School.

Shmerling proposes several hypothetical situations in which the "first, do no harm" dictum is hard to apply due to the uncertainty of estimates of risk and benefit. He sums it up beautifully: "Ultimately, it is a reminder that doctors should neither overestimate their capacity to heal, nor underestimate their capacity to cause harm."

GERMINATION

This book arose from my knowledge of a small number of doctors who were not behaving in a professional or proper manner. As I read about them, I found that, more and more, I was astonished at the extent of some offenders. The book, as far as I can tell, is fact. It is from numerous sources, including library records of medical journals, newspaper reports, manuals and law case records, internet publications, and occasionally, my observations. Other than the last-mentioned, everything can be found through the references given with each chapter. Names have been changed only sometimes where the individual's privacy required protection and did not affect the core of the tale.

ACKNOWLEDGEMENTS

I acknowledge contributions to the manuscript from Mrs Janette Anderson, Mr David Russell, Dr Raema Lancaster, Dr Paul Lancaster, Mr David Rittie, Ms Patricia Lewis, Dr Peter Crowe, Dr Brian MacGregor, Mr Keith Weinel, Mr Ian Anderson. In particular, I wish to acknowledge, as my co-author, Mrs Helen Weinel, for her assistance with the bibliographies, editing and as the author of Chapter Thirteen. Without her enthusiasm and industry the book would never have been completed.

THE CO-AUTHOR

Helen Weinel

Born in Sydney, Australia, Helen studied Nursing at Charles Sturt University (CSU) – Mitchell, Bathurst gaining a Diploma of Applied Science (Nursing), R.N. Certificate between 1987 and 1990. Moving back to Sydney, she undertook her graduate year at Repatriation General Hospital (RGH), Concord, N.S.W., before joining the Royal Alexandra Hospital for Children (RAHC), Camperdown, N.S.W., to gain experience as a first year Registered Nurse in a Level IV 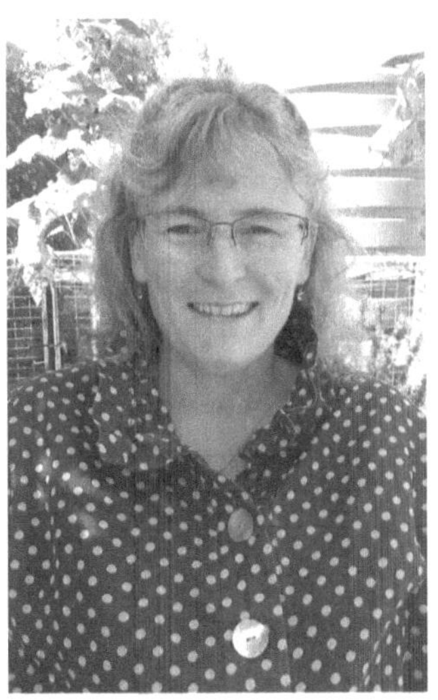 Neonatal Intensive Care Unit as part of a multi – disciplinary team caring for infants with life – threatening medical and surgical conditions. This led to the completion of the Neonatal Intensive Care (NICU) course through Royal Alexandra Hospital for Children (RAHC) Royal Prince Alfred Hospital (RPAH), Camperdown NSW, with clinical placements at King George V Hospital (KGV) for Mothers and Babies, where she was born twenty-two years earlier. Helen was accepted into the Certificate in Midwifery course at Royal Hospital for Women (RHW), Paddington, inner city Sydney, NSW., the last hospital-based course before the training moved to tertiary institutions.

After moving to South Australia in 1994, Helen joined the staff of a busy hospital in the north suburbs of Adelaide, in an especially low socio- economic area on a year- long Graduate Midwife Program as a means of consolidating midwifery knowledge and practise.

A longstanding interest in Childbirth Education led to her applying for her current role, of Antenatal / Parenting Educator, completing the two-year part-time Graduate Diploma in Childbirth Education (Grad Dip CBE) through Birth International, Sydney, in 2006. Calmbirth® training seemed an obvious next step. Once accredited, in 2010, as a Calmbirth® educator through Australian Calmbirth® organisation run by midwife, Peter Jackson, Helen built a business that drew upon her antenatal and parenting education knowledge and continued for seven years.

CHAPTER ONE

DR. RICARDO ASCH— EGG THIEF

Prologue

Renee Ballou hardly slept that night in 1987, but she woke early the next day. It was a bright and calm morning, but Renee did not notice. She did not care. She was very excited because at last she was booked for the gamete intrafallopian transfer (GIFT) procedure, which would be carried out by the famous *Dr. Ricardo Asch* himself, the inventor of the technique. She had endured days of painful injections, blood tests, and ultrasounds in preparation for this day and had fasted from the previous midnight, so there was no need for breakfast. She was to report to the Garden Grove Hospital Medical Center in Orange County, California, by 7:00 a.m. for the laparoscopy to collect eggs from her ovaries and place them in her fallopian tubes along with her husband's sperm, collected previously. Renee was there in plenty of time, and the GIFT procedure was carried out at 11:00 a.m. After the operation, as Renee was awakening in the recovery room, Dr. Asch was by her bedside, and he leaned over her and, with a gentle pat on her head, whispered, "Renee, I just know that you are pregnant."

Renee learned a few days later that she was not pregnant.

Eight years later, Renee Ballou discovered that at least one egg of the seventeen that Asch took that day had been given without her permission to another woman who had a baby boy. Renee Ballou was furious. "He basically took my hopes and dreams and gave them to someone else," she fumed. "He was playing God." Now she is haunted by the possibility that some of the other seventeen eggs that he took that day have been given to other women. "And I never questioned him. I wanted a baby. To me, he was a god," she lamented, her voice cracking.[1]

Dr. Ricardo Asch

I first met Ricardo Asch in Kyoto, Japan, at the International Society for In Vitro Fertilization Scientific meeting in 1993, where he was an invited speaker and I was a humble delegate. Ricardo was at the height of his academic fame and widely recognized. Delegates at the meeting were hosted by the Japanese organizers at their courteous and generous best. We were taken to the best venues, bathing houses, and restaurants. I was privileged to dine with Ricardo on several occasions, and I found him to be charming, amusing, even humble. I admired him greatly. Little did I know what he was doing. In retrospect, I am not sure that he knew either.

Ricardo Hector Asch was born on October 26, 1947, in Buenos Aires, Argentina. His parents were academically high achievers, his mother being a lawyer and his father a successful orthopedic surgeon. Both were professors. Asch graduated in medicine at the University of Buenos Aires in 1971. The peer-reviewed medical literature shows that Asch's first scientific paper was published in the *Journal of Reproduction and Fertility* in 1972 although it had been accepted for publication by that journal on November 2, 1971.[2] He had gone into print almost as soon as he graduated, and it is interesting that even at that early stage his interest was in reproduction, albeit in the rat. In 1980, Asch was granted a visa to live in the USA and subsequently furthered his studies with internships at the Department of Endocrinology and Human Reproduction at the University of Georgia under the supervision of the eminent Canadian *Dr. Robert B. Greenblatt* who had been at the forefront of the development of the sequential oral contraceptive pill. Later, Asch moved to the University of Texas Health Science Center at San Antonio under *Dr. Carl J. Pauerstein*, one of whose principal research interests was the mechanism by which the human egg travels down the fallopian tube. This, perhaps, sparked Asch's later interest in developing the technique known as gamete intrafallopian transfer (GIFT).

By 1998, he was credited with 201 peer-reviewed scientific papers (although he claims 225 in his CV on his website). Fifty-one of these were as the first author between 1976 and 1993 and 105 as last author between 1972 and 1998. The English-language scientific literature shows no more publications since then. Curiously, in medical literature, the first author is usually regarded as the one whose concept it may have been but who also carried out most of the work or was its driving force. Most of Asch's papers as first author occurred earlier in his career and as last author later in his career. The last author is usually the head of the department or the supervisor. The practice of adding the senior person's name as the last author is known as gift authorship, and it reflects the rising status as one's career advances.

Artificial Reproductive Technology

The treatment of human infertility took a huge leap forward when the first babies were born in 1979 from the treatment known as *in vitro fertilization* (IVF).[3] One of the common causes of infertility is damage to or blockage of the fallopian tubes, and IVF was developed to overcome this as it bypasses the fallopian tubes. Fertilization occurs typically in the fallopian tube when the oocyte (egg) is met by a sperm. With IVF, the egg is collected surgically and placed together with prepared sperm in an incubator usually for two to five days. Great care must be exercised handling the gametes (eggs and sperm) when they are outside the body. The atmosphere, temperature, and culture medium in which they are kept must be tightly controlled. Much research has gone into identifying the constitution of the culture medium required to care for the gametes and embryos in the incubators. When an egg is seen to have been fertilized, it is called a zygote, and it can be returned to the uterus through the cervix without an anesthetic or to the fallopian tubes by laparoscopy. If implantation follows, the patient becomes pregnant. Unfortunately, pregnancy often does not follow no matter how much care is taken or how many cycles are undertaken. Repeated failures often end up in despair.

Many women whose fallopian tubes appear normal and indeed have no known cause for their infertility still do not conceive, and it was in this scenario that Ricardo Asch may have found his knowledge of tubal transport of gametes and embryos so useful. The theory was that the egg would have the best chance of being fertilized if it met the sperm in the environment of the fallopian tube where it would also be at the correct temperature. The GIFT technique involves the collection of sperm in advance by masturbation so that it can be prepared for transfer. The ovaries are stimulated by injecting fertility drugs so that more eggs than usual will be available for collection. When a girl is born, her ovaries contain many hundreds of thousands of undeveloped eggs. Most decay even before she reaches puberty, and likewise, most of the remainder die after puberty as they lose an internal hormonal struggle to become dominant and make themselves available to be fertilized. Only about four hundred eggs reach maturity in the life of a woman; the remainder dies and is, therefore, lost. Fertility drugs are designed to prevent this loss of eggs by blocking the hormonal struggle that causes the loss so that more are available for fertilization. In gamete intrafallopian transfer, a general anesthetic is required so that laparoscopy can be performed to collect eggs. After inspection, under the same anesthetic, a small number of eggs is selected and returned to the fallopian tubes along with prepared sperm. Any eggs not returned during one cycle can be saved after fertilization with stored sperm, hopefully, to be frozen for future use. It was not possible in those days to freeze unfertilized eggs.

Gamete Intrafallopian Transfer

In 1984, Dr. Ricardo Asch reported his success with the new technique called gamete intrafallopian transfer, conveniently abbreviated to the acronym GIFT.[4] Further successes followed shortly with a successful birth.[5] The pregnancy rates from GIFT in most clinics exceeded those from IVF, so many women were offered GIFT in preference to IVF, provided their fallopian tubes were normal. As the same laboratory facilities were not required for GIFT as for IVF to care for embryos, fertility clinics everywhere switched to GIFT as the preferred procedure. GIFT became standard practice for those couples who had failed IVF cycles, provided they had normal fallopian tubes.[6]

GIFT also appeared to be consistent with Catholic doctrine because fertilization occurs within the body, and there is no decision required about whether to discard or to keep eggs. Asch and *Balmaceda*, a colleague, visited the Vatican in November 1986. While in Rome, Asch consulted *Dr. Nicolas Garcia*, professor of gynecology and obstetrics at a Catholic university and helped the Gemelli Hospital at the Vatican to start a GIFT program. Asch reported that they treated thirty-five to forty women and that Catholic Church officials were "very much in favour of the GIFT technique."[7,8,9] Nobody seems to have been concerned that collection of sperm for GIFT is usually by masturbation, which is generally disapproved of by the Catholic Church. Asch, however, reassured couples who wished to respect the Catholic Church doctrine that they could collect the sperm in a perforated condom during sexual intercourse and he would keep it separated from the egg with an air bubble until they were placed in the fallopian tubes, thereby ensuring that fertilization occurred within the body.[7,8]

Always the entrepreneur!

Dr. José Balmaceda

At the time of his publication on GIFT in *The Lancet* in 1984, Asch was working in San Antonio, Texas. Coincidentally, Dr. José Balmaceda was employed there also. They were later to become partners in the Center for Reproductive Health (CRH) at the University of California Irvine Medical Center along with *Dr. Sergio Stone*.[10]

José Pedro Balmaceda was born on August 22, 1948, in Santiago, Chile. His mother, Juanita, owned a women's boutique in the city; and his father, José, was a successful businessman, owning several timber mills. He grew up with five sisters who remained in Santiago all their lives. Balmaceda attended the San Ignatius College Preparatory School where he met Sergio Stone, his future partner at the Center for Reproductive Health fertility clinic in the University of California Irvine Medical Center.[10]

In 1974, Balmaceda graduated from Catholic University Medical School and became a resident at the University of Chile Hospital in obstetrics and gynecology.[10] In 1975,

Balmaceda and his wife, Veronica, were accused of hiding political dissidents in their home and were forced with their two children to flee into political exile from the totalitarian rule of *General Augusto Pinochet*. They escaped to Denmark, and one year later, the University of Texas recruited Balmaceda to its medical facility in San Antonio where he completed his obstetrics and gynecology residency in 1980.[10] The following year, the Rockefeller Foundation awarded him a fellowship in reproductive endocrinology, and he began a close working relationship with fellow Dr. Ricardo Asch. Balmaceda's reputation soared, and he was invited to present his fertility research in places as diverse as Kenya, Switzerland, Israel, France, Italy, Indonesia, Korea, and Venezuela.[10]

Asch and Balmaceda opened a clinic in 1986 at the American Medical International Facility in the Garden Grove Hospital Medical Center in Orange County, California, staffed by the university, and they opened another at Saddleback Memorial Medical Center in Laguna Hills, also in Orange County, in 1989.[11]

Dr. Sergio Stone

Hilary Gilson in *The Embryo Project Encyclopedia* reports that a year later (1990), Asch and Balmaceda closed the Garden Grove clinic and, to the university's delight, opened a new clinic, the Center of Reproductive Health (CRH) at the University of California at Irvine (UCI) where they were joined by Dr. Sergio Stone who was previously known to Balmaceda. They had gone to school together at the San Ignatius Jesuit School in Santiago.[10,11] Stone was from a family of lawyers; his father was a judge. He had arrived at UCI in 1978 as the recipient of a Ford Foundation scholarship and was already established in the field of reproductive endocrinology.[10] Stone had organized for all three of them to become partners in the Center for Reproductive Health (CRH) at University of California at Irvine (UCI).[10,11] The university gave the trio space in a new medical pavilion, providing all the staff.[12]

Life Was Good

They soon became extremely busy, handling five hundred to seven hundred cycles a year. Couples came from all over, some with bundles of cash, buoyed by the hope of dreams fulfilled by the new technique. Earnings were reported to reach $4.5 million between January 1992 and August 1994, of which 10 percent went to the university.[12] The university was delighted to have this prestigious group move into their hospital. It would improve the reputation of the hospital, but more than that, it would bring much-needed cash. It was no secret at the time that the hospital was grossly short of cash, mainly because it was treating a substantial proportion of Orange County's indigenous population. Indigent patients were sometimes turned away on the grounds of overcrowding. The hospital administrator, *Mary Piccione*, made it clear to the UCI regents that the hospital was in financial trouble. It would not be unusual for patients at the CRH to be responsible for doctor's fees to be over $10,000 for a treatment cycle. Under an agreement with the doctors, 10 percent of their income would be paid to the university as well as $2,000 for each use of the operating theater. The university was therefore delighted to offer favorable contracts to the doctors. Under the agreement, the university paid almost all the doctors' costs of their private practices. It was an arrangement that suited all parties.

Asch carried out most of the procedures at CRH, while Balmaceda worked mostly at Saddleback and filled in at CRH when on call. Dr. Stone did not carry out any operative procedures but did share in profits. When Asch was not in the clinic, he was traveling or lecturing, attracting business to his clinic. He bought mansions in Del Mar and in the gated community of Big Canyon in Newport Beach where he lived with wife Silvia, four daughters, and an adopted son. Dr. Asch owned at least five cars, including a BMW convertible, and rode around town in a red Ferrari with a number plate "DR GIFT." He indulged a lifelong passion with racehorses and valuable artworks, including a Salvador Dalí sculpture. He rubbed shoulders with heads of state and celebrities. He was personally friendly with *Andre Agassi* and has been seen in his private box at Wimbledon.[12]

In 1992, Asch started a company called Asch Entertainment to manage the horse business and, in addition, to produce sports apparel and videos, with projected sales by Dun and Bradstreet of $500,000 per annum. Along with Agassi and others, the company produced a video named "Attack: Andre Agassi and *Nick Bollettieri*."[12] In January 1994, he was named among the seventy top doctors in Orange County from a nationwide survey by doctors themselves.[12] He was mentioned again in the *Orange County Register* that year. Another report describes how a patient with leukemia had her eggs collected by Asch, fertilized with donor sperm and frozen for use later, after recovering from leukemia and chemotherapy. It is a glowing description of how reproductive technologies could be used by Asch to help couples with little hope.

A very much abbreviated curriculum vitae of Dr. Ricardo Asch is quoted below from his own website:

In 1991 Dr Asch returned to his native Argentina to receive the title of Honorary Professor at the Universidad de Buenos Aires. In 1993 he was named Professor of the Department of Reproductive Medicine at the University of California in San Diego. In 1994 he was privileged to be named Doctor Honoris Causa in Medicine at the University of Genoa, Italy.

As a Principal Investigator, Dr Asch, successfully obtained for the Universities where he worked multiple levels of support for research from governmental agencies, private organizations and pharmaceutical companies, amounting to over 2,550,737 U.S. dollars. The NIH (National Institutes of Health of the USA) awarded individual research grants to Dr Asch to investigate the effects of drug abuse in reproduction and pregnancy.

During his professional career, Dr Asch is proud to have educated and trained over 100 fellows from over 20 different countries. This global connection has created a network of internationally recognized fertility specialists. Many occupy major positions in a variety of health organizations.

Dr Asch has been a prolific researcher and a scientific author. He has published six books, 225 scientific articles in peer-reviewed prestigious international journals, 349 abstracts and posters in International Scientific Conferences, 25 invited manuscripts and authored 60 chapters in books of Biology of Reproduction.

Among the thirty-seven prizes and awards received by Dr Asch nationally and internationally, the following stand out: One of the top 37 physicians in Orange County, California in 1993 and 1994. In 2003 he received the A PART (Association of Private Clinics of Assisted Reproductive Techniques) award in Tokyo, Japan. In 2004 he was named as an Extraordinary member of Cecolfes in Bogota, Colombia.

Dr Asch has obtained licenses to practice medicine in Argentina, Mexico, Italy and USA.[13]

Although it is from his own website, it is an impressive CV even if only half of it were correct. Again, from his website:

> Dr Asch also developed other essential techniques for the treatment of both male and female infertility such as MESA (microsurgical epidydimal sperm aspiration). This technique aspirated the sperm from infertile men directly from his testes; something never thought possible before. Another technique created was ZIFT (zygote intrafallopian transfer), one of many methods he designed to stimulate ovarian function to produce healthy oocytes, particularly with the use of GnRH analogues.[13]

Developments in Artificial Reproductive Technologies

There is no doubt that Ricardo Asch had a brilliant mind and was always on the lookout for new developments. He was among the first to help men who were infertile due to congenital absence of the vas deferens by aspirating sperm microsurgically and using the sperm to fertilize the egg. Since IVF was first successfully described, numerous technical developments have occurred to improve the results.[14] Eggs can be fertilized before transfer to the fallopian tubes. This can be done by placing them together to fertilize the oocyte, which becomes a zygote, and transferring it to the fallopian tube (ZIFT) or by intracytoplasmic sperm injection where a single sperm is captured under a microscope and injected directly into an egg (ICSI).[14] These techniques make it more difficult for us to understand what might have happened in the clinic. Asch was among the first to use (allegedly donated) eggs to treat menopausal women. His reputation was spread not only in the United States through the popular press but also internationally through the scientific literature. But not all was well in the clinic.

Audits

After a theft of $4,600 from the center, an employee who was suspected of taking the money told university auditors in February 1992 that "there are problems with the eggs." The audit also disclosed severe failings in financial record-keeping and security. But university *executive vice chancellor Sidney H. Golub* said auditors were unable to confirm the "vague, unsubstantiated" rumor about the eggs.[12] "The auditors had asked the doctors, who stated that it was not true." Another audit in 1993 found weaknesses in operating procedures, internal accounting, and inadequate staff supervision. Auditors also found that documents and some files were missing, and employees were unable to locate them.[12]

Then in February 1994, office manager *Marilyn Killane* challenged the use of Massone, a fertility drug that had not been approved by the Food and Drug Administration (FDA). It had been imported by Asch from Argentina where it was approved. She accused Asch of importing Massone from Argentina and giving it to patients. She also noted that center doctors were keeping cash receipts that should have been reported to the university. When university auditors investigated, they again heard rumors of exchanging of patients' eggs. Again, Golub explained that the auditors found "no specific information that could be investigated."[12] The university seemed reluctant to listen to the auditors.

Still, the rumors persisted, and on July 18, 1994, there was another complaint. This time the warnings came from a much higher level: *Debra Krahel*, the senior associate director of ambulatory care at UCI. But Golub claimed that Krahel's letter alleging numerous problems at the center made only "vague" references to egg misuse and she did not appear to have firsthand knowledge.[12]

Rumblings of Discontent

Meanwhile, life could not be much better for Ricardo, and as is so often the case when people in power think of themselves as untouchable, he did not notice that his staff were slowly becoming disgruntled by his repeated delays in attending to patients, sometimes leaving them anesthetized in theaters for up to forty-five minutes while he took phone calls from his horse trainer *Robert Hess Jr.*[15] On other occasions, he failed to attend to his patients altogether by canceling treatment cycles without notice to attend to his passion on the racetrack. *Norbert Giltner*, one of Asch's theater nurses, said of Asch, "He once told us that he was already famous for GIFT. Now he wanted to be famous for winning the Kentucky Derby." The staff sarcastically described his horses as the "Alpo Express" because they lost so often. Stone, too, was unpopular because of his explosive temper, sometimes accusing them of being "complete imbeciles," throwing charts and pounding his fists on the table.[15]

It soon became apparent that irregularities had been occurring as far back as 1987 at Garden Grove where it was estimated two-thirds of the egg swapping occurred.[15] As early as 1991, funds had gone missing, and audits revealed that there had been money handling and procedural irregularities. This motivated Giltner to divulge his suspicions of egg transfers to *Toula Batshoun*, the clinic manager, who informed the auditor of improper egg use. She alleged that Asch had destroyed the evidence when she had confronted him, but the formal reports of the audit dismissed the claims and emphatically approved of the clinic. These were the first failures of the university to take definitive action about serious ethical lapses.[15,16]

Krahel was sent on leave as she could not be dismissed under California whistleblower laws.[11] In 1995, she signed a confidentiality agreement with the university and was paid almost $500,000 for alleged distress caused by the university. Two other whistleblowers were paid almost $350,000,[11,17,18,19] but she and other whistleblowers had already contacted the *Orange County Register* with their complaints. It was too late; the cat was out of the bag. Asch was mentioned in the *Orange County Register* only twice in 1994, but he was mentioned 169 times in 1995 in the *Register* and over fifty times in the *Los Angeles Times*.

Another Audit

In late 1994, UCI Medical Center requested an independent audit of "clinical, fiscal and management practices." They were concerned about a discrepancy in the financial returns to which they were entitled under their agreement.[20,21]

In October 1994, the auditors *Peat Marwick* found that

1. Asch and Stone had failed to report cash income,
2. Asch and Balmaceda submitted false insurance claims,
3. the clinic required employees to work at non-UCI facilities but charged the university for their time, and
4. Asch, Stone, and Balmaceda operated a nonlicensed operating room at the UCI clinic.

Many patients attended the clinic for treatment with bundles of cash. According to at least four former employees, those payments were not recorded as income on logs known as day sheets. Instead, they were recorded as "adjustments" rather than payments, an accounting device that auditors stated enabled the doctors to reduce the amount of their reportable income to the university and keep the difference. At the end of the day, either Dr. Asch or Dr. Stone was given an envelope of cash, which they would sign for. The auditor stated, "Each month the physicians would split the cash amongst themselves." Balmaceda's lawyer, *Patrick Moore*, said the doctors began taking the cash after a break-in at the office and that all the money had been accounted for. "The reason that the doctors started to take the cash in 1992 was that $4,600 had been stolen from the office while under the care of the University. The policy of taking the cash was so that no university employee could touch it." When auditors checked the day sheets provided for January 1992 to December 1993, they determined that about $167,000 was collected in cash and given to the doctors. From January 1992 to August 1994, $5.4 million was deposited in the first account but only $4.6 million was reported as income to the UCI according to the auditors. The doctors explained that the apparent $800,000 discrepancy might have included funds the university was not entitled to under an agreement that obliged doctors to pay UCI about 11 percent of their professional fees. In January 1995, the auditors noted that the doctors took in an additional $1 million that they did not report to the university.[20] It seems that instead of the staff taking the cash, the doctors took it!

The auditors also found when they examined the records that most procedures were described as cyst aspirations rather than egg removals—even when, in some cases, a patient's chart listed the number of eggs harvested. Cyst aspirations, which are manually like egg removals, attract an insurance rebate, whereas egg harvesting did not. This, therefore, would represent an offense against the insurance company.[10,15,17,20,21]

Egg Theft

Then in September 1994, things really began to heat up when university officials received yet another complaint. This time it was a letter from an attorney representing three whistleblowers, showing officials how eggs were allegedly being stolen at the center and details of other misdeeds.[22] Only then, Golub caved in and admitted that UCI had enough information to appoint a clinical panel of three UC doctors to investigate.[23] So far, questions of impropriety had mostly concerned fiscal matters; and until now, whispers of illegal drug misuse and egg mishandling were rumors only until National Institutes of Health investigators found alleged violations of human research protocols. Research at the clinic was suspended by UCI. In March of that year, the three independent physicians in committee confirmed that, in at least two instances, doctors at the clinic had taken human eggs without consent and transferred them to other women also without their consent or knowledge. They found, however, that there was evidence in a three-week period that approximately thirty more patients at the two clinics had been involved in unapproved egg transfers. Inappropriate procedures may have occurred back as far as 1988 at the Garden Grove clinic.[23] We now know, it was before that.[1] "What happened is serious," announced *Dr. Stanley Korenman* of UCLA, one of the panel members. "It strikes at the heart of the doctor-patient relationship on several levels and could have a major nationwide impact."[12]

He was right.

The panel reported in March that Asch, Balmaceda, and Stone had committed a host of research and clinical violations, including conducting large-scale laboratory studies of patients without their consent.[12]

On April 26, 1995, Asch and Balmaceda took laboratory records of many egg transfers and arranged for a large shipment of frozen embryos and sperm donations to be moved from the Irvine clinic to the California Cryobank in Los Angeles, presumably in anticipation of the closure of the clinic. During this time, it became evident that the doctors had made fictitious insurance claims for work that they had never done. Also, they had failed to report cash payments owed to the university.[20]

These observations had already been made by the auditors Peat Marwick in their audit in October 1994, but nothing had been done. They could no longer be ignored. UCI officials proposed that the doctors quietly resign, but when they refused, the UCI ordered that the clinic be closed on April 28, 1995.

More Audits

After a January 1995 visit to the campus, the NIH threatened to pull UCI's funding for human research unless the school rapidly revamped how it oversaw human research. The university rushed to comply. Shocked federal investigators had discovered that the three fertility doctors did not seem to recognize the seriousness of the concerns or to understand the difference between standard medical practice and experimentation.[11] Faced with losing up to $14 million, university officials admitted that the system of oversight had suffered an "unacceptable" breakdown at the fertility center.[11] After launching multiple internal investigations, UCI officials made the controversy public on May 15, 1995, by severing ties with the clinic, giving it three weeks to move. The clinic moved to Fountain Valley.[12]

The next day, the university sued the three doctors and the clinic, seeking to stop the doctors from destroying or altering patient records and alleging that the physicians had blocked efforts to get at the truth.[12] The lawsuit also accused Asch of attempting to strong-arm a former patient the previous week into signing a retrospective consent form allowing eggs extracted from her in 1993 and 1994 to be used for research. The woman, whose identity was not revealed, filed a legal claim against the university and the doctors, alleging that Asch used her eggs to make another woman pregnant.[12]

The Challenders

In May 1995, two reporters from the *Orange County Register* visited *John and Debbie Challender* in their home in Corona, California, with photocopies of their medical records. These showed that the eggs taken from Debbie had been given to other women without Debbie's consent.[16,21] The records showed that in November 1991, Dr. Ricardo Asch had collected forty-six eggs from Debbie Challender and placed five of them back into Debbie's fallopian tubes. Debbie had been trying to conceive for a decade using assisted reproductive technology without success.

This time she conceived and delivered a son on August 24, 1992. Debbie's delight could hardly be contained. Her husband, John, said, "He was great, gentle, wonderful—an excellent salesman."

Debbie exclaimed, "He is a gift from God." Whether she was talking about the baby or Dr. Asch is not known. But her delight was not to last. When she was shown the medical records brought by the reporters from the *Register*, she saw that ten of her eggs had been given to another woman. That woman also received eggs or embryos from yet another woman, and the records show that this woman had twins.

John Challender declared, "The embryos they took were our children. The embryos they stole were our children."[16]

Then later, after finding out a woman had given birth to Debbie and John's twins, "When we saw the records, we just sat there and wept," says John. "It was the loss of three of our children, children that had yet to be born. We felt betrayed."[21] Now John does a double take when he is in a supermarket and sees a child who resembles Debbie or himself, wondering if it is their child.[16]

Not surprisingly, the Challenders were horrified. They denied emphatically that they had ever given permission to donate their eggs, primarily as they had never achieved a pregnancy themselves. They decided to go public, so they consulted a lawyer, *Theodore S. Wentworth*, who was experienced in dealing with the media. Wentworth claimed that he was aware of five other clinic patients who were confirmed or possible victims of egg or embryo swapping. He thought that there might be as many as six others. This proved to be well short of the mark. Finally, there were over one hundred legal cases of whom about thirty-five to seventy were thought to involve egg switching.[22]

The Porters

In late 1991, *Budge Porter* and his wife, *Diane*, visited the fertility clinic at UCI. Porter was once a college football star who was severely paralyzed after a football injury. He was in a wheelchair, and the doctor told him that it would take two operations, one for him to obtain sperm by microsurgery and one for his wife to collect eggs.[18,24] The eggs would be fertilized by intracytoplasmic sperm injection and returned to the fallopian tubes to give the Porters a chance of becoming parents. The cost would be $35,000.[22,25]

Later, the Porters discovered from records obtained by the *Orange County Register* that Dr. Asch had collected twenty-six eggs from Diane, told her that he had collected twenty-two, and fertilized three of them with sperm from her husband and returned them to her fallopian tubes. The other four of Diane's eggs were inseminated with another man's sperm and given to a Newport Beach woman who was also trying to conceive. The eggs from Diane Porter did not fertilize, so the Newport woman for whom they were reserved was given three embryos from the Challenders and three from another unidentified source. The Newport woman had twins whose parentage is unknown without DNA testing. Diane Porter declared emphatically that at no time had she given permission to donate her eggs.

The Challenders Go Public

On May 19, 1995, Asch resigned from the UCI Medical Center, and the university placed all three doctors on leave from the faculty. The following Thursday, the university issued a blistering amendment to its legal complaint, expanding the allegations to include egg-stealing and drug misuse.[12]

In the same month, the *Orange County Register* published an article entitled "Baby Born after Doctor Took Eggs without Consent." It won the Pulitzer Prize for Investigative Reporting for the authors *Susan Kelleher* and *Kim Christensen*.[26] They claimed that they had copies of records from 1991 showing that fourteen eggs had been harvested from one woman and four had been returned to her fallopian tubes along with her husband's sperm. The remaining eggs were to be fertilized and frozen for later use, but three of the resulting embryos were not frozen and instead, without the donor mother's consent, were transferred to another patient two days later. A baby boy was born nine months later. The donor mother failed to conceive. The patient and clinic employees, interviewed by the *Register*, were adamant that consent to donate eggs had not been given; and *Della Morrison*, a medical assistant, insisted that the consent form had been altered by Asch two days after the surgery by ticking a box marked "Yes" against a line "Donation."[27] It would be most unusual for a patient who is trying to conceive to donate eggs before her family is complete. The typical decision is to fertilize eggs and to store them frozen for future use.

On June 6, 1995, the Challenders went public at a press conference attended by over two hundred journalists. This opened a can of worms involving the doctors, the clinic patients, the university, and the lawyers. Some argued that it was simple theft, while others claimed that it was unethical. Some men wondered what all the fuss was about as, personally, they would donate sperm to treat infertile patients and would not worry or wonder what the outcome might be because they had been giving it away all their lives, hundreds of millions at a time, but others pointed out that women had only a few hundred eggs at their disposal and that the removal was not so straightforward.[10,16,20]

Staff Gather Evidence

Late in 1991, a fresh sperm sample had arrived in a sealed plastic cup at the Center for Reproductive Health. This delivery was unexpected, and the clinic staff was puzzled. This sperm was from the husband of a former patient, Mrs. A, but she was not booked for surgery and had no eggs waiting to be fertilized. Dr. Asch told a medical assistant, "Just keep it fresh." The same afternoon, Mrs. B arrived and underwent an egg harvesting procedure. The scientist *Teri Ord* was told to set aside three eggs from Mrs. B for Mrs. A. Shortly afterward, Teri Ord became concerned because she could find no consent from Mrs. B to donate her eggs. She told Medical Assistant Della Morrison that she had been ordered to inseminate "donor" eggs on at least fifty occasions since 1986 but could recall hardly any in which an infertile patient had consented to donate eggs. Della Morrison said, "That's when it really clicked. From then on, we just started figuring things out and putting it together." Norbert Giltner, the theater nurse, also expressed his anxiety and repeatedly told Medical Center officials of his anxieties, but nothing ever happened. However, in 1994, he told his story to Debra Krahel, the medical center's ambulatory care director. They all started meeting secretly in a building across the street to compare notes. They soon included an auditor who asked for documentation to go with the egg sheets. Giltner located the records in a cabinet in Asch's office but did not make copies. Two days later, they had gone. Giltner reported that he did not know who took them.[15]

Another Audit

In December 1994, Medical Center officials showed up to examine patient charts. Dr. Asch was worried and ushered admissions employee Yvonne Alexander into his office and handed her a handwritten list of patient charts he wanted to be brought to him. She recognized the names as those whom she believed were involved in egg diversions. "Once I looked at the first three names, I knew what it was about." Dr. Asch was frantic, pleading with her not to show the UCI officials the list of names. "Don't show it to anybody. Don't tell anybody, please, Yvonne. Please, Yvonne" she remembered him saying as the investigations went on for several weeks. Asch started waiting around to debrief employees after they had talked to auditors. She revealed this to the auditors and reported that sometimes he would call her at home and ask what she had told them. UCI investigators then suspected that at least forty women had been unwitting donors or recipients of eggs or embryos taken at clinics and Garden Grove and CRH.[15] The numbers increased much higher than that.

As news spread that eggs or embryos had been given away, more and more women worried that their eggs had been used to produce a child for another couple and that a child might be walking around out there who was genetically theirs. Women would look at other people's children and wonder, if they looked physically similar, whether they were really their own. Many former patients were in limbo, wondering whether the children they were raising were really their own and wondering whether their own genetic children were being raised in someone else's house. As many as sixty-seven women were now thought to be victims of egg or embryo theft.

Eggs Had Been Collected from Diagnostic Laparoscopies

Asch is also alleged to have collected eggs from women undergoing diagnostic laparoscopies to investigate the cause of their infertility after giving them fertility drugs typically used to stimulate ovarian function. The eggs were then given to other women on his GIFT program.[27] One of the earliest examples of alleged egg theft occurred in 1987 at the Garden Grove fertility clinic. During a diagnostic laparoscopy, three eggs were removed from the ovaries of a woman from Laguna Hills. These eggs were transferred to the fallopian tubes of a woman from Laguna Niguel along with sperm from that woman's husband. They later had a boy who was born prematurely but who is now well. The records show that Ricardo Asch performed the procedure, and the records were shown anonymously to each of the parents separately. They were horrified. The woman who underwent the diagnostic laparoscopy was adamant that she had never given permission to donate eggs. She stated categorically that there was no doubt that Asch stated that the procedure was carried out to see why she was unable to bear a child. However, before the procedure, she was given a powerful fertility drug, which is only given to patients wanting to produce multiple eggs for their own use. "This is unbelievable," she raged. "They put me under just to take my eggs." The birth mother, who was unable to produce her own eggs, was always grateful to the woman whom they thought had donated the eggs.[27] Like other couples who have discovered that their children have been born using eggs unknowingly taken from other women, they have lived in the fear that one day someone will turn up demanding parental rights. Those couples, whether biological or birth parents, who have been victims of egg swapping have been devastated by these revelations but have decided in the best interests of the child not to press for biological parental rights but to leave the children to grow up in the house that they have always known. There were only occasional cases of couples who wanted to pursue DNA testing to establish paternity if the court would only allow.[1,28,29]

The End Cometh

In June 1995, Asch, Balmaceda, and Stone were subpoenaed to appear before a State Senate Select Committee, where they all denied any part in the fertility scandals. Asch took the Fifth Amendment. Balmaceda sold his Corona Del Mar property in July and left the United States for Chile to visit his mother in August 1995. He closed his medical office in Laguna Hills in November that year. Asch sold his Big Canyon home for about $1 million in July and his $2 million Del Mar property shortly afterward. When they heard about these sales, officials became worried that they might not return. They were correct. Asch and Balmaceda never returned.[30] Ironically, because Asch and Balmaceda were tenured and officially on leave, the university was obliged to pay them until January 1996, although in the meantime they had fled the country, Asch to Europe (for a speaking tour) and thence Mexico and Balmaceda to Chile.

Asch Washes His Hands of It All

In January 1996, after leaving the United States, Asch testified by deposition under oath from a hotel in Tijuana, Mexico. He stated that he had not made errors in egg transfers. "Any errors were made by technical staff, as I was not responsible for egg selection but only for performing surgery." He declared that he did not match donors and recipients and did not obtain patients' consents, so he had no way of knowing how many mistakes were made, according to those who attended.[31]

If he was not responsible, who was?

Life seemed to have gone on normally after he returned to Mexico where he continued his reproductive research and fertility work at the Grupo de Reproducción y Genética AGN y Asociados clinic at the Hospital Angeles near San Angel. Later he changed to private practice and was employed as the director at the Reproducción Asistida de México. As of 2003, Asch had opened multiple fertility clinics throughout Mexico, including the cities of Cancún, Acapulco, and Puebla. He was collaborating with specialists in Barcelona trying to perfect preimplantation genetic diagnosis that could theoretically screen embryos for over ten chromosomal abnormalities, with techniques that nowadays are routine. He flew from Mexico City to Argentina in 2004 where Argentine officials arrested him when he arrived, but he was released the next day after he posted bail of $8,000. It was presumably during this trip that he was charged with and found not guilty of insurance fraud, cash theft, and egg theft.

However, he received a severe jolt when he was arrested in Mexico City on November 3, 2010, about fifteen years after he had fled from the United States, on an Interpol Red Notice.[32,33] US prosecutors worked frantically to get the required extradition papers together, but a Mexican federal judge released Asch on bail of MEX $1 million (about $85,000) in January 2011. In March, the judge ruled that Asch's extradition would amount to double jeopardy as he had already been tried and found not guilty on the same charges in Argentina (vide supra).[34,35] On March 15, 2011, Dr. Ricardo Asch was freed in Mexico City and trumpeted on his Facebook page a message to his followers: "today is freedom day … Enjoy it with me please." He went on, "Many thanks to all who celebrated the triumph of justice and my freedom."[35] His wife (Silvia), four daughters, and adopted son all reside in the US and frequently visit him in Mexico.

Balmaceda Washes His Hands of It All

When news of the fertility clinic's scandals hit the headlines, Balmaceda distributed a letter to the UCI College of Medicine condemning the administration for accusing all three doctors of having equal responsibility in the wrongdoing. Balmaceda contended that the misappropriation of eggs was mainly Asch's doing, facilitated by laissez-faire management by the university. In September 1995, Balmaceda visited his mother in Santiago, Chile, and never returned to the United States to face his charges. The following year, he was labeled a fugitive, indicted in absentia on twenty counts of mail fraud for insurance billing, and his faculty salary at the University of California Irvine was terminated.[12]

In Chile, Balmaceda began work at one of the country's most prestigious private practices, the Clinica Las Condes in Santiago. Most of his colleagues celebrated his return to Chile and dismissed the clinic scandal as gossip. However, his new life in Chile was disrupted by personal tragedy when his wife committed suicide in 1999, leaving him with four children. On January 17, 2001, he was arrested at the Ezeiza Airport in Buenos Aires, Argentina, and held for extradition to the United States on charges of mail fraud and tax evasion. He was released on bail with orders not to leave Argentina but failed to attend his court hearing that February. Balmaceda returned to Chile, maintaining it would be impossible to find justice under Argentine law.

Since 2003, Balmaceda has served as the director of the Latin American Network of Assisted Reproduction. The group reports success rates for fertility clinics in Chile, Peru, and Bolivia and, ironically, standardizes patient consent forms. Balmaceda continues to place blame for the California scandal on the university administrators for not acting sooner and claims to be innocent of any illegal egg transfers. He also laments the prosecution of his ex-associate *Sergio Stone*, whom Balmaceda claims never participated in any assisted reproduction procedures. Balmaceda has given many interviews and made appearances on television programs professing his innocence, but the fertility clinic scandal remains a blot on his reputation and that of others.[36]

The University

The UCI had consistently ignored warnings from auditors and others about irregular occurrences since the CRH opened. They did not want to kill the goose that laid the golden egg. That policy came back to haunt them. In 2006, UCI advised that it had tried to contact all patients affected, but it had not been able to do so. Some patients had moved, others had not realized that they might be involved, and some could not be found. In truth, some probably did not want to be involved for fear of what they might hear. Regardless, in 2009, UCI settled a dozen lawsuits stemming from fertility fraud nearly fifteen years before. The last three cases were settled in 2011 when they paid a total of $4.23 million. The total payments, ranging up to nearly $1 million, from UCI to 137 couples in which eggs or embryos were either unaccounted for or given to another woman without consent came to $27 million.[37,38]

It is evident now that the use of other women's eggs and other men's sperm contributed to much of Dr. Asch and Dr.

Balmaceda's clinical success. It has been claimed that the physicians preferred to take eggs from women with blond hair and blue eyes or to take them from women in return for discounted fertility treatment to give them to well-to-do couples or couples who were friends of Ricardo.[1,15] They seemed to run an egg bank as a sperm bank except that the eggs were taken without asking. It is apparent that the source of the eggs and the sperm became a matter of convenience without regard to whether the prospective parents cared how they conceived a child, and most of the recipient patients were not told that the eggs were donated without consent. Some children might not be related to either of those whom they regard as their parents, and some children might be biologically related only to the woman whom they see as their mother while some might be related only to the man whom they see as their father. As far as Asch was concerned, the use of eggs and sperm belonging to others was simply a routine clinical matter directed at achieving the highest success rates for his own satisfaction.

In November 1995, on *Primetime Live*, Asch told the interviewer, *Diane Sawyer*, "I think this society is entirely obsessed with genes." He went on, "Genes are not important even for IQs or athletic ability or any of that." But Asch did not stop there. He went on to say in the interview taped on ABC somewhere outside the United States that the patients and their lawyers were greedy and unscrupulous, only interested in "opportunism."[39] Clinicians and ethicists alike were aghast. This man could not possibly believe in what he was saying. Indeed, he was later known to be collaborating with workers in Barcelona attempting to develop a preimplantation genetic diagnosis. His attempt to discount the importance of genes might have been aimed at minimizing the damage that he had caused.

The eggs and sperm were simply a convenient resource, like a syringe or petri dish, to be used by the physicians on a whim.

Yet Asch knew he was doing wrong. Otherwise, he would not have become so anxious when he thought the auditors were going to expose him. His audacity was breathtaking. It is regrettable that it took greed, an ethical catastrophe, and dozens of devastated couples to expose this brilliant man to the English-speaking world.[40,41]

Epilogue

Before they left the US for the last time, Asch and Balmaceda transferred many patients' data and frozen embryos from CRH to the California Cryobank, but about two thousand frozen embryos remained in the clinic at the Saddleback center. These were "adopted" by *Dr. Robert Anderson* at his clinic at Newport Beach, California, in November 1995. Dr. Anderson "adopted" the "orphans" as what he thought was an act of goodwill. He undertook to care for the orphans, perhaps not realizing what an enormous task it would be. His staff tried to contact the parents of these orphans to ask what they would like done with them. The owners are invited to donate them to another couple who are trying to conceive or to give them to research if they do not wish to use them themselves. Alternatively, they can be discarded as medical waste. But fifteen years later, Dr. Anderson still had about one thousand embryos from Saddleback to care for.[42] Of course, as with all these cases, there are some supporters who will deny the undeniable. *Ginger Canfield*—who, with Asch's help, gave birth to a daughter in 1988—said when she heard of the charges against Dr. Asch, "It was like somebody had told me the Pope was a serial killer, I love Dr Asch."[21] None are so blind as those who will not see.

Summary

Dr. Ricardo Asch is now over seventy years of age, and his interests in clinical life have evolved but are still related to reproduction. He still lives in Mexico and can be found on YouTube, having made a movie about the photography of quarks, which are subatomic particles that are so small that they cannot be identified alone. He seems to have found another interest in life.[43]

Whether the drive to use eggs and embryos without consent was to bolster success rates for academic glory or financial greed, Asch's serial ethical misconduct ruined his record of achievement, and he remains a fugitive from US justice and a shame to the medical profession—at least in the English-speaking world. Asch's reputation as a scientist and an innovator has long since been lost beneath the waves of disgrace. Like so many others in this book, he came to think of himself as godlike, omnipotent and untouchable. One of life's great mysteries is what drives a person who has achieved so much to discredit himself when he already had everything to gain without doing any more.

Notes

1. Brandon, K. "Emerging Fertility Clinic Scandal Has California Rapt." *Chicago Tribune* (internet). 1996; Available from http://articles.chicagotribune.com/1996-03-24/news/9603240208_1_egg-or-embryo-transfers-dr-ricardo-asch-fertility-treatment.
2. Schuchner, E., A. Paczy, and R. Asch. "Subcellular Distribution of Some Inorganic Cations in the Vaginal Epithelium of the Rat." *Journal of Reproduction and Fertility*. 1972; 30(2): 283–286.

3. Edwards, R., P. Steptoe, J. Purdy. "Establishing Full-Term Human Pregnancies Using Cleaving Embryos Grown in Vitro." *BJOG*: An International Journal of Obstetrics and Gynaecology. 1980; 87(9): 737–756.

4. Asch, R., L. Ellsworth, J. Balmaceda, P. Wong. "Pregnancy after Translaparoscopic Gamete Intrafallopian Transfer." *The Lancet*. 1984; 2(8410): 1,034–1,035.

5. Asch, R., L. Ellsworth, J. Balmaceda, P. Wong. "Birth Following Gamete Intrafallopian Transfer." *The Lancet*. 1985; 2(8447): 163.

6. Burfoot, A. *Encyclopedia of Reproductive Technologies*. Boulder, Colo.: Westview Press; 1999.

7. Dodson, M. "Fallopian Tube Technique for Conception Has Papal Blessing." *Los Angeles Times* (internet). 1967; Available from http://articles.latimes.com/1987-03-14/local/me-9688_1_fallopian-tubes.

8. Catholic Infertility—Catechism (internet). CatholicInfertility.org. Available from http://www.catholicinfertility.org/catechism.html.

9. Dodson, M. "Event, Possibly in Garden Grove, Would Be World's Second Such Happening: Infertility Pioneer Awaits Birth of Special Twins." *Los Angeles Times* (pre-1997 full text)—Los Angeles, Calif (Orange County Edition). 1986; start page 1 Metro: Metro Desk.

10. Dodge, M., G. Gies. *Stealing Dreams: A Fertility Clinic Scandal*. 1st ed. Boston: Northeastern University Press; 2003.

11. Gilson, H. "Center for Reproductive Health (1986–1995)" | The Embryo Project Encyclopedia (internet). Embryo.asu.edu. 2008. Available from http://embryo.asu.edu/handle/10776/1946.

12. Weber, T., J. Magius. "In Quest for Miracles, Did Fertility Clinic Go Too Far? Medicine: Allegations of Egg Stealing at UC Irvine Expose Lack of Regulations."

Los Angeles Times (internet). June 3, 1995. Available from http://articles.latimes.com/1995-06-04/ news/mn-9521_1_uc-irvine-fertility-clinic.

13. Asch, R. Biographies.net (internet). STANDS4 LLC, 2014. Web, September 9, 2014. 2014. Available from http://www.biographies.net/people//en/ricardo_asch>.

14. Kamel, R. "Assisted Reproductive Technology after the Birth of Louise Brown." *J Reprod Infertil* (internet). 2013; 14(3): 96–109. Available from http://www.jri.ir/article/535.

15. Kelleher, S., K. Christensen, C. McGraw. "A view from Inside the Fertility Clinic." *Orange County Register*: Pulitzer Prize for Investigative Journalism (internet). 1995; Available from http://www.pulitzer.org/winners/staff-37.

16. Nicolosi, M. "Corona Parents Make Ordeal Public." *Orange County Register*: Pulitzer Prize for Investigative Journalism (internet). 1995; Available from http://www.pulitzer.org/winners/staff-37.

17. Kelleher, S., K. Christensen, D. Parrish, M. Nicolosi, E. Slone. "Clinic Scandal Widens." *Orange County Register.* 1995; Available from http://www.pulitzer.org/winners/staff-37.

18. Nicolosi, M., D. Parrish, E. Slone. "UCI Offers Secret Deal to Doctors." *Orange County Register*: Pulitzer Prize for Investigative Journalism (internet). 1995; Available from http://www.pulitzer.org/winners/staff-37.

19. Kelleher, S., D. Parrish. "Workers: UCI Hushed Us Up." *Orange County Register*: Pulitzer Prize for Investigative Journalism (internet). 1995. Available from http://www.pulitzer.org/winners/staff-37.

20. Christensen, K., S. Kelleher, J. Grimaldi. "UCI Probes: Doctors Mishandled Eggs, Cash." *Orange County Register* (internet). 1995. Available from http://www.pulitzer.org/winners/staff-37.

21. Sanz, C. "A Fertility Nightmare" (internet). PEOPLE. com. 1995. Available from http://people.com/ archive/a-fertility-nightmare-vol-44-no-4/.

22. Kelleher, S., P. Love. "A Legacy in Limbo: Couple Say Transferring Eggs to Someone Else Robbed Them of Their Genetic Heritage." *Orange County Register* (internet). 1995. Available from http://www.pulitzer.org/winners/staff-37.

23. Marquis, J., T. Weber, M. Wagner. "Egg Misuse May Have Involved 30 More Patients, UCI Reports: Scandal: The Scope of the Fertility Clinic's Alleged Improprieties Is Widened Dramatically, Touching a Third Hospital and Including Patients Treated as Long Ago as 1988." *Los Angeles Times* (internet). 1995; July 6. Available from http://articles.latimes. com/1995-07-06/news/mn-20673_1_fertility-clinic.

24. Patrizio, P., S. Silber, T. Ord, J. Balmaceda, R. Asch. "Two Births after Microsurgical Sperm Aspiration in Congenital Absence of the Vas Deferens." *The Lancet*. 1988; 332(8624): 1,364.

25. Temple-Smith, P., G. Southwick, C. Yates, A. Trounson, D. de Kretser. "Human Pregnancy by In Vitro Fertilization (IVF) Using Sperm Aspirated from the Epididymis." *Journal of In Vitro Fertilization and Embryo Transfer*. 1985; 2(3): 119–122.

26. Kelleher, S., K. Christensen, M. Nicolosi, T. Saavedra. "Baby Born after Doctor Took Eggs without Consent." *Orange County Register*: Pulitzer Prize for Investigative Reporting (internet). 1995; May. Available from http:// Baby Born after Doctor took Eggs Without Consent.

27. Kelleher, S., K. Christensen, D. Parrish, M. Nicolosi, E. Slone. "Egg Thefts during Exams Alleged: Records and Interviews Show that Eggs Were Stolen during Routine Procedures at the UCI Fertility Clinic."

Orange County Register (internet). 1995. Available from http://www.pulitzer.org/winners/staff-37.

28. Kimi, Y. "UC Irvine Fertility Scandal Isn't Over." *Los Angeles Times* (internet). January 20. Available from http://articles.latimes.com/2006/jan/20/local/me-uci20.

29. Marocq, L., R. Gibson. "'Truth and Consequences of Genetic Revolution' DNA on Trial Senate Select Committee on Genetics and Public Policy Informational Hearing." (Internet). May 9, pp. 14–16. 1996. Available from https://play.google.com/books/rea der?id=gYQkNB5gRBYC&printsec=frontcover& output=reader&hl=en&pg=GBS.PA16.w.0.3.0.

30. Marquis, J. "Key Figure in O.C. Fertility Clinic Scandal Sells Home." *Los Angeles Times* (internet). 1995; October 24. Available from http://articles.latimes.com/1995-10-24/ news/mn-60646_1_fertility-clinic-scandal.

31. Marquis, J. "Fertility Doctor Denies Role in Errors." *Los Angeles Times* (internet). 1996; January 20. Available from http://articles.latimes. com/1996-01-20/news/mn-26676_1_fertility-doctor.

32. Saillant, C. "Fugitive in UC Irvine Fertility Scandal Arrested in Mexico City: U.S. Hopes to Extradite Him." *LA Times* Blogs—LA Now (internet). 2010; December 27. Available from http://latimesblogs. latimes.com/lanow/2010/12/uci-fertility-scandal- ricardo-asch-arrest-mexico-city-extradition.html.

33. "Doctor Arrested in California Fertility Scandal." NBCNews.com (internet). Women's Health: Associated Press. 2010. Available from http://www. nbcnews.com/id/40827964/ns/health_wom.

34. Christensen, K. "Mexico Won't Extradite Jew Embryo Thief." *Los Angeles Times* (internet). 2011. Available from https://vnnforum.com/showthread.php?t=125841.

35. Christensen, K. "Doctor Linked to UC Irvine Infertility Scandal Released from Custody in Mexico." *Los Angeles Times* (internet). 2011. Available from http://articles.latimes.com/2011/mar/23/local/la-me-0323-asch-20110323.

36. Gilson, H. "Jose Pedro Balmaceda (1948–)" | The Embryo Project Encyclopedia (internet). Embryo.asu.edu. 2010. Available from https://embryo.asu.edu/pages/jose-pedro-balmaceda-1948.

37. Kim, Y. "UCI Settles Dozens of Fertility Suits." *Los Angeles Times*. 2009; September 11.

38. Anderson, N., E. Schrader. "50 Couples to Get $10 Million to End UCI Fertility Clinic Suits." *Los Angeles Times* (internet). 1997; July 19. Available from http://articles.latimes.com/1997/jul/19/news/mn-17879.

39. Slone, E. "Asch's Remarks on TV Stir Outrage Reaction: Doctors and Ethicists Decry His Discounting of the Importance of Genes and His Attacks on Clinic Patients." *Orange County Register*. 1995; news section page a10 OCR646261.

40. Granberry, M., R. Trounson. "Charges Impact Worries Many in Fertility Field." *Los Angeles Times* (pre-1997 fulltext)—Los Angeles California (Orange County Edition). 1995; start at page 1. Part-A Metro Desk.

41. Creator unknown. "Egg Swapping at Birth Clinic Brings Change." *New York Times* (internet). 1995; p. 17. Available from http://hdl.handle.net/10822/885797.

42. Newsweek staff. "Doctor Who Adopted Thousands of Abandoned Embryos." Newsweek (internet). 2009. Available from http://www.newsweek.com/doctor-who-adopted-thousands-abandoned-embryos-80525.

43. Quarks; Ricardo Asch Y. Luzma (internet). YouTube. 2018. Available from YouTube Dr. Ricardo Asch quarks—Bing video (internet). Bing.com. 2014. Available from

https://www.bing.com/videos/search?q=youtube+dr+ri
cardo+asch+quarks&qpvt=youtube+dr+ricardo+asch+
quarks&view=detail&mid=3FB8B25FD1F04EA9750
E3FB8B25 FD1F04EA9750E&&FORM=VRDGAR.

Suggested Further Reading

Dodge, M., G. Gies. *Stealing Dreams: A Fertility Clinic Scandal*. 1st ed. Boston: Northeastern University Press; 2003.

CHAPTER TWO

DR. JAYANT PATEL— DOCTOR DEATH

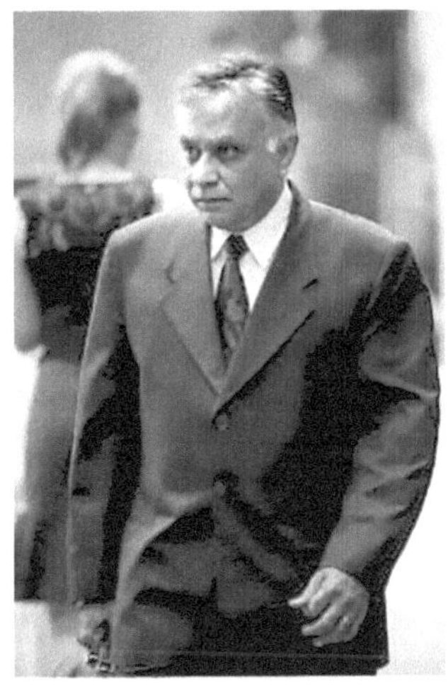

Photo: Patrick Hamilton / AFP via Getty Images

Prologue

Dr. Jayant Patel was only the tip of the cancerous iceberg that concealed the incompetence of the Medical Board of Queensland, the Bundaberg Base Hospital, the Area Health Services of Queensland, the Queensland Department of Health, and the Queensland Government itself. Patel was an impostor who falsified his history to qualify himself for a license to practice medicine with the Oregon Medical Board of Examiners and to ingratiate himself with his future employers, the Kaiser Permanente Health Maintenance Organization (HMO) in Oregon, USA, then the Bundaberg Base Hospital (BBH) to secure a position of surgeon at that hospital. He proceeded to operate on about one thousand patients over a period of two years in Australia with unacceptable complications, including death, until he was exposed by the efforts of *Ms. Toni Hoffman*, nursing unit manager of the intensive care unit; the *Hon. Rob Messenger, MP*; *Mr. Hedley Thomas*, investigative journalist of the Brisbane *Courier Mail*; and others. As Mr. Thomas demonstrated, Patel's fraudulence could have been uncovered by a simple Google search. If any of the bodies responsible for his registration had thought to do such a search, the subsequent disastrous outcomes might have been avoided.

In the Beginning

Jayant Mukundray Patel was born on April 10, 1950, in Jamnagar in the state of Gujarat, western India.[1] On March 11, 1973, at the age of twenty-two, he graduated from the M. P. Shah Medical College–Jamnagar with Bachelor of Medicine and Bachelor of Surgery (MBBS) degrees. These bachelor degrees are the usual degrees awarded to graduates in medicine in the British system and are common where that system has had influence as it did at that time in India. They equate to an MD (Doctor of Medicine) degree in the United States of America and do not suggest an inferior qualification. Neither do they suggest, however, that the candidate has any specialized training as a surgeon. What is more important is the standing of the university awarding the degrees. Of the universities in India, I doubt that the M. P. Shah Medical College was among the most prestigious.

On March 20, 1976, Patel was awarded a Master of Surgery (MS) degree by the M. P. Shah Medical College only three years after he graduated MBBS at the same college.[2] It would be almost unknown for a surgeon to be awarded specialist status within five years of graduating as a medical practitioner, whether that be in the USA, Australia, the UK, Canada, South Africa, Ireland, or New Zealand. One cannot help but wonder then what standing an MS at the M. P. Shah Medical College had when compared with the requirements for a specialist surgeon who had been granted fellowship with one of the learned colleges in any of the countries just mentioned, but on August 8, 1976, he was certified as a resident surgeon, Irwin Group of Hospitals, Jamnagar, India.

Buffalo, New York

It was with this background in 1977 that he successfully applied for a position as a surgical resident at the University of Rochester–New York. On September 25, 1978, he was certified by the Educational Commission for Foreign Medical Graduates and entered the surgical residency program at the University of Rochester.[3] During the next five years, his performance was substandard; and the Office of Professional Discipline, after a lengthy investigation ending on May 10, 1983, found him guilty of professional medical misconduct for "failing to examine patients before surgery," "moral unfitness to practice," "abandoning or neglecting a patient in need of immediate professional care," and "harassing, abusing or intimidating either physically or verbally." He was fined $5,000 and suspended for six months, the sentence held over pending the completion of three years' probation.[4]

During the investigation, his defense included glowing references from four eminent medical practitioners: *Dr. James*

S. Williams, *Dr. Marguerite Dynski*, *Dr. William G. Farlow*, and *Dr. James R. Hinshaw*. These references were to be treasured by Patel and reserved for future use. The evidence from those who spoke against him was to be ignored by Patel and not to be given much weight by the committee. He was, therefore, free to go back to work after paying the $5,000, which he did. During that time, he was certified as an assistant surgical resident and later as chief surgical resident at the Erie County Medical Center–Buffalo, New York. It seems extraordinary that, with this history, on November 1, 1988, he was certified by the American Board of Surgery–Philadelphia, Pennsylvania; and in early 1989, he was granted a full license to operate as a surgeon by the American Board of Surgeons.[1]

Portland, Oregon

Under the circumstances and while the going was good, he must have thought that the smart thing to do was to get away as far as possible from New York, and the next best thing within the USA other than Alaska or Hawaii was Portland, Oregon, so he then popped up in Kaiser Permanente Northwest Health Maintenance Organization (HMO) in 1989. It staggers the imagination how Dr. Jayant Patel came to be appointed to the Kaiser Permanente with a record as disgraceful as his. But appointed he was. According to *Roger Sandall* in the *Quadrant*, the executive director of the Oregon Board of Medical Examiners (BME), Katherine Haley, held his references from New York in higher regard than his disastrous professional history.[4] When she required some reassurance, however, Patel presented her with a second reference from the eminent Rochester surgeon *Dr. James Raymond Hinshaw* who wrote to the Oregon Board of Medical Examiners that Patel showed "technical and professional brilliance"; and when asked for more detail, Hinshaw responded that Patel's application for the post of surgeon "was being obstructed by harassment of a brilliant young surgeon whom I would recommend without reservation."[4] He and Dr. Jayant Patel nonetheless neglected to mention Patel's history of malpractice or that he had been dismissed from the surgical residency program in the University of Rochester in 1981 so his application to Kaiser was successful.[5] After commencing there in 1989, he soon became swamped, operating on the most challenging cases—indeed, as it turned out, many of which were too complicated and which he was not qualified to do.

However, he clearly impressed those around him, so much so that he was promoted within three years at Kaiser Permanente as a trainer of younger surgeons. In 1995, Kaiser Permanente doctors voted him Distinguished Physician of the Year.[5] Considering his incompetence, he must have been some sort of magician to fool those watching. Maybe they were impressed by his bravado. But that came at the expense of his patients.

Kaiser Permanente, 1989–2001

The system for licensing, certifying, and monitoring medical practitioners in Oregon was different from the system as it is today. In those days, it was a requirement that all cases of malpractice or negligence that resulted in settlement of over $100,000 by an insurance company were to be reported to the legislators. The details were then reviewed by a medical tribunal consisting of experts who would decide whether further action should be taken by the medical board. In this way, if there were sufficient cases, the performance of the surgeon would come to the attention of the officials who might take some corrective or punitive action. If the circumstances were not reported, they would not be detected. What made it even more challenging to expose inferior or incompetent care was that in Oregon, as in many other states, a doctor's performance was confidential.[6,7]

Once installed at Kaiser Permanente, Dr. Jayant Patel sank himself into his work. He soon became busy, tackling the most difficult cases with aplomb. He and his wife, Kishore, also working as a doctor at Kaiser, bought a large home at Beaverton, and Jayant took on extra responsibilities such as screening of surgeons for national certification.

Life Was Good for Jayant Patel

About 1995, around the time when he was awarded Distinguished Physician of the Year, suspicions started to arise that the rate of complications following his operations was greater than that of his colleagues. One patient on whom he operated to fashion a new colon using the stomach had his urethra severed and later started urinating from his rectum. Another patient with a history of bowel cancer had a sigmoidoscopy instead of a colonoscopy and subsequently developed cancer of the bowel from which she died when the cancer was missed because the sigmoidoscopy was the wrong investigation. The family sued for malpractice, and Kaiser settled the case for $1.4 million. In another case, Patel accidentally cut the ureter (the tube from the kidney to the bladder) and failed to recognize the damage despite being warned by his surgical assistant. The patient required three further operations and lost a kidney. Kaiser settled the malpractice claim confidentially in 1997.

Another patient was scheduled for an outpatient hernia repair. When she awoke after the surgery, her femoral vein had been severed accidentally and a repair was attempted, but a life-threatening blood clot developed at the site. The patient was in pain for six months. Another surgeon who reviewed the case said that the injury to the vein was so far away from the site of the hernia that Patel must have been operating in the wrong place. Kaiser settled the claim confidentially. Another patient had his colon removed for alleged ulcerative colitis, but the diagnosis was later shown to be Crohn's disease, which can have similar symptoms but seldom requires surgery. The patient had lost his colon for nothing. More cases followed, some with complete wound dehiscence (breakdown) and some with massive bleeding and even death. Several similar cases resulted in malpractice suits. Kaiser settled many of these, some for over $1 million. The total was in the millions, but Kaiser did not report them to the legislators, claiming there was no requirement for them to do so as they were self-insured, so they went unnoticed.[6,7]

Surgery itself is a risky business, and complications can occur in the most straightforward of cases. It may have been felt that the high number of complications in Patel's case was due to the complicated nature of the surgery itself, and consequently, many of the adverse outcomes did not result in malpractice suits. Even so, of those that resulted in malpractice claims, none was notified to the legislators because Kaiser regarded itself as a self-insured association and therefore claimed to be outside the law that required that malpractice cases be notified to the Oregon Board of Medical Examiners. In this way, Patel's incompetence went unnoticed until Kaiser itself had a closer look at his performance because of the huge compensation payments.[7]

In late 1997, Kaiser reviewed seventy-nine of Patel's operations. After six months, when the review was finished in June 1998, there were so many complications that the HMO prohibited him from operating on the pancreas, liver, and colon. It also required Patel to get a second opinion before any major surgery and insisted that he attend classes on communications and preventing malpractice cases. Then the Oregon Board of Medical Examiners published a biennial report that showed that he had been prohibited from a wide range of surgery.[5] Finally, Kaiser reported this disciplinary action to the National Practitioner Data Bank and the state board. Kaiser placed Patel on probation in late 1999. To Dr. Jayant Patel, who regarded himself as the Great Achiever, this must have been galling. By late 2000, he was essentially no longer performing inpatient surgery. In April 2001, his license had been revoked in New York State. Patel resigned from Kaiser on June 20, 2001, the day before the hospital's medical board was scheduled to discuss his dismissal.[4,6]

Australia, Here I Come

So what now for Dr. Jayant Patel? Somehow, despite being disciplined by the New York State Board for professional misconduct, Patel had managed to have himself certified by the American Board of Surgery and had been granted a full license as a surgeon by the American Board of Surgeons.[8]

He had secured a position as a surgeon with Kaiser Permanente in Oregon. He had been awarded Distinguished Physician of the Year, and he had been given the responsibility of screening surgeons for national certification, but the game was up in Oregon. That meant that the game was up in the USA, including Alaska and Hawaii. Where could he go? He had to make a living, and he was used to being king. He had to go somewhere they might not look too closely at his credentials.[9]

Australia was a long way away, and it was south of the equator. It was a vast land, about three million sq. mi. (7,618,000 sq. km.) with a relatively small population, about twenty-three million. Queensland is one of six states and a territory of Australia. It occupies the northeastern part of the continent and has an area of about 715,000 sq. mi. (1,853,000 sq. km.) and has a population of about five million, so it was sparsely populated. That's not even three people per square kilometer. That was even better. They might not notice. Indeed, they did not notice.

Whatever the causes, there are fewer doctors per head of population in Queensland than in any other state or territory in Australia.[10] Because of the chronic and severe shortage of doctors in Queensland, large regions were declared as "areas of need."[9] Once declared an area of need, a region could advertise outside the usual restrictions that applied to other areas such as metropolitan regions. In these areas of need, if the employing authority was unable to fill the position locally or nationally, it was permitted to advertise internationally. In 2002 to 2003, the Queensland government's average recurrent expenditure on health was the lowest in the nation, at 20 percent below the national average. Salaried medical officers were remunerated at the second-lowest rate in the country. Queensland, therefore, was mainly dependent on overseas trained doctors (OTDs), who accounted for one in four doctors in the state.[10,11,12] Australia's immigration laws are quite specific, but when a skill is in short supply, admission can be allowed and a work permit on a special visa issued, usually for one year in the first instance, for a specific position. Employers tended to favor candidates on these visas as they had more control over the employee who might be afraid of having his visa canceled and often a lower salary could be arranged.

Wavelength Consulting P/L was an employment agency based in Sydney that advertised principally for overseas trained doctors (OTDs) because local positions were usually already filled by trained Australian doctors. *Dr. John Bethell*, a director of Wavelength, said that he was first contacted by *Dr. Nydam*, the director of medical services at Bundaberg Base Hospital (BBH), with a request to refer a surgeon for the senior medical officer (SMO) position at the Base on November 14, 2002. Soon afterward, he received the position description for the job, and he recorded the position on Wavelength's database. Back in Oregon, Dr. Jayant Patel was trolling the websites of employment agencies looking for a position that might suit him. When he spotted the advertisement, he immediately approached Wavelength through its website, expressing an interest in working as a general surgeon in Australia.

Dr. Bethell then telephoned Dr. Patel in Portland, Oregon, in the United States. Dr. Patel described himself as a general surgeon with experience in pediatric, vascular, and laparoscopic surgery. On December 13, 2002, Dr. Bethell sent Dr. Patel generic information about Bundaberg Base Hospital by email; and on the same day, Dr. Patel sent his *curriculum vitae* (CV). Dr. Bethell considered Dr. Patel to be very well qualified, so he forwarded the CV to Dr. Nydam. He noted that Dr. Patel claimed that he had held a position as staff surgeon at the Kaiser Permanente hospital in Oregon for some twelve years, had held academic postings, been the head of a surgery residency program, and was widely published in well-recognized journals.[11] (A search of the medical literature through PubMed reveals none.)

Dr. Nydam received Dr. Patel's CV and spoke by telephone to him twice. The CV repeated the claims already made by Dr. Patel. It stated, among other things, that Dr. Patel was a US citizen, that he was a Fellow of the American College of Surgeons, and that he was aged fifty-one. He provided six open references addressed "To whom it may concern," and they dealt with the authors' experiences in Oregon with Dr. Patel over the last ten years rather than match him to any given position. It was Wavelength's policy to check a minimum of two verbal references. Dr. Bethell spoke to Dr. Patel about this, and Dr. Patel nominated three referees, being three of the doctors who had provided the open recommendations. Dr. Bethell spoke with two of them, *Dr. Peter Feldman* and *Dr. Bhawar Singh*, an anesthetist; they both spoke very favorably about the applicant. It is quite surprising that an anesthetist should be so impressed by a surgeon's ability as they, more than anyone, have had the opportunity to observe the surgeon's technique.

Patel's References

The references were effusive in their praise for the skills, knowledge, and industry of Dr. Patel, even by the usual standards of such documents.

Dr. Edward A. Ariniello, former chief of surgery at the Kaiser Permanente hospital in Portland, wrote that Dr. Patel had demonstrated that "he is one of the most well-read and well informed of all our surgeons, and his superior skill was also demonstrated in the operating room. He is entirely selfless in his determination to be available for call, consultations and problems … He will be difficult or impossible to replace. I can recommend Dr Patel without any reservations whatsoever."

Dr. Peter M. Feldman, staff surgeon at Kaiser Permanente, wrote, "I have many good things to say about Dr Patel. He has been a wonderful colleague over the years and has been a very hard worker. He has a well above average interest in his work, and a well above average knowledge of surgery. I would judge Dr Patel to have very high moral standards."

The anesthetist from the Kaiser Permanente Hospital, *Dr. Bhawar Singh*, wrote, "Dr Patel's balanced judgment, surgical skills and decisive steps, especially in the management of high-risk, complex procedures has always been appreciated by anaesthetists and other members of the OR Team. Dr Patel's professional expertise, passion and energy for quality patient care coupled with ethical and best practice advocacy won him the vote of his colleagues for a Distinguished Physician Award."

There were also glowing tributes from *Dr. Wayne F. Gilbert* of Portland, *Dr. J. T. Leimert* (chief of the Department of Hematology-Medical Oncology at Kaiser Permanente), and *Dr. Leonora Dantas* of the Department of Internal Medicine at Kaiser Permanente.

It is hard to understand how these leading medical practitioners could be so misguided about a deficient surgeon.

Neither Dr. Bethel nor Dr. Nydam noticed that the references were dated 2001 before he left Kaiser or that they claimed that he had been employed by Kaiser until 2002. Patel finished with Kaiser in 2001 and had been unemployed for fifteen months.

Documentation

Dr. Patel's application for registration with the Medical Board of Queensland stated that he had been employed by Kaiser Permanente until September 2002. That was false.

The application also included the following questions:

1. "Has your registration under the Medical Practitioner's Registration Act 2001 or equivalent of a foreign country, been affected by an undertaking, the imposition of a condition, suspension or cancellation in any other way?" Patel answered no.
2. "Has your registration as a health practitioner ever been cancelled or suspended or is your registration currently cancelled or suspended because of disciplinary action in any State or Territory or in another country?" Again, Patel answered no. They were both false.[9]

Dr. Patel faxed a certificate of good standing to Wavelength on January 19, 2003, and Wavelength forwarded the certificate to the board on January 29, 2003. The document carried the following words:

Limitations: None
Extensions: None

However, it also included a sentence that read as follows:
Standing: *Public Order on File See Attached:*

The public order was not attached to the document provided by Dr. Patel, and Wavelength did not notice that critical omission.[9,13]

Patient Has the Wrong Procedure

Patel started work on April 1, 2003. It was not long before the first complaint occurred, on May 14, 2003. A patient was admitted to the Day Surgery Unit at the Base so that Dr. Kingston could perform a right epididymectomy (removal of the epididymis, which is the tiny coiled tube in the scrotum that carries sperm away from the testicle—Ed). While the patient was waiting for that procedure, Dr. Patel "inadvertently" conducted a gastroscopy upon him, a procedure for which he had not consented and for which he had not been scheduled. The patient must have been astonished when he awoke. Dr. Kingston apologized on behalf of the hospital, and it seems that no harm was done. *Dr. Darren Keating*, who had replaced Dr. Nydam as medical director, investigated and found that there were inadequate checks in the transfer of the patient from the day surgery unit to the operating theater.[14]

The First Esophagectomy

The second complaint concerned a forty-six-year-old man called *James Phillips*. He had a potentially curable lesion in the esophagus so that an esophagectomy (in which a portion of the esophagus is surgically removed) was one treatment path for consideration. The circumstances were complicated, however, by his renal condition. Mr. Phillips was being dialyzed through a graft, but the graft itself was suffering from the stenosis (that is, it was closing over), and there was a "very good chance" that major surgery would lead to a blood clot, preventing dialysis. In those circumstances, the operation was "as difficult an esophagectomy as one could envisage," and a question arose as to whether the patient should be transferred to Brisbane. The transfer might have been attractive because the Brisbane hospital had a sophisticated renal unit, staff that included specialist esophagectomists, and much better facilities for postoperative intensive care.

Dr. Patel, however, performed an esophagectomy on Mr. Phillips at the Base Hospital on May 19, 2003, and he survived that operation briefly. The nurse unit manager of the intensive care unit in BBH, *Ms. Toni Hoffman*, was involved in the postoperative care for Mr. Phillips. Ms. Hoffman had held her position as the most senior nurse in the intensive care unit for almost three years, and she had been a nurse in intensive care for twenty-two years. She was present when the operating theater staff handed over Mr. Phillips to the intensive care unit. Ms. Hoffman found that the patient was unstable and that his blood pressure was so low it could not be recorded, and the anesthetist commented that "this is an expensive way to die." Mr. Phillips was given large amounts of Adrenalin and was maintained on ventilator support. The course of treatment was complicated by the fact that he required constant dialysis, and there was some conflict between the doctors as to how the patient should be managed. Ultimately, Mr. Phillips progressed to brain death.

There were several aspects to the case that caused Ms. Hoffman great concern, and consequently, she approached her line manager—the director of nursing, *Glenys Goodman*—who made an appointment for them to visit Dr. Keating in his office where all three met. Ms. Hoffman raised three areas of concern with Dr. Keating.

First, she said that Dr. Patel was habitually "rude, loud, and did not work collaboratively with the ICU medical staff." She said that he did not seem to be on the same "wavelength" as other staff who were working in the intensive care unit, that there was a "whole bravado about things and things didn't match up," and that his choice of drugs and treatment seemed to be "twenty years behind" contemporary thinking. Ms. Hoffman said that she attempted to paint an overall picture of the problems encountered in the intensive care unit with Dr. Patel. Dr. Keating said that they had to allow that Dr. Patel was from another country. Ms. Hoffman replied to Dr. Keating that it was more like they were from two different planets.

The second issue Ms. Hoffman raised was that while in intensive care, Mr. Phillips was obviously extremely unwell and the nursing staff told the family this, but Dr. Patel told the family and wrote in the chart that the patient was stable. Ms. Hoffman knew that this was untrue and that it caused unnecessary tension.

Thirdly, Ms. Hoffman expressed the view that esophagectomies were outside the scope of services that could be offered at Bundaberg.[14]

The cascade of disasters continued. In early June 2003, a man with cancer of the ear had the wrong part of his ear removed. He realized this when he looked in the mirror after the operation and complained. Dr. Keating apologized, and the correct part of the ear was removed by another surgeon. Nothing more came of that matter.[15]

Another Esophagectomy

Another esophagectomy was carried out in June 2003, and the wound broke down twice. The patient was returned to the theater three times and eventually, despite protests by Dr. Patel, was transferred to Brisbane where surgeons questioned whether Bundaberg was an appropriate place to have undertaken such surgery. Surgeons at Brisbane contacted Dr. Keating at Bundaberg and challenged the decision not to transfer. Ms.

Hoffman questioned whether esophagectomies should ever be carried out at the Base when it lacked appropriate intensive care facilities for patients undergoing major surgery. She pointed out that the Base's intensive care unit lacked an intensive care specialist, had only three ventilators, and did not have an adequate nursing staff to cope with more than two ventilated patients at the same time. Ms. Hoffman said that the issue of transferring esophagectomies to Brisbane was explicitly addressed during a second meeting with Dr. Keating who told her that Dr. Patel "is a very experienced surgeon, very used to doing surgery of this type. It is important that we keep him in the hospital, so we need to work with him and do what he wants, basically." Dr. Keating, however, undertook to discuss the matter with the Credentialing and Privileges Committee. No such committee existed at the time, so the esophagectomies continued.[4]

Dehiscence

Several cases of wound dehiscence followed.[16] Among them, a patient who underwent an operation called a sigmoid colectomy (removal of the sigmoid colon—Ed) for diverticulitis, and his wound burst open after twelve days.[17]

Operating on Another Doctor's Patient

Another patient—who was not a patient of Dr. Patel but rather a patient under a physician, *Dr. Smalberger*—was in the radiology department for a CT scan ordered by Dr. Smalberger. Dr. Patel came across him and decided he had a ruptured spleen and that he should be taken to theater for removal of the spleen. An altercation followed. Dr. Smalberger said that the patient had recently had a heart attack and was not suitable for surgery and, in any case, did not have a ruptured spleen, so the patient was sent to Brisbane where it was found that his spleen was not ruptured.[18]

Lack of Hygiene

Other problems seemed to follow Dr. Patel around. But then he seemed to generate them. He moved from patient to patient changing dressings and inserting catheters without washing his hands or putting on gloves. On one occasion, he said, "Doctors do not have germs." He left the theater and went to the car park in his theater scrubs to smoke a cigarette and then returned to the theater wearing the same theater gown. He inserted peritoneal dialysis catheters without gloves. These frequently moved, blocked, or became infected, requiring further treatment. The complications were so common that the nurses arranged for the catheters to be inserted in a private hospital elsewhere in Bundaberg. Patel's complication rate and reputation became so bad that *Dr. Peter Miach*, the director of medicine, refused to allow any of his patients to be operated on by Dr. Jayant Patel, the director of surgery![15]

Further cases occurred toward the end of 2004. A patient with inoperable cancer of the esophagus was operated on by Dr. Patel and died within a day. A fifteen-year-old boy was admitted with an injury to the femoral vein in his leg, and after four operations, he was transferred to Brisbane where he lost his leg.[16]

Ms. Toni Hoffman's Letter

Eventually, Ms. Hoffman, the nursing unit manager for ICU, became so frustrated that she wrote to *Mr. Peter Leck*, the district manager of the Bundaberg Health Service on October 22, 2004. The letter was tabled at the Queensland Public

Hospitals Commission of Inquiry, 2005, and an edited version is reproduced here because it exposes so many issues:

Dear Peter,

I am writing to inform you officially, of the concerns I have for the patients in ICU in relation to the behaviour and clinical competence of one of the surgeons, Dr Patel.

Dr Patel first voiced his displeasure with the ICU around the 19th May 2003.

Patient 1. A patient came to the ICU post esophagectomy. This patient had multiple comorbidities, and for the last 45 minutes of surgery, had no obtainable blood pressure. The anaesthetist stated that this was "an expensive way to die." He required 25 ug of Adrenaline and 100% Oxygen. Dr Patel stated the patient was stable. The nursing staff who were communicating with the patient's family told the patient's mother that he was extremely ill. Indeed, he progressed to brain death. Dr Patel continued to say the patient was stable. The course of treatment for this patient was challenging, he required dialysis, and there was constant conflict between the anaesthetists, Dr Patel and the physicians about his care. The Direct of Anaesthetics and ICU was away, and Dr Younis was left in charge, he was reluctant to question whether we should be doing such large operations here at Bundaberg. Dr Jon Joiner and I went to see Dr Keating to voice our concerns. We both believed we could not offer adequate post-op care for oesophagectomies. The literature stated a hospital should be doing at least 30 per year to maximise outcomes. At this time, I first stated my concern that Dr Patel could describe a patient on maximum Inotropes and ventilation as stable. I voiced these concerns to Dr Keating. After this incident, Dr Patel and I had a conversation where I told him that the ICU wished to have an excellent professional working relationship with him. I tried to tell him that we were a level one ICU and that our staffing levels and scope of practice meant that we could only keep ventilated patients for 24–48 hours, before transferring them to Brisbane. Dr Patel stated that he would not practice medicine like this and he would go to "Peter Leck and Darren Keating and care for his own patients." This incident was repeated relatively soon after the first. Dr Patel would threaten the staff with his resignation when it was suggested it was time to transfer out a ventilated patient.

Ms. Hoffman went on:

He continually stated he was working in the "third world" here. He would use "Peter Lecks" and "Darren Keating's" names as a type of intimidation and threat to the staff. He stated on several occasions he would go straight to Peter Leck as he had made him "half a million dollars this year." Every time we had a ventilated patient in the ICU that required inotropes, he would argue with the anaesthetists about which inotrope to use. His choice of inotropes did not reflect best practice guidelines in Australia. He refused to speak to the writer [myself] All requests for a bed would go through either another nurse or doctor. He would yell and speak in a loud voice, denigrating the ICU and myself and at times the anaesthetists. The nursing staff felt they were often the "meat in the sandwich." He would harass them and ask them "whose side they were on." At times he would actively try to denigrate my ability as a NUM to the nursing staff and other doctors. (See attached documentation). Soon after Dr Patel started operating here, the nursing staff observed a high complication rate amongst the patients. Several patients had wound dehiscence and several experienced perforations. This is a list of patients I believe require formal investigation. This is taken from our ICU stats, and they are not a full and comprehensive review as there are no stats from OT or Surgical Ward.

For example: -

Patient 2: 6/6/03 post-op oesophagectomy

12/6/03 wound dehiscence [in other words, surgical wound burst open—Ed]

15/6/02 2nd wound dehiscence suffered a third wound dehiscence was transferred to Brisbane on 20/6, had a J tube leak and peritonitis. A bed had been obtained earlier for this man, but Dr Patel went up to Dr Keating who advised our anaesthetist to keep him for a few more days, in which time the bed was taken, and he stayed several more days whilst another bed was sourced. The doctors at RBH questioned why we were doing such surgery here when we were unable to care for these patients.

Patient 3: post-op oesophagectomy ventilated for 302 hours

Patient 4: ventilated for many days: transferred to Brisbane after many arguments in the ICU with Dr Patel who refused initially to transfer this patient.

Patient 5: issue with transferring patient to Brisbane

Patient 6: Bowel Obstruction Resection and Anastomosis on 7/2/04 T/F to Brisbane on 11/2/04 on the 12/2/04 laparotomy showed perforation and peritoneal soiling [in other words, perforated bowel in Bundaberg—Ed]

Patient 7: Wound dehiscence and complete evisceration 8/4/04. Booked for sigmoid colectomy and found to have ovarian ca.

Patient 8: 27/4 Wound dehiscence

Patient 9: 29/6 Insertion of Vascath perforated ® IJ

Patient 10: Delay in Transfer to Brisbane, see attached report, Pt died.

Patient 11: 10/7 laparotomy for ventral hernia, developed haematoma in the ward and attempted evacuation done without any analgesia. Drs notes consistently say that the patient is well when Pt was experiencing large amounts of pain and wound ooze.

Patient 12: patient had Whipples [a major and technically very difficult operation suitable for some cases of cancer of the pancreas—Ed] death cert stated he died of Klebsiella pneumonia and inactivity

Patient 13: death cert stated patient died of malnutrition. Had been operated on 31/7/04

Several conversations were had with other doctors, Acting Directors of Nursing and NUMs Dr Miach refused to allow Dr Patel to care for his patients as he stated he had 100 percent complication rate with Peritoneal Dialysis insertion. This was stated in a Medical Services forum as well as in a private conversation with me. This data was shown to the Acting Director of Nursing Mr Patrick Martin.

Ms. Hoffman continued:

On the 27th July 2004, Patient 14 returned to ICU in extremis with a chest injury. The events of these 13 hours are well documented. Dr Patel interfered in the arranged transfer of this patient to Brisbane, and the patient died after it was thought the retrieval team were on their way to retrieve this patient. The subsequent events of this intervention and the traumatic pericardial tap (described by the nurse caring for the patient as repeated stabbing motions) resulted in the ICU staff requesting advice from the nurses' union. The staff involved in this situation described it as the worst they had ever seen. They were acutely distressed. An attempt was made to seek EAS support, but they were unable to assist due to their workload. One staff member accessed Psychological support privately. I was requested to fill in a sentinel event form, by the then QI Manager Dr Jane Truscott. The events of this incident were discussed at length with the union, who offered support to the staff. They also offered me several ways I could report the long-standing concerns I had with the current situation in ICU. The day after the patient's death, when I thought he had safely been transferred to Brisbane, Dr Strahan came to talk to me in the office and found me very distressed. He offered to talk to some of the other doctors and get back to me as the representative of the AMA in Bundaberg. He did state "there is widespread concern, but now no one is willing to stick their neck out." He urged me to keep stats on my concerns. I spoke with Dr Dieter Berens and informed him the nursing staff were going to report their concerns with Dr Patel to an official source. He stated he would support us, by telling the truth, but he was concerned he would lose his job, and Dr Patel would be the one left behind. It is widely believed amongst the medical and nursing staff that Dr Patel was compelling, that he was wholeheartedly supported by Peter Leck and Darren Keating and was untouchable. Anyone who tried to alert the authorities about their concerns would lose their jobs. This perception was indeed perpetrated by Dr Patel daily. Many of the residents and PHO's have expressed their concerns, Dr Alex Davis and Dr David Risson, were unsure of what to do because of the widespread belief Dr Patel was protected by the executive. The Nurses union have offered advice in that there are several ways these concerns can be reported if not dealt with internally, after my conversation with Peter Leck and Linda Mulligan on Wed, I believe they were not in receipt of the full concerns, but now that they are they will deal with them.

Ms. Hoffman concluded:

Dr Miach has reiterated he has dealt with the issue by not letting Dr Patel near his patients. These concerns were openly discussed at the medical services forum. A peripheral concern is the reports the junior doctors have voiced about forms not being filled out correctly, of being told not to use certain words in discharge summaries, and various other chart irregularities.

Toni Hoffman.

Further Documentation

Documentation from Karen Stumer, Karen Fox, Kay Boisen (x 2), Karen Jenner, and Vivienne Tapiolas was included.[19]

Peritoneal Dialysis Catheters

Dr. Miach provided a report to Dr. Keating on peritoneal dialysis catheter insertions. It showed that peritoneal catheter insertions had a complication rate of 100 percent when inserted by Dr. Patel. Consequently, Dr. Miach did not allow Dr. Patel to see any of his patients. It seems that Dr. Keating had difficulty understanding the ramifications of the report, but nevertheless, he refrained from mentioning it to Dr. Miach.

On October 22, 2004, Mr. Leck provided Dr. Keating with a copy of the Hoffman letter. He said he asked Dr. Keating to arrange meetings with some of the doctors mentioned in the letter because Dr. Keating maintained that it was "all personality-based conflict," and Mr. Leck wanted him to hear what other doctors had to say. Subsequently, Dr. Keating approached *Drs. Dieter Berens, David Risson*, and *Martin Strahan* and met with them over the next fortnight. The doctor, in each case, was interviewed by Mr. Leck and Dr. Keating, and the latter made notes of the meetings.[20]

At those meetings, Dr. Berens said that Dr. Patel's critical care knowledge was not up to date in relation to the choice of some drugs and fluids, plus the application of some physiology principles to care for critically ill patients. He was also aware that Dr. Patel had a complicated working relationship with the intensive care unit nurses. He accepted that Dr. Patel's manual skills were excellent and that the patients being admitted to the Base were, as a group, older and sicker than several years ago. He questioned Dr. Patel's judgment in undertaking some procedures in relation to his currency and made mention of vascular surgery and the Whipple operation. He also said that Dr. Patel's attitude to other professionals made him hard to work with on occasions and that he made categorical statements that were inflexible and he refused to discuss other clinical options.

Dr. Risson was concerned about the number of postoperative complications, including infection. He said that his relationship with Dr. Patel was amicable, but he appreciated that he could be flighty and unpredictable and that resident staff considered that he could be severe in his reprimands. He had never been told to refrain from writing or mentioning anything on a discharge summary.

Dr. Strahan was concerned by a case in which he was performing a gastroscopy but he could not advance the scope further after multiple attempts. Dr. Patel operated and found carcinoma of the pancreas. The patient was sent home and later readmitted for a Whipple operation, but she died. Dr.

Strahan wondered whether Dr. Patel should be doing Whipple operations.[20]

One might have expected some reaction on the part of Mr. Leck or Dr. Keating after the letter from Toni Hoffman and these interviews, especially as it recorded that Dr. Patel had a 100 percent complication rate from peritoneal dialysis catheter insertion. It also recorded that Dr. Miach, the director of medicine, refused to allow Dr. Patel, the director of surgery, to see any of his patients. It seemed that Mr. Leck had formed the opinion that the trouble was entirely personality-based and none of it was Dr. Patel's fault. In the meantime, on November 15, 2004, the tilt train disaster occurred in Bundaberg, and that may have taken some time on the part of the administration.

The Chief Medical Officer

Mr. Leck was becoming unsettled because of the continuing grumbling, and on December 14, 2004, he finally called *Dr. Gerry Fitzgerald's* office and requested a review. Dr. Fitzgerald, the chief medical officer, was scheduled to take leave over the Christmas and New Year period, but the tsunami struck in the Indian Ocean on December 26, so his return from holiday was delayed until January 17, 2005, and he decided to visit Bundaberg on February 14, 2005. His brief, he said, "would be more of a clinical review rather than a serious disciplinary visit." When he returned, he reported that he had formed no opinion of Dr. Patel. Meanwhile, Dr. Patel was still happily operating as usual. In early February 2005, Dr. Patel came into the ICU and announced that his contract was to be extended for a further three months. That was the straw that broke Toni Hoffman's back. She determined to take her complaint to the Hon. Rob Messenger, MP.

The Hon. Rob Messenger, MP

Mr. Messenger was a member of the National Party, which was in opposition at the time, but he had a longtime interest in Queensland Health and was aware of its problems. On March 18, 2005, he listened sympathetically to Toni Hoffman in his office for about two hours with her letter in front of him. After she had left, he consulted some of his colleagues and made a couple of phone calls to confirm what Ms. Hoffman had told him.[8] He decided to table the letter in parliament where, of course, it would be public and privileged. The letter was tabled on March 22, 2005, and that was the end of Dr. Patel's time at Bundaberg. Even then, the staff was called together and given a severe lecture about teamwork and cooperation by an enraged Mr. Leck, but it was too late. The cat was out of the bag. Dr. Jayant Patel was on his way back to the USA on March 31, 2005, courtesy of a business class ticket funded by Queensland Health.

A Commission of Inquiry and Surgeon's Review Panel

Queensland Health ordered a Commission of Inquiry into the Queensland Public Hospital System on April 26, 2005 and implemented an arrangement whereby former Patel patients were invited to see one of a panel of surgeons, at Queensland Health's expense, for a second opinion or follow-up surgery. The review panel also commenced on April 26, 2005 and completed its findings on June 30, 2005. Dr. Geoffrey de Lacy saw over 150 patients and carried out more than one hundred procedures. *Dr. Barry O'Loughlin* saw forty-two patients, and *Dr. Peter Woodruff* reviewed the notes from 221 patients, including eighty-eight deaths. The review panel found that thirteen deaths might have been caused or contributed to by Dr.

Patel. The report of the Surgeon's Review Panel was included in the inquiries of the commission, which issued its final report on November 30, 2005.[21]

The Commission's Findings—Dr Patel

a. Dr. Patel knowingly misled the Medical Board of Queensland and Queensland Health by failing to disclose disciplinary action brought against him in the United States of America and by falsifying his work history for the two years prior to December 2002.

b. Dr. Patel repeatedly performed surgical procedures at the Base that he had been restricted from performing in the United States of America.

c. Dr. Patel performed surgical procedures at the Base that were beyond his competence, skill, and expertise; beyond the capacity of the hospital and its staff to provide adequate postoperative care; and unnecessary.

d. As a result of negligence on the part of Dr. Patel, thirteen patients at the Base died, and many others suffered adverse outcomes.

e. Dr. Patel unreasonably failed to transfer patients to a tertiary referral hospital within an appropriate time frame, causing adverse consequences for many of those patients.

f. On many occasions, Dr. Patel failed to record adequately in patients' files the exact details concerning material facts, including the surgical procedures undertaken, complications arising from surgery, wound dehiscence, infections, the course of postoperative care, and reasons for postoperative return to surgery.

g. As the director of surgery at the Base between April 1, 2003, and April 1, 2005, Dr. Patel failed to ensure that the Department of Surgery conducted appropriate surgical auditing, including the holding of effective morbidity and mortality meetings.

h. Dr. Patel failed to refer thirteen reportable deaths to the coroner.

i. Dr. Patel held himself out as a general surgeon when he lacked any specialist registration in Queensland.[22]

Commission's Recommendations—Dr. Patel

The commission recommended that

a. the conduct of Dr. Patel in relation to securing registration with the Medical Board of Queensland and a position at the Base Hospital be referred to the Queensland Police Service for further investigation with regard to fraud and attempts to procure unauthorised status;

b. with respect to the matters found by Dr. Woodruff, Dr. O'Loughlin, and Dr. de Lacy (the Surgeon's Review Panel), Dr. Patel's conduct be referred to the Queensland Police Service for further investigation in relation to the offenses of assault, assault occasioning bodily harm, grievous bodily harm, of negligent acts causing harm and manslaughter;

c. the conduct of Dr. Patel in holding himself out as a general surgeon be referred to the Medical Board of Queensland for further investigation in relation to the Medical Practitioners Registration Act 2001.[23]

The Commission's Findings—Dr. Nydam, Dr. Keating, Mr. Leck

The commission made adverse findings against Dr. Nydam, Dr. Keating, and Mr. Leck ranging from incompetence in the case of Dr. Nydam to more serious matters extending to the *criminal code* in the case of Dr. Keating and Mr. Leck.

The Commission's Recommendations—Dr. Nydam, Dr. Keating, Mr. Leck

The commission made no recommendations regarding Dr. Nydam but did recommend the referral of Dr. Keating and Mr. Leck to Queensland Police or the Australian Federal Police for further investigation of a string of administrative offenses.[24] Dr. Keating was banned from ever working as a senior medical administrator in public or private hospitals again. Mr. Peter Leck later graduated as a doctor and, like Dr. Keating, now works in Western Australia.

Dr. Jayant Patel's Trial

The commission's recommendations were referred to the Director of Public Prosecutions who decided that Patel should be charged with three cases of manslaughter and one of grievous bodily harm, these being the most likely to secure a conviction.[25] One of the first problems that faced the prosecution was that Dr. Patel was not around, having left for Oregon six months before the commission issued its findings. He had to be extradited from the USA before he could be tried. Queensland Police commenced proceedings in March 2008, and under an extradition treaty with the USA, he arrived back in Brisbane on July 21, 2008. He was released on bail the next day awaiting trial.

The trial, under *Judge John Byrne*, charged Dr. Patel with the unlawful killing of three patients and grievous bodily harm of a fourth as well as for administrative offenses such as fraud and misconduct. He was found guilty of all charges on June 30, 2010. The next day, he was sentenced to seven years in prison. Under the law, as a nonviolent offender, he would have been eligible for release in three years and six months.[25] Patel appealed his sentence to the appeals court, but the appeal was dismissed. He then appealed to the high court. On August 24, 2012, the high court unanimously allowed the appeal and quashed Patel's convictions, claiming prejudicial evidence had probably influenced the jury. Patel argued that by the time prosecutors admitted forty-three days into the trial that they could not prove Patel was guilty of incompetence, the jury had already heard testimony and evidence about his unusual behavior. The high court declared a miscarriage of justice and granted Patel a new trial.

The Next Trial

Prosecutors decided that their best chance of a successful prosecution would be to charge Patel with one case at a time. One of the great difficulties of successfully charging a surgeon with manslaughter is the absence or lack of a precedent. Another problem is that complications, including death, will happen in any surgeon's practice. For a case to succeed, it would have to be clearly shown that one surgeon's rate of complications is statistically much higher than that of his peers. This can be difficult to prove, as the defense will argue that the "offender" has operated on more complicated cases. Patel operated on over one thousand patients in his two years in Bundaberg, so it was to be expected that he would have complications. The Davies Commission connected Patel to eighty-eight deaths, the Surgeon's Review Panel thought he was likely the cause of thirteen deaths, and the prosecutors charged him with three; but even these charges could not be proven and were overturned by the high court.

The next trial began in November 2012, and this time Patel was charged with only one count of manslaughter, and he was found not guilty. Prosecutors realized that they might never get a guilty verdict. Consequently, they entered into a plea bargain whereby they would drop the remaining manslaughter charges in return for a guilty verdict of dishonestly gaining registration and two counts of dishonestly gaining employment in Queensland. He was sentenced to two years in prison for these offenses, wholly suspended as he had already spent two years in jail, and he walked out of court a free man.[26]

In the End

When released by the court, Patel announced that Australia had a very fair legal system and that it had been a very traumatic four years but now "I can get back to work." In May 2015, the Queensland Civil and Administrative Tribunal banned him from the practice of medicine ever again in Australia, so (hopefully) he will not be there.[27,28]

Ms. Toni Hoffman

Ms. Toni Hoffman, the senior nurse who blew the whistle on Jayant Patel, received the Order of Australia medal and the 2006 Local Hero Award for her part in exposing Dr. Jayant Patel. She later received financial compensation from the Queensland Government for damages suffered during her employment there.[29]

Epilogue

Dr. Jayant Patel was an enigma. On the one hand, he was industrious, and he could be charming, humorous, and was obviously intelligent; but he was a megalomaniac who could be bombastic, patronizing, and was without empathy for his patients—or "victims" as Roger Sandall of the *Quadrant* called them.[4] There is evidence that he was dexterous and had potential to be an excellent surgeon, but like others in this book, he never cared about realizing that potential, and he regarded himself as above others.

Patel was also an unrepentant fraud from the outset. He was disciplined in Buffalo, New York, not long after emigrating from India. His license to practice in New York State was canceled in 2001. He deliberately concealed those of his documents that revealed his unfitness to practice in New York to legislators in Oregon and then those documents that revealed his history in Oregon from officials in Queensland, Australia. The Board of Medical Examiners and Kaiser Permanente in Oregon, as well as the Medical Board in Queensland and the Bundaberg Base Hospital, were all derelict in their duty to ensure that Patel was qualified to do the things that he was doing, so he was not entirely to blame.

If others had been more meticulous and double-checked Dr. Patel's CV, it would have prevented many medical disasters.

Notes

1.   *The Australian.* "The Life and Times of Rogue Surgeon Jayant Patel." June 30, 2010.
2.   Associated Press. "A Look at the Career of Dr. Jayant Patel." (Online). 2005. (Accessed June 22, 2018). Available from https://web.archive.

org/web/20050620233637/http://asia.news.
yahoo.com/050520/ap/d8a6pvn83.html.

3. Associated Press. "Beyond the Headlines: US Doctor
    Charged." *Democrat and Chronicle*. April 21, 2009.
    (Accessed June 22, 2018). Available from https://
    www.newspapers.com/image/137719363/.

4. Sandall, Roger. "Doctor Death in Bundaberg." *Quadrant*
    (online). 2005. (Accessed June 30, 2018). Available from
    http://www.rogersandall.com/doctor-death-in-bundaberg/.

5. Thomas, Hedley. *Sick to Death*. Sydney:
    Allen & Unwin, 2007. pp. 30–31.

6. Goldsmith, Susan, and Don Colburn. "Patel's
    Disturbing Record at Kaiser Stayed Hidden for Years."
    The Oregonian. 2005. p. first part. November 6.

7. Woodward, Steve, and Susan Goldsmith. "State
    Let Kaiser, OHSU Escape Oversight." *The
    Oregonian*. 2006. p. second part. November 7.

8. Colburn, Don, and Susan Goldsmith. "Australia Ready to
    Charge Patel." *The Oregonian*. 2006. p. 22. November.

9. Bundaberg Hospital Commission of Inquiry. Interim
    Report. June 10, 2005. para. 11. http://www.case-
    watch.net/foreign/patel/interimreport.pdf.

10. Queensland Public Hospital Commission of Inquiry.
    Final Report 2005. para. 2.21. http://www.qphci.
    qld.gov.au/final_report/Final_Report.pdf.

11. Ibid. para. 3.75.

12. Queensland Health Systems Review Final Report. p. 19.
    September 2005. http://www.parliament.qld.gov.au/docu-
    ments/tableOffice/TabledPapers/2005/5105T4447.pdf.

13. Queensland Public Hospitals Commission of
    Inquiry. 2005. paras. 3.91–3.109. http://www.
    qphci.qld.gov.au/final_report/Final_Report.pdf.

14. Ibid. paras. 3.184–3.192.

15. Ibid. para. 3.195.

16. Ibid. para. 3.272.

17. Ibid. para. 3.208.

18. Ibid. paras. 3.214–3.216.

19. Ibid. para. 3.331.

20. Ibid. paras. 3.335–3.338.

21. Ibid. para. 3.418.

22. Ibid. para. 3.424.

23. Ibid. para. 3.425.

24. Ibid. paras. 3.426–3.430.

25. Oberhardt, Mark. "Dr. Jayant Patel Sentenced to Seven Years in Jail." *Brisbane Courier Mail* (online). 2010. (Accessed July 12, 2018). Available from https://www.couriermail.com.au/news/dr-jayant-patels-sentencing-underway/news-story/853286fd1d27ec4638146da6a5070a66.

26. Duys, Ted. "Miscarriages of Justice." MiscarriagesofJustice.com.au (online). 2014. (Accessed July 13, 2018). Available from http://www.miscarriagesofjustice.com.au/jayant_patel.html.

27. Jabour, Bridie. "Dr. Patel Tells of Traumatic Four Years." *Brisbane Times*. 2012.

28. Marks, Kathy. "'Doctor Death' Jayant Patel Escapes with Fraud Conviction and Plans to Return to Work." *News World Australasia* (online). 2013. (Accessed July 13, 2018). Available from https://www.bing.com/search?q=doctor+death+jayant+patel+escapes+with+fruad+conviction+kathy+marks&form=EDGTCT&qs=PF&cvid=12d268ec90324db2ac44287c00f791c0&refig=3c2e423fd813409a9bb98900db92db97&cc=AU&setlang=en-US&elv=AY3%21uAY7tbNNZGZ2yiGNjfM01*VotiCqR*J2oQAk1sXG2tJa0fEg0IK08dTctPsFWtluTFQUu1ICN-GAGEg7PmSerZvTcBoawdULVA0YDQmfr&PC=DCTS.

29. *The Courier Mail*. "Dr. Jayant Patel Nurse Ms. Toni Hoffman Settles Claim with Queensland Health."

(Online). 2012. (Accessed July 16, 2018). Available from https://www.couriermail.com.au/news/queensland/patel-nurse-queensland-health-settle-claim/news-story/0e9f044c09d7c653663645d2fffb8bf5.

Suggested Further Reading

Sandall, Roger. "Doctor Death in Bundaberg." *Quadrant* (online). 2005. (Accessed June 30, 2018). Available from http://www.rogersandall.com/doctor-death-in-bundaberg/.

Thomas, Hedley. *Sick to Death*. Crows Nest, NSW: Allen & Unwin, 2007.

CHAPTER THREE

YOSHIKI SASAI—STEM CELL SENSEI

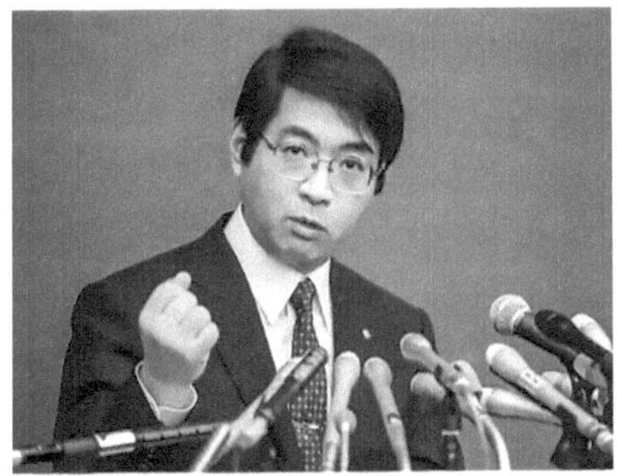

Photo: Toru Yamanaka / AFP via Getty Images

In the Beginning

Yoshiki Sasai, known in Japan as *Sensei* (teacher) was born on March 5, 1962, in the prefecture of Hyogo, Kansai, Japan. He was said to be healthy physically and played baseball and kendo (Japanese martial art using bamboo swords).[1] In 1986, he attained his medical degree from the Kyoto University, which is also in the Kansai region of Japan. While at medical school, he played American football.[2] After graduation, he became a resident at the Kobe Municipal General Hospital where he completed his residency in 1988. He was awarded his PhD from Kyoto University in 1993.

Career

Sasai soon became interested in molecular biology, especially stem cell biology. He quickly established a name for himself and, in 1993, was appointed to a position as a research fellow in *Dr. Edward De Robertis's* laboratory in Los Angeles at the University of California. Arriving in California was memorable when his and his wife's passports and some thousands of dollars were stolen at the airport while collecting his baggage. The next few days were busily occupied arranging new passports at the Japanese Embassy. Nonetheless, he remained at Dr. Robertis's laboratory from 1993 until 1996, where he completed many stem cell experiments.[2] He was appointed as associate professor at Kyoto University back in Japan in 1996. The importance of his work became so well-known that he was dubbed "the Brainmaker" for showing how to direct stem cells into brain cells. From 1995 until 2017, he had approximately 142 publications in respected scientific journals, of which he was the first author in about twenty-four. He became a full professor at Kyoto University in 1998 and group director at the government-funded RIKEN Center for Developmental Biology in Kobe, Japan, in 2000, a position that he held until his death. In 2010, he was awarded the Osaka Science Prize for his work on mechanistic study and in vitro recapitulation of brain development.[3,4] He was indeed a remarkable, gifted scientist. His future was assured.

Stem Cells

There are various types of stem cells. The most primitive are the least differentiated but have the greatest potential to develop into other cell types. They originate from the fertilized egg after dividing to form a blastocyst until about four or five days after fertilization (around 120 cells). These cells have the capacity to develop into any body tissue (or a whole body) and the required placental tissue or identical twins if some cells split off and implant separately. These cells are called totipotent because of their ability to differentiate into any tissue type, body cells, or placental cells. These are the cells that are used for cloning. Of the other types of stem cells, perhaps the most important are pluripotent stem cells, which are in the next level down, because they have undergone some degree of differentiation. These also have the ability to turn into almost any type of body tissue other than placental cells. They can also be used for cloning but only after extensive manipulation in the laboratory. Unipotent stem cells at the other end of the scale can only replace themselves because they have been wholly differentiated. For example, muscle stem cells can only replace damaged muscle, and skin stem cells can only replace skin cells, and that is what they do.

Stem Cell Manipulation

It has been known for some years that unipotent cells could be dedifferentiated or reprogrammed, at least partly, but the methods are sophisticated, involving genetic manipulation, exposure to enzymes and hormones, and therefore challenging to replicate.[5] Yoshiki Sasai's unique skill lay in his ability to sense the conditions required to care for cells in the laboratory, allowing them to develop from embryonic stem cells into retinal cells or brain cells. The potential for stem cell research is unlimited.

Haruko Obokata

Perhaps Yoshiki Sasai's greatest mistake was his appointment of *Haruko Obokata* to the RIKEN institute and his subsequent coauthorship with her of two papers in the journal *Nature* in

2011.[6,7] Haruko was born in Chiba, Japan, in 1983. She had a promising early career, earning her Bachelor of Science in 2006 and following this up with a Master of Science in applied chemistry in 2008 at the Waseda University. Rowan Hooper, the news editor of *New Scientist* magazine, reports that young female scientists are rare in Japan, making her career all the more exciting and her subsequent announcement of STAP cells so extraordinary.[8] A search of the scientific literature shows that she had eleven publications in prominent journals between 2008 and 2014. Unfortunately, the two most recent were retractions. Seven of these were as the first author, including the retractions. Obokata spent two years in Harvard under *Dr. Charles Vacanti* working toward her PhD, which would be awarded by the University of Waseda. Her interest in the development of pluripotent stem cells commenced in Vacanti's laboratory at Harvard University in Cambridge, Massachusetts.

STAP Cells

Haruko noticed that some mammalian cells, having been stressed, became smaller, about the same size as stem cells. She might have thought that the change in response to stress was nature's way of dealing with the repair of injuries. She followed this up by subjecting other cells to numerous different stressors, one of which was to a slightly acid solution. To prove that the resulting cells were new pluripotent cells, she had to use newborn mice cells tagged with colored fluorescent cells. This produced a completely green-colored mouse embryo, regardless of the source, demonstrating that all the cells in the green mouse were pluripotent. Furthermore, Haruko claimed that some of the STAP cells produced were capable of producing placental cells as well as all other cell lines, such as brain, liver, lung, and spleen. This meant that there were endless implications for cloning as well.

The whole idea was revolutionary, and according to Haruko, "It was a difficult time" because her experiment was rejected repeatedly by the scientific journals. It was not surprising as it turned out. Rowan Hooper thought that it was too good to be true, and he was right.

Eventually, in January 2014, the journal *Nature* accepted the two articles on the amazing process, which the authors named STAP, which stood for stimulus-triggered acquisition of pluripotency. The authors were Haruko Obokata, Yoshiki Sasai, Teruhiko Wakayama, and nine others. They claimed that by dipping healthy animal body cells in a weak acid solution (pH 5.7) for about half an hour, the cells would acquire pluripotent properties. The theory was that the mild acid would remove whatever regulators or triggers were on the outside of the cell wall, allowing the STAP cells to be reprogrammed. "No longer," they said, "would nuclear transfer or the introduction of transfer factors be required." In other words, the complex processes previously required would be redundant. The implications were mind-blowing.[6,7,8,9]

The Minister for Education for Japan gave her great credit, saying that "the groundbreaking research led by such a young female is something of which Japan can be proud." He went on, "The government wants to support favourable working environments for young, female researchers." He also added, "We want to do all we can to make Japan one of the world's best places for scientific and technological innovations to nurture more scientists like Obokata."[10] Not long after the paper was published, however, suspicions arose that it might have been partly plagiarized even from her own doctoral work at Waseda.[11] It seemed too good to be true, and of course, it was.

The trouble began shortly after publication when questions were asked about the methods used. Others who tried to replicate them were unable to do so.[12] Some authors noted that the images appearing in the article from *Nature* had already been used in

Haruko's doctoral thesis, which was not from the same work. When Professor Wakayama, who was also a senior author of the paper, proposed withdrawing the article until its findings could be reproduced, RIKEN launched an investigation and found Haruko guilty on two counts of scientific fraud.

The investigators said, "In manipulating the image data of two different gels and using data from two different experiments, Dr Obokata acted in a manner that can by no means be permitted. This cannot be explained solely by her immaturity as a researcher. Given the poor quality of her laboratory notes it has become clearly evident that it will be extremely difficult for anyone else to accurately trace or understand her experiments, and this, too, is considered a serious obstacle to healthy information exchange. Dr. Obokata's actions and poor data management lead us to the conclusion that she sorely lacks, not only a sense of research ethics but also integrity and humility as a scientific researcher."[13,14]

Stern Stuff Indeed

She was given three months to revise it but to no avail. The university withdrew her doctoral degree in 2015, and she was given until the end of the year to replicate her results but was unable to do so. Dr. Obokata resigned from RIKEN in December 2014.[15]

Dr. Charles Vacanti

Dr. Charles Vacanti was famous for his part in the development of the mouse lacking an immune system with an engineered ear on its back. His family—including his brother Joseph, who was the director of the unit—were all in the business of tissue engineering. Dr. Charles Vacanti, unfortunately, was one of the contributing authors to the fraudulent STAP science. He was based at the Brigham and Women's Hospital–Boston, USA, where his brother was director of the unit.

He was not available to be interviewed by the RIKEN investigation, and he stepped down from his position, saying, "I plan to take a one-year sabbatical to contemplate my future goals, redirect my efforts and spend time doing some of the things that I enjoy most. When I return in September 2015, I hope to focus a significant portion of my academic efforts on regenerative medicine and mentoring the next generation of anesthesiologists."[16]

Another scientist bites the dust. But that was not the end of this sad saga.

Retraction of the Paper

Haruko Obokata resisted the criticism of her science despite the controversy that blew up around it. She refused repeatedly, even on television, denying that the science was fraudulent, but agreeing that she may have made errors in the data and used incorrect images. She attributed her mistakes to inexperience until June 2014 when the pressure became too great, and she agreed to retract the papers. The authors were accused of falsifying the data, and even Dr. Yoshiki Sasai, deputy director of RIKEN, said, "It has become increasingly difficult to believe that STAP is even a promising hypothesis."[17,18]

Suicide

On August 5, 2014, Yoshiki Sasai, Ms. Obokata's supervisor and mentor at RIKEN, was found hanging from the stairwell in the institute. He had committed suicide.[19,20] Sasai had left five suicide notes, which have not all been made public for the sake of the family. In one, he urged Obokata to continue her work and prove that her detractors were wrong. This would suggest that he thought that she was correct. Death by suicide is not viewed in the same context in Japan as it might be in some Western countries. In Japan, there is a feeling among some that he did the right thing. There may be a cultural attitude that he had corrected the error of a junior, for whom he was responsible, in an honorable way.[19] The RIKEN investigation found that Yoshiki was accountable for failing to oversee Ms. Obokata at the cellular level, but it found that he did not have a direct influence on the science. Arguments raged in the popular press for months about the reasons for his failure. Some claimed that Yoshiki was so motivated by a desire to eclipse the work of another Japanese group that had led the way in the inducement of cells to become pluripotent (iPC) in 2006 and that his judgment was clouded, causing him to skip some steps in the process.[5] Some said that he also omitted some steps in the appointment of Ms. Obokata to the RIKEN, and others blamed supposed events in his life that had troubled him in the past. It was known that he had spent some time in a hospital environment being treated for depression. One report suggested that RIKEN should be shut down. At any rate, there was a great storm in the media; and in one suicide note, Yoshiki said that he was "worn out by the unjust bashing in the mass media and the responsibility he felt towards RIKEN and his laboratory."[21]

He ended his life by wasting it.

Epilogue

The scientific studies that concern stem cell research and molecular biology are so complex that only those who are involved in the business can spot fraudulent science. Even then, perhaps only those who are involved in the experiment itself might see the fraud. In the case of Obokata, she was required to subject herself to close supervision and video monitoring when given a chance to repeat the study. Even then, video monitoring can be edited. It seems that subjecting oneself to video monitoring and personal supervision will be required to confirm that stem cell research is real and to be trusted. Obokata must have gone to some lengths to conceal the fraud in her laboratory work. Watching cells grow on one side or another in a ninety-six well dish and reporting it to a scientific journal gives the editor and the peer-reviewers a severe challenge. Who to believe? When the editor reads the paper, the subject matter should be reported as quickly as possible if it is essential. Pressure comes from the authors who do not know whether others are going into print elsewhere and they want to be first or whether to wait and be sure. In this case, Obokata wanted to get in print, as her career was on the line. Scientists will sometimes try to find ways around fraud when their career is on the line without waiting to be sure.

She did not wait to be sure, and now her work will never be trusted, and her boss is dead.

Notes

1. Piccolo, S. "Yoshiki Sasai: Stem Cell *Sensei*."
    Obituary; *Development*. 2014; 141: 3,613–3,614.
2. De Robertis, E. "Yoshiki Sasai 1962 2014."
    Obituary; *Cell* 158. September 2014; 1,233–1,235.
3. Cyranoski, D. "Tissue Engineering: The Brainmaker."
    Nature. August 23, 2012; 488: 444–446.
4. "Osaka Science Prize Awarded to Yoshiki
    Sasai." *Riken* News. September 17, 2010.

5. Takahashi, K., S. Yamanaka. "Induction of Pluripotent Stem Cells from Mouse Embryonic and Adult Fibroblast Cultures by Defined Factors." *Cell*. 2006; 126(4): 663–676.

6. Obokata, H., T. Wakayama, Y. Sasai, K. Kojima, M. P. Vacanti, H. Niwa, M. Yamato, C. Vacanti. "Stimulus-Triggered Fate Conversion of Somatic Cells into Pluripotency." *Nature* 505. January 30, 2014: 641–647. Retracted July 2, 2014.

7. Obokata, H., Y. Sasai, H. Niwa, et al. "Bidirectional Development Potential in Reprogrammed Cells with Acquired Pluripotency." *Nature* 505 (7485). January 30, 2014: 676–680.

8. Hooper, R. "Stem-Cell Leap Defied Japanese Norms." *The Japan Times*. News. February 15, 2014.

9. Cyranoski, D. "Acid Bath Offers an Easy Path to Stem Cells." *Nature*/News. January 29, 2014.

10. Profile of Riken scientist Obokata. *NHK Online World Newsline*. January 29, 2014.https://web. archive.org/web/20140203035652/http://www3.nhk. or.jp/nhkworld/english/news/20140130_19.html.

11. Johnson, Carolyn Y. "Review Finds 'Discrepancies' in Papers on Stem Cells." *The Boston Globe*. Saturday, March 15, 2014.

12. Hawkes, N. "Scientist Concludes that Easy Stem Cell Production Published in *Nature* 'Does Not Work.'" *BMJ*, 2014; 348: g3,229.

13. Ishii, Shunsuke, et al. "Report on STAP Cell Research Paper Investigation." Riken.jp. March 31, 2014. http://www3.riken.jp/stap/e/f1document1.pdf.

14. Schlanger, Zoe. "Haruko Obokata, Who Claimed Stem Cell Breakthrough, Found Guilty of Scientific Misconduct." *Newsweek*. April 1, 2014.

15. Fackler, Martin. "Scientist Resigns over Stem Cell Results." *The Journal News* (Hamilton, Ohio). Saturday, December 20, 2014.
16. Johnson, Carolyn. "Brigham Researcher in Flawed Stem Cell Study Will Step Down." *Boston Globe*. August 12, 2014.
17. Osterath, B. DW. "From Stem Cells to Physics, Fraudulent Science Results Are Plenty but Hard to Find." *Science.* June 6, 2014. https://www.dw.com/en/from-stem-cells-to-physics-fraudulent-science-results-are-plenty-but-hard-to-find/a-17687505.
18. Associated Press. "Scientists Withdraw Stem Cell Report." *Odessa American* (Odessa, Texas). July 3, 2014.
19. Spitzer, K. "Science Scandal Triggers Suicide, Soul-Searching in Japan." *Time*. August 8, 2014.
20. Johnson, C. Y. "Scientist Takes Own Life after Scandal." *The Boston Globe*. August 6, 2014.
21. Cyranoski, D. "Stem-Cell Pioneer Blamed Media 'Bashing' in Suicide Note." *Nature*. August 13, 2014.

Suggested Further Reading

Hovanky, V. Stanford University. "The Mutation of Altruistic Intents in Scientific Research." *Intersect.* vol. 10, no. 2 (2017).

CHAPTER FOUR

DR. HWANG WOO-SUK— CLONE CELL FAKE

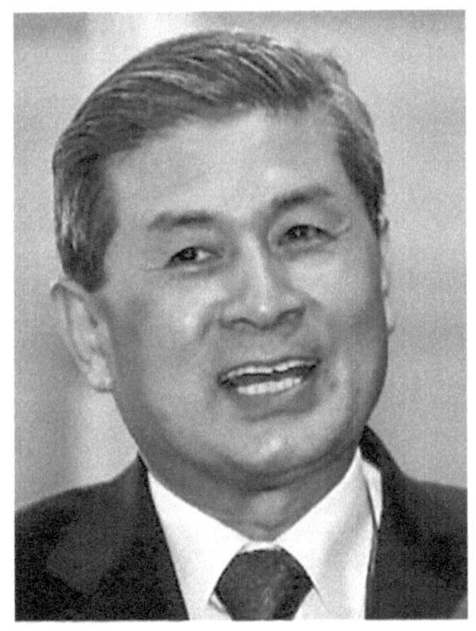

Photo: Jung Yeon-JE / AFP via Getty Images

Prologue

Dr. Hwang Woo-Suk is a South Korean veterinarian who specialized in theriogenology, which is the study of the reproductive process in animals. He was born in Buyeo, South Korea, on December 15, 1953, and graduated in veterinary medicine from the College of Veterinary Medicine in the Seoul National University in 1977, receiving his master's degree in theriogenology in 1982. Two years later, he transferred to the

Hokkaido University in Sapporo, Japan, where he remained until taking a post as a research fellow in the Seoul National University in 2006.[1]

Career

Somatic cell nuclear transfer (SCNT) is the technique used to clone a species of animal. The DNA in the somatic (body) cell is taken from the cell of an adult animal who is to be cloned (say, a sheep), who is the donor after being extracted from the cell (of a mammary gland in the case of Dolly, the first mammal to be cloned).[2,3,4] The DNA from the donor will be a copy of its DNA and genetic material from the somatic cell of the adult who donated it. It is then inserted into an egg cell from another animal (sheep in the case of Dolly) after the egg cell has had its nucleus removed. The result will be that the DNA from the donor is in the care of the cytoplasm of another sheep. It will then copy the DNA of the donor cell (Dolly in this case). A current of electricity is then passed through the resulting embryo to trigger its multiplication by division so that it becomes a blastocyst. It is then implanted into another ewe's uterus (the surrogate). If it survives, the resulting newborn will be an identical genetic replica to the donor sheep. In other words, it is similar to the actions of the cuckoo bird, which kicks out the egg of another bird in order to use its nest to nurture its own chick, except that in the case of the cuckoo, the egg is not a clone and is placed in the same nest, not that of another bird! This might not be a good analogy, but hopefully, it will explain some of the difficulties of cloning.

Dr. Hwang's initial attention was directed at cloning of pigs, cows, beagle dogs, and other animals, including threatened and extinct species.[3,4,5,6] He is credited with cloning the first dog, a black Afghan hound named Snuppy in 2005.[1] This was a great achievement, as cloning of dogs was thought to be difficult due to the canine's complicated reproductive cycle and the fragility of its eggs in culture. Dr. Hwang's renown as a scientist spread throughout the world and sparked a flame of national pride in South Korea, where they were worried about advancing technological developments in China.

Cloning of a Human

After having cloned Snuppy, Dr. Hwang turned his attention to the cloning of a human. He formed an association with *Dr. Moon Shin Yong*, an obstetrician and gynecologist who had extensive experience in IVF techniques in humans. Together in 2004, they announced that they had cloned human embryos and that one of these cells had produced a human stem cell line.[5] This resulted in great excitement through the scientific community and the world at large. It was also highly controversial due to the implications that the cells could be used for therapeutic or reproductive purposes.[6] A tense public debate ensued regarding the ethical implications of using the cells for therapeutic purposes, such as the investigation of new treatments for human disorders, for example, Alzheimer's and Parkinson's diseases. Drs. Hwang and Moon both made it known that they were not in favor of the cells being used for reproductive purposes.[7,8]

When asked how they succeeded where so many others had failed, Drs. Hwang and Moon claimed that they had used a new technique of squeezing the egg to reduce damage and had access to a large number of human cells but that they only needed fewer than twenty to produce each stem cell line. This last was going to come back to haunt them. After repeatedly denying the use of eggs from staff, in November 2005, Hwang admitted to the use of eggs taken from two of his own laboratory workers but claimed that they were voluntary donations. This was a contradiction of ethical behavior, even if it was not technically illegal at the time. Then later that year, *Sung-Il Roh*, a whistleblower from Dr. Hwang's own laboratory, came forward and advised that Dr. Hwang's claims on human cloning were fabricated.[1]

Investigation

A committee was formed by the Seoul National University to investigate the claims. It reported in early 2006 that both papers published in *Science* (in 2004 and 2005) were fabricated and that they had not cloned human stem cells.[9,10] The committee did confirm, however, that Snuppy the dog was a clone. As far as the claim to have cloned human cells was concerned, the committee remarked, "The scientific basis for claiming any success is wholly lacking." Further to the claim that eggs from staff that were voluntary donations about which Dr. Hwang knew nothing, a staff member came forward and stated that Hwang had personally accompanied her to the MizMedi Hospital for the oocyte (egg) harvesting procedure. Staff members later stated that they had been asked to sign forms volunteering to donate eggs. The committee also established that claims that only 427 oocytes had been used for the work described in the two papers were incorrect and that 2,061 had actually been used from four different hospitals in 2005 alone. It is not known who the donors of these eggs are or whether they gave consent for the procedure, which is uncomfortable, even painful.[11,12]

Epilogue

Dr. Hwang was dismissed from Seoul National University in March 2006. He was charged, and his trial lasted three years.

He was found guilty of buying human oocytes and human embryos that were smuggled into his laboratory to give the impression that he had cloned human stem cells.[12] He had also accepted private donations worth $2.1 million and embezzled government research funds of up to $856,000.[13,14] He was given a two-year prison sentence, wholly suspended.[15] His claim that he had produced human stem cells from them has long since been discredited. The judge said he could not believe that Hwang had taken so many eggs for monetary gain and found that he had committed embezzlement but not fraud.[16,17,18] In spite of his spectacular fall from grace, Dr. Hwang enjoyed enormous popular support from people reluctant to accept the "Pride of Korea" was a fraud. One freezing evening in winter in central Seoul after his downfall, one thousand people gathered in a grand show of support.[19] More than seven hundred women offered to donate eggs.[20]

He then took employment with an American technology company in Tripoli. They specialized in cloning dead pets, but he had to leave Libya shortly afterward due to the rising violence there. Lately, he was said to be working in South Korea again where he has cloned coyotes using eggs from a domestic dog and, it is said, hoping to clone another woolly mammoth.[14]

The enthusiasm gradually waned, however, leaving the world to wonder why such a talented scientist who had already achieved fame would risk it all by falsifying his work. As with so many others in this book, the answer is blowing in the wind!

Notes

1. Craine, A. Hwang Woo-Suk | South Korean scientist (internet). *Encyclopedia Britannica*. 2019 (cited October 29, 2019]. Available from https://www. britannica.com/biography/Hwang-Woo-Suk.

2. BBC. Dolly Cloned sheep (internet). 2019. Available from https://www.britannica.com/topic/Dolly-cloned-sheep.

3. Dyer, O. "Sheep Cloned by Nuclear Transfer." *BMJ*. 1996; 312(7032): 658.

4. BBC: On This Day. "Dolly, the Sheep, Is Cloned." BBC News. 1997.

5. Lee, B., M. Lim, W. Hwang, et al. "Dogs Cloned from Adult Somatic Cells." *Nature*. 2005; 436(7051): 641.

6. Kim, M., G. Jang, H. Oh, F. Yuda, H. Kim, W. Hwang, et al. "Endangered Wolves Cloned from Adult Somatic Cells." *Cloning and Stem Cells*. 2007; 9(1): 130–137.

7. Hossein, M., Y. Jeong, S. Park, J. Kim, E. Lee, K. Ko, et al. "Birth of Beagle Dogs by Somatic Cell Nuclear Transfer." *Animal Reproduction Science*. 2009; 114(4): 404–414.

8. Hwang, W. "Evidence of a Pluripotent Human Embryonic Stem Cell Line Derived from a Cloned Blastocyst." *Science*. 2004; 303(5664): 1,669–1,674.

9. Normile, D., G. Vogel, J. Couzin. "Cloning: South Korean Team's Remaining Human Stem Cell Claim Demolished." *Science*. 2006; 311(5758): 156–157.

10. "High Interest Clones." *Nature*. 478, 5 (2001). Available from http://doi.org/10.1038/478005a.

11. Hwang, W. "Patient-Specific Embryonic Stem Cells Derived from Human SCNT Blastocysts." *Science*. 2005; 308(5729): 1,777–1,783.

12. Hwang, W., B. Lee, C. Lee, S. Kang. "Cloned Human Embryonic Stem Cells for Tissue Repair and Transplantation." *Stem Cell Reviews*. 2005; 1(2): 99–110.

13. Hwang, W., B. Lee, C. Lee, S. Kang. "Human Embryonic Stem Cells and Therapeutic Cloning." *Journal of Veterinary Science*. 2005; 6(2): 87–96.

14. Hwang, I., Y. Jeong, J. Kim, H. Lee, M. Kang, K. Park, J. Park, Y. Kim, W. Kim, T. Shin, S. Hyun, E.

Jeung, W. Hwang. "Successful Cloning of Coyotes Through Interspecies Somatic Cell Nuclear Transfer Using Domestic Dog Oocytes." *Reproduction, Fertility and Development*. 2013; 25(8): 1142-8.

15. CNN News. "Disgraced Cloning Researcher Convicted in South Korea." 2009.

16. Kim, H. "Disgraced Cloning Expert Convicted in S. Korea." Independent Assoc. Press (internet). 2009 (cited October 28, 2019). Available from https:// www.independent.co.uk/news/world/asia/disgraced-cloning-expert-convicted-in-s-korea-1809648.html.

17. Cyranoski, D., E. Check. "Clone Star Admits Lies over Eggs." *Nature* (internet). 2005; 438(7068): 536. Available from https://www.nature.com/articles/438536a.

18. Cyranoski, D. "Woo Suk Hwang convicted, but Not of Fraud." *Nature*. 2009; 461(7268): 1,181.

19. Scanlon, C. "Korea's National Shock at Scandal." BBC News (internet). 2006. Available from https://www. google.com/search?q=Korea%27s+national+shock+ at+scandal&rlz=1C1GCEAenAU776AU776&oq=K orea%27s+national+shock+at+scandal&aqs=chrom e..69i57.5500j0j7&sourceid=chrome&ie=UTF-8.

20. Parry, J. "Korean Women Rush to Donate Eggs after Research Pioneer Resigns." *BMJ*. December 2005; 331(7528) :1,291.

CHAPTER FIVE

DRS. FUJII, BOLDT, AND REUBEN—THE GREAT PRETENDERS

Prologue

All three of these doctors were anesthetists, and all three were frauds.

Dr. Yoshitaka Fujii was an anesthetist but was not just any old fraud; he was the mother of all fraudsters. Fujii was born in the city of Hatogaya-Honcho in Saitama, just northwest of Tokyo in Japan in 1960 and went to medical school in Tokai University. He was first registered as a doctor in 1987 and qualified as a specialist anesthetist in 1994. He then spent two years in Canada before returning to Tokyo, Japan, in 1997 where he worked as an anesthetist at the University of Tsukuba and then the Toho University until his employment at that institution was terminated in 2012.[1]

Life was good for Dr. Yoshitaka Fujii, and it is hard to believe that, from 1991, he published dozens of papers on his chosen subject while happily making a living as an anesthetist.

Dr. Fujii's main area of interest (and his imagination) initially was the prevention and treatment of nausea and vomiting after a general anesthetic. He published extensively and frequently on the subject, especially on the use of a drug called granisetron as a preventative or curative for postoperative nausea or vomiting. Fujii's studies purported to show that granisetron was more effective at higher doses than at lower doses. Studies from other groups failed to show this difference; however, Fujii published works in many other subjects as well, such as muscle relaxants, the response of the heart to having a tube inserted in the throat, and pain when an intravenous anesthetic called propofol was injected. He was a prolific publisher, usually describing his studies as "double-blind placebo randomised controlled trials" (RCT). In this type of study, there are two (usually large) groups, in one of which everyone has an inactive (sugar) tablet and everyone in the other group has an active tablet (granisetron in this case). Nobody knows which is which until the study is over. This method generally results in a meaningful answer. Unless, of course, the data entered is false. As they say regarding computers, "Put rubbish in; it will put rubbish out." It was so over the years, Dr. Fujii put lots of rubbish in and got lots of rubbish out. When he finished, he claimed to have used fourteen thousand human subjects in RCTs as well as seven hundred mongrel dogs.

Although it must have been a phenomenal amount of work, it was not wasted, as it opened opportunities to Dr. Fujii for personal advancement and employment at professorial level, as well as access to public research money.

His scientific publications on granisetron, propofol, scopolamine (a muscle relaxant), and several other drugs influenced their use around the world. But not all anesthetists accepted his findings without critical thought.

Three anesthetists—*Peter Kranke*, *Christian Apfel*, and *Norbert Roewer*—from Würzburg, Germany, wrote a letter to the editor of *Anesthesia & Analgesia*. It was titled "Reported Data on Granisetron and Postoperative Nausea and Vomiting by Fujii et al. Are Incredibly Nice!"[2] Its clever use of the word *nice* is especially remarkable, as the author's first language is German. Most native English speakers have difficulty knowing how to use *nice* properly. One of its correct meanings would be "fine," in the sense that "it is fine work" as by a watchmaker. In this case, it is used dripping with sarcasm and by no means should be read as fine work. The authors are not in praise of Fujii's work. Quite the opposite. Their letter goes on to imply that they are not impressed without actually saying so. They commented on twenty-one articles from 1994 to 1999 in which Fujii had reported headache as a side effect of granisetron. In thirteen of the articles, the incidence of headache was reported as the same; and in the other eight, there was only a difference of one from patient to patient. Kranke and colleagues analyzed the results and found that they were unlikely to be true. Statistically, the number of headaches in each group should have varied more. In other words, the chance of a headache in the population studied would be expected to vary more than Fujii had allowed. His study population was just too perfect. This was not surprising, as it did not exist! The letter from Kranke et al. finishes by saying, "We have to conclude that there must be an underlying influence causing such incredibly nice data reported by Fujii et al."[2] Another masterpiece in sarcasm! The "underlying influence" being Fujii.

Then in 2001, Kranke et al. published again, this time on granisetron specifically, and again they challenged the findings of Fujii, but again their warnings were ignored. Instead of taking note of this criticism, the University of Toho employed Dr. Fujii as an anesthetist, and he continued publishing figments of his imagination.[3]

Regardless of this remarkable piece of detective work, Dr. Fujii's scientific studies were largely ignored, and he continued publishing fabricated data for another ten years. However, perhaps due to the articles by Kranke et al., Dr. Fujii directed more of his contributions to less noticeable journals such as

Ophthalmology. Suspicions arose though, and Dr. Fujii's colleagues became anxious. Then in 2012, *Dr. John Carlisle*, an anesthetist from Torbay Hospital in England, who had developed a comfortable grip of the mathematics of statistics, published a paper seventeen pages long in the journal *Anaesthesia*.[4] The paper was an analysis of 168 of Fujii's randomized controlled trials over twenty years from 1991, and it systematically demolished Fujii's work. He showed that in the case of some variables, the likelihood of such an event might be as low as 1 in 10^3, which, for most of us, is nil.

Fujii was interviewed by the university committee and asked to explain himself, but he denied everything, saying that his findings could not be wrong as "so many journals have accepted them"! The statistical analysis by Carlisle was the nail in Fujii's coffin. Toho University Hospital dismissed Dr. Yoshitaka Fujii.[5]

The online blog Retraction Watch by *Adam Marcus* and *Ivan Oransky* provides some fascinating information. Their "Leaderboard" has Dr. Yoshitaka Fujii as the number 1 fraud in the world by a country mile. He is credited with 183 retracted (withdrawn) scientific papers in the twenty years from 1991. Marcus and Oransky point out that their "Leaderboard" will change from time to time (as it does in golf). Fujii is unlikely to lose the lead any time soon.[6]

In 2012, the Toho University found him guilty of failing to get ethics committee approval in eight cases and retracted them. Probably because of this, later that year the Japanese Society of Anesthesiologists took more interest in Fujii and set up a Special Investigation Committee (SIC) to inquire into his publications. It credited Fujii with 212 original papers. Of these, 172 were fabricated (including 126 that were randomized double-blind trials), and thirty-seven were indeterminate.[5] Only *three* publications were confirmed as reliable scientific studies!

Fujii had covered his tracks in several ways:

1. He reported randomized controlled trials. This made it difficult to detect fraud.
2. He reported some of them as though they occurred at other institutions.
3. He reported some that had occurred when he allegedly had a part-time job.
4. He did not report the sources of his studies, making it difficult to check.
5. He reported some as multihospital (meta-analysis) studies.
6. He used existent authors who did not know that they were included or nonexistent coauthors.
7. He forged the signature of supposed coauthors who were unaware of their collaboration.

Moreover, finally, 172 of them were figments of his imagination, and the other thirty-seven may have been when he was dreaming as well.[7]

Dr. Fujii was last thought to be working part-time at several hospitals in Tokyo.[8]

Dr. Fujii is well ahead of second on the Leaderboard—Dr. Joachim Boldt with ninety-seven retractions.

DR. JOACHIM BOLDT

Dr. Joachim Boldt is an anesthetist and a fraud, like the others in this chapter, but unlike the others, he was born in Germany on September 29, 1954. He became an extremely well-known, respected, and admired anesthetist employed in the Klinikum Ludwigshafen, a hospital in the Rhineland-Pfalz.

Colloids are commonly occurring substances. They consist of tiny, microscopic particles suspended in a diffuse continuous (usually liquid) phase. Homogenized milk is a good example. It contains microscopic particles of fat suspended in a solution of milk. Perhaps because they are so small, the particles in a colloid do not settle but remain in suspension even when standing in storage. They are often used to thicken the solution of which they are part, for example, in a meringue. Dr. Joachim Boldt was interested in colloids—particularly one called hydroxyethyl starch (HES). Hydroxyethyl starch has had many uses in medicine, especially as a plasma (volume) expander in critically ill patients who might have suffered much blood loss. When whole blood is lost, the patient not only loses red blood cells that carry oxygen but also plasma, which carries the red blood cells. The red blood cells and the plasma can be replaced with donated blood, but donated blood is not always available in unlimited supply. In that case, a volume expander such as saline (water and salt) or Hartmann's or Ringer's solution containing water and electrolytes and known as crystalloids may be used. Other solutions that have been used include albumin (a protein) and various colloids (including HES). Dr. Joachim Boldt used it to prime cardiac bypass machines before they underwent open-heart surgery. He also published widely on the benefits of HES for that and other purposes.

It was not long before he had accumulated almost one hundred publications, many of which compared HES with other colloids such as human albumin (HA) to prime cardiac bypass machines. Ironically, he made comparisons as late as 2010.[9,10] His hospital, the Klinikum Ludwigshafen, when it later conducted an inquiry, found that HA had not been available in the hospital since 1990, and the suppliers of HA confirmed that none had been delivered to the hospital since that year. How he made the comparison without the albumin, only he knows.

Many of Boldt's papers recommended the use of HES or HES-related substances as a primer in cardiac bypass pumps, regardless of the fact that the FDA had recommended as long ago as 2003 that HES should not be used as a bypass primer. Boldt claimed several advantages for it, including reduced tissue damage to blood vessels and kidneys and increased control of blood coagulation, regardless of many other studies suggesting the opposite.[11]

In 2009, Boldt and others published a paper in the journal *Anesthesia & Analgesia* comparing HES with an albumin-based primer. That was curious, as he had no albumin. However, that is not what drew attention to the article, as readers did not know that he had no albumin. What did attract the attention of some readers was how perfect was the reported acid-base balance of the patients after their operation. The editor of the journal, *Dr. Stephen Shafer*, received several emails within weeks of publication, drawing his attention to the unusual consistency of the findings. He read the paper again and came to the conclusion that the fluid balance was not possible, saying, "There appeared to be a perfect acid-base balance after surgery. No one has ever seen this in the history of the world. And once I saw that I thought that this had to be fake." In other words, this is too good to be true. Dr. Shafer tried repeatedly to contact Dr. Boldt over the next few weeks without success.[12]

Eventually, Shafer asked the Landesärztekammer Rheinland-Pfalz (LÄK-RLP), the state medical association, which is the Institutional Review Board (IRB), to investigate. The IRB is the body responsible for clinical research at the Klinikum Ludwigshafen, where Boldt worked. Unfortunately, they were only empowered to investigate whether Dr. Boldt had IRB approval to carry out the research. In October 2010, the IRB reported that Boldt did not have ethics committee approval to conduct the study. This allowed Shafer to retract the article.

Dr. Shafer's retraction of the article sparked a joint investigation of all Boldt's papers by the IRB and the hospital. The committee reported in 2011 that

- there were no data to support the findings,
- albumin had not been used in the studies reported,
- Boldt had forged the signatures of supposed coauthors,
- there was no evidence that the studies had been carried out in some cases,
- there was no evidence of ethics committee approval in sixty-eight of seventy-four articles reviewed,
- he had claimed payment for operations he had never performed.[13]

As a result, the editors of eighteen well-known medical journals agreed to retract eighty-eight articles for which they could find no evidence of ethics committee approval.[14] Further investigations established that many other studies of Boldt's had incomplete or manipulated data, and Boldt was dismissed from the hospital.

HES is much more expensive than most of the other plasma expanders. It was in the interests of the manufacturer that HES continued to be used. Dr. Boldt was remunerated by the manufacturers of HES and paid to speak at many international symposia. Boldt's support of it resulted in many anesthetists continuing to use it.[15]

The authorities followed up 455 of Boldt's patients and could find no evidence that any had come to harm, although many had comorbidities. That would be reassuring except that a study by Schierhout and Roberts in 1998 at University College Hospital in London suggested that the mortality rate using colloids or HES was 4 percent higher than with other primers—in other words, eighteen deaths in 455 patients.[15] So there was no increase in morbidity noted, just an increase in mortality!

Results of the investigations were handed to the prosecutor, and at the time of writing, Boldt's whereabouts are unknown, although it is rumored that he is working as an anesthetist in the Czech Republic.

DR. SCOTT REUBEN

Dr. Scott Reuben is the third of our fraudulent anesthetists.

He was born in 1958 and graduated in medicine from the State University of New York in Buffalo in 1985. His first year as a doctor was at Mount Sinai Medical Center before moving to Boston, Massachusetts, in 1991. Later, in 2008, he became professor of anesthesiology and head of the acute pain service at the Baystate Medical Service in Tufts University–Boston.[16,17]

Cyclooxygenase-2 is an enzyme that causes pain and inflammation. The COX-2 inhibitors target this enzyme in an effort to reduce pain, and they do not carry the risk of peptic ulceration as do aspirin and ibuprofen. COX-2 inhibitors (celecoxib and rofecoxib) are in a group of pain relievers called nonsteroidal anti-inflammatory agents (NSAID). The COX-2 inhibitors are claimed to be superior to others in the NSAID group for pain relief. Reuben was said to be interested in a multimodal approach to the relief of pain. This meant that he directed his studies at pain relief at different levels using different recipes of drugs. Additionally, he was interested in relieving pain without resorting to the opiates. The USA was in the grip of an opiate epidemic at the time (and still is). Unfortunately, celecoxib and rofecoxib were found to be associated with heart attacks and strokes. Rofecoxib (sold as Vioxx) was removed from the market entirely in 2004 for this reason. Celecoxib is still available but with conditions. There is some evidence that it may delay bone healing and, therefore, should not be used for orthopedic patients.

It was with this background that Dr. Reuben based his interest and his research. Among other attributes, he suggested that his multimodal method using COX-2 inhibitors resulted in

- reduced postoperative pain,
- reduced reliance on opiates,

- less nausea and vomiting, and
- they did not hinder the rate of bone healing.

Animal studies were done by others, on the other hand, and suggested that the use of these COX-2 inhibitors could slow the recovery rate of bone. This would be a major disadvantage to their use in orthopedic patients.[18]

Dr. Scott Reuben had been merrily going along for eleven years publishing his findings on postoperative pain.[19] He happily went along to clinical meetings and symposia spouting the benefits of celecoxib (sold as Celebrex) and downplaying the benefits of other pain killers while being supported by Pfizer. In 2005, he formed a working association with an orthopedic surgeon, *Dr. Evan Ekman*, and together they published several articles on pain relief. Dr. Ekman was asked to peer-review an article that Dr. Reuben had written on surgery to the knee, but when he asked for the name of the surgeon, Reuben did not respond.[20,21] Two or three years later, at a conference, Dr. Ekman saw the same article published with his own name on it. His signature had been forged![22]

Things started to become really unstuck for Reuben when, in 2008, a routine audit of the Baystate Institutional Review Board noted that two of Reuben's studies did not have approval to carry out research on humans. This led to further investigation, and it was found that in twenty-one studies that he had authored or coauthored since 1996, the data had been fabricated. In many cases, the work that he had published had never been done and was a figment of his imagination. In other cases, he had forged the signatures of imagined coauthors who had no knowledge that their names were being used. The editors of the affected journals were asked to retract the work. *Dr. Steven Shafer*, editor in chief of the journal *Anesthesia & Analgesia*, considered retracting every article that had been submitted by Reuben.[18,19,20]

In 2010, Dr. Reuben was charged with health-care fraud. He pleaded guilty and was sentenced to six months in prison and fined $420,000, most of which had to be repaid to the pharmaceutical companies who had supported him with grants.[10,11,16] They seem to have been the great winners, as they were also the beneficiaries of the sale of billions of dollars' worth of the COX-2 inhibitors.

Influence of Fujii, Boldt, and Reuben's Fraudulent Work

PubMed shows that Reuben has seventy-two publications to date, of which fifty-five are as first (or only) author. Twenty-four of them were withdrawn, but even so, his work has been referred to 3,079 times from 1991 until 2019. Of them, 2,808 were before 2009, after which they dropped off. There were still twenty-nine citations in the year 2019 alone in spite of his jail term. Dr. Reuben's citations are uncommon now, and some of them are of retracted articles, but if twenty-four studies are withdrawn because of fraud, how can the reader trust any of the researchers' other forty-eight publications? Nonetheless, this number of citations must have affected the practice of anesthesia worldwide and changed the method of pain relief given to millions of patients, possibly to their detriment.[16,17] Fujii and Boldt together had 290 articles withdrawn, but not before an enormous amount of damage had been done.

An analysis of the 304 combined works of Fujii, Boldt, and Reuben showed that 11 percent of those eligible for retraction had still not been retracted until the journal authors were contacted in 2018, and even then, 6 percent were still not withdrawn in 2019, six years after publication.[23] In other words, even after six years, the cat was still not entirely back in the bag.

If an article has been accepted from a scientific journal and printed, it means that if the subscriber to that journal incorporates that information into clinical practice, it may become clinical practice forever. If the findings are subsequently retracted and the subscriber is unaware of the retraction, the effects will carry on forever. Later issues of the journal will carry advisories that the piece has been withdrawn, but users may not see this, and inappropriate practices might carry on. Thus, the damage might last for decades.

Notes

1. "Dr. Geoff: Yoshitaka Fujii—Japanese Anaesthetist and Record-Breaking Research Fraud." Available from https://drgeoffnutrition.wordpress.com/2017/04/05/yoshitaka-fujii-japanese-anaes-thetist-and-record-breaking-research-fraud/.
2. Kranke, P., C. Apfel, N. Roewer. "Reported Data on Granisetron and Postoperative Nausea and Vomiting by Fujii et al. Are Incredibly Nice!" *Anesthesia & Analgesia.* 2000,90: 1,000.
3. Kranke, P., C. Apfel, L. H. Eberhart, M. Georgieff, N. Roewer. "The Influence of a Dominating Centre on a Quantitative Systematic Review of Granisetron for Preventing Postoperative Nausea and Vomiting." *Acta Anaesthesiol Scand.* July 2001; 45(6): 659–70.
4. Carlisle, J. B. "The Analysis of 168 Randomised Controlled Trials to Test Data Integrity." *Anaesthesia.* 2012, 67: 521–537.
5. Sumikawa, Koji. "The Results of an Investigation into Dr. Yoshitaka Fujii's papers." The Japanese Society of Anaesthesiologists. June 29, 2012.
6. Marcus, A., I. Oransky. Retraction Watch: The Retraction Watch Leaderboard. Available from https://retrac-tionwatch.com/the-retraction-watch-leaderboard/.

7. Miller, D. R. "Retraction of Articles by Dr. Yoshitaka Fujii." *Can J. Anesth. / J. Can. Anesth.* (2012) 59: 1,081. Available from https://doi.org/10.1007/s12630-012-9802-9.

8. McNeill, David. "Japanese Fraud Case Highlights Weaknesses in Scientific Publishing." *The Chronicle of Higher Education.* October 8, 2012. Available from http://www.ruppweb.org/CHE_The-Great-Pretender_Oct_8_2012.pdf.

9. Boldt, J., S. Suttner, C. Brosch, A. Lehmann, K. Röhm, A. Mengistu. "Cardiopulmonary Bypass Priming Using a High Dose of a Balanced Hydroxyethyl Starch versus an Albumin-Based Priming Strategy." *Anesthesia & Analgesia.* 2009; 109(6): 1,752–1,762.

10. Boldt, J. "Use of Albumin: An Update." *British Journal of Anaesthesia.* 2010; 104(3): 276–284.

11. Geoff, D. "Joachim Boldt—German Anesthesiologist Who Faked Data Relating to the Management of Critically Ill Patients." (Internet). 2019 (cited September 22, 2019). Available from https://drgeoff-nutrition.wordpress.com/2017/11/09/joachim-boldt-german-anesthesiologist-who-faked-data-relating-to-the-management-of-critically-ill-patients/

12. Wise, J. "Boldt: the Great Pretender." *BMJ.* 2013; 346(Mar 19, 2013):1,738

13. Blake, H., H. Watt, R. Winnett. "Millions of Surgery Patients at Risk in Drug Research Fraud Scandal." *The Daily Telegraph* (internet). 2011 (cited September 23, 2019). Available from https://www.telegraph.co.uk/news/health/8360667/Millions-of-surgery-patients-at-risk-in-drug-research-fraud-scandal.html.

14. Editor. "Editors-in-Chief Statement Regarding Published Clinical Trials Conducted without IRB Approval by Joachim Boldt." *Minerva Anestesiologica* (internet).

2011 (cited September 23, 2019); March 12 (vol. 77, no. 5): 562–563. Available from https://www.minervamedica.it/en/getfreepdf/9wTwh%252Fc7m58rqO Kh3fZsbvoJl4IezrFh%252Bqq%252BuGNAccCD ysHBUTcq38ZqAruBNkRtPutdeUwK3wi4YdLPIj GGdw%253D%253D/R02Y2011N05A0562.pdf.

15. Schierhout, G., I. Roberts. "Fluid Resuscitation with Colloid or Crystalloid Solutions in Critically Ill Patients: A Systematic Review of Randomised Trials." *BMJ*. 1998; 316(7136): 961–964.

16. Webb, G. "Scott S. Reuben—Anesthesiologist Who Went to Prison for Faking Pain Control Trials." Dr. Geoff (internet). 2017 (cited September 25, 2019). Available from https://drgeoffnutrition.wordpress. com/2017/11/19/scott-s-reuben-anesthesiologist-who-went-to-prison-for-faking-pain-control-trials/.

17. Borrell, B. "A Medical Madoff: Anesthesiologist Faked Data in 21 Studies." *Scientific American* (internet). 2009 (cited September 25, 2019). Available from https://www.scientificamerican.com/ article/a-medical-madoff-anesthestesiologist-faked-data/.

18. Barry, S. "Dr. Scott Reuben, Former Chief of Acute Pain at Baystate Medical Center in Springfield, Pleads Guilty to Health-Care Fraud." Blog (internet). 2019 (cited September 24, 2019). Available from https://www.masslive.com/news/2010/01/ dr_scott_reuben_former_chief_o.html.

19. Harris, G. "Doctor's Pain Studies Were Fabricated, Hospital Says." *The New York Times* (internet). 2009 (cited September 24, 2019). Available from https://www.nytimes.com/2009/03/11/ health/research/11pain.html?ref=us.

20. Kowalczyk, L. "Doctor Accused of Faking Studies." *The Boston Globe* (internet). 2009 (cited

September 24, 2019). Available from https://web.
archive.org/web/20090316053206/http://www.
boston.com/news/health/articles/2009/03/11/
doctor_accused_of_faking_studies/?page=2.

21. Reuben, S., E. Ekman. "The Effect of Initiating a
Preventive Multimodal Analgesic Regimen on Long-
Term Patient Outcomes for Outpatient Anterior
Cruciate Ligament Reconstruction Surgery."
Anesthesia & Analgesia. 2007; 105(1): 228–232.

22. Reuben, S., E. Ekman, D. Charron. "Evaluating the
Analgesic Efficacy of Administering Celecoxib as a
Component of Multimodal Analgesia for Outpatient
Anterior Cruciate Ligament Reconstruction Surgery."
Anesthesia & Analgesia. 2007; 105(1): 222–227.

23. McHugh, U., S. Yentis. "An Analysis of Retractions of
Papers Authored by Scott Reuben, Joachim Boldt and
Yoshitaka Fujii." *Anaesthesia.* 2018; 74(1): 17–21.

DR. GEOFFREY EDELSTEN—A BRILLIANT CAREER

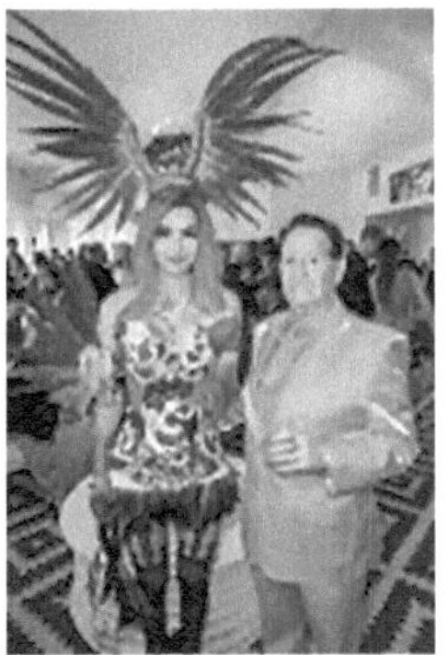

Photo: Scott Barbour / Getty Images

Prologue

Geoffrey Walter Edelsten has certainly lived life to the full. Writing about him is not difficult because he has chronicled his own life through his websites and the printed and electronic media. He had one scientific article published in the *Medical Journal of Australia* in 1970 on computers in general practice, so he was well ahead of his peers in that era.[1] Another article was published under his name in the same journal on the legislation of tattoos in 1983.[2] Again, at that time he was much involved in removing tattoos.

Geoffrey Edelsten was a Melbourne boy. He was born and grew up in the inner-city suburb of Carlton, home of the famous Carlton Australian rules football (AFL) club. His love of AFL probably started there. His mother (Esther) and father (Hymie) ran a store for women's underwear called Linda Leigh after Hymie returned from WWII. The family later moved from Carlton to Burwood, also in Melbourne, where Geoffrey went to school at the Mount Scopus Memorial College, the first coeducational school in Australia. Geoffrey was said to be a high achiever even at that age. He was captain of the first football team and cricket team as well as the fastest over the one-hundred-yard sprint.

Geoffrey was awarded a Commonwealth Scholarship to attend medical school at the University of Melbourne. In those days, Commonwealth Scholarships were easy to get as there was still a shortage of doctors in Australia. Nonetheless, his progress through medical school was said in his website to be that of a high achiever, and he graduated on December 17, 1966.[3]

It is abundantly clear that from the time of his graduation in Melbourne in 1966 until 2004, Geoffrey was devoting himself to academic improvements and achievement, attaining seven master's degrees, diplomas in aviation medicine and family medicine, two law degrees, a PhD, and an MBA—all this while recovering from brain surgery. He gives himself the titles of "professor doctor" but does not say which institution awarded the title of professor.

All this would be a daunting task for a lesser man. But Geoffrey was not such a man. After graduation, he worked in several rural family practices in New South Wales and Queensland before settling in Coogee in the coastal suburbs of Sydney.

Before long, Dr. Edelsten had opened a general practice in George's Hall and later in Liverpool, suburbs close to Bankstown Airport (about fifteen to twenty kilometers west of Coogee and the Central Business District of Sydney) and, therefore, a likely source of pilots who required annual medical checks.

Dark clouds were gathering on the horizon, however. Some irregular patterns were noted in his style of administering his practice. He was charged by the Medical Tribunal of New South Wales with several serious complaints.

Not of Good Character—Soliciting a Hit Man

The first complaint was that he was not of good character. It was alleged that Dr. Edelsten had a conversation with a person whom he knew to be a criminal and a murderer to obtain his assistance in attempting to intimidate a former patient. Dr. Edelsten appealed this decision.[4]

On January 26, 1984, *Mr. Christopher Dale Flannery* attended Dr. Edelsten in his surgery at George's Hall, a Sydney suburb close to Bankstown Aerodrome. Mr. Flannery requested removal of some tattoos, so Dr. Edelsten arranged his admission to Bigge Street Private Hospital–Liverpool on January 28 to have the tattoo removed. Mr. Flannery remained in hospital until February 2, 1984, during which time he told Dr. Edelsten that he was due to stand trial on February 1 on a charge of murder. He requested a medical certificate, the effect of which would be to excuse him from attendance at court before a particular judge. The medical certificate was presented to the court by Sergeant Duff (also known to be a patient of Dr. Edelsten), and the case was adjourned. The medical certificate was written for one or two weeks, but as it turned out, Mr. Flannery was discharged after one day.[5]

On March 1, 1984, Dr. Edelsten was harassed by someone whom he thought was a previous patient, a Mr. Evans. Dr. Edelsten received a bullet with his name engraved on it as well as a death threat. On March 3, Edelsten spoke by telephone with his secretary, Ms. Bissaker. The call was illegally intercepted and recorded by an amateur. During this telephone call to his secretary, when it was clear that Dr. Edelsten was talking about Mr. Flannery, he said, "I want this guy [Evans] found and got off my back." On April 15, 1984, Dr. Edelsten had another call, which was also intercepted and taped. This call was to his fiancée, *Ms. Leanne Nesbitt*. On this occasion, it was clear that Dr. Edelsten understood that Christopher Flannery was a professional killer. During the conversation, the price that Flannery charged was freely discussed. His price to beat somebody up was $15,000, and to kill somebody would be $50,000.[6] Counsel for Dr. Edelsten challenged the admissibility of the tapes used to record telephone conversations, but the court found that the tribunal was within its rights to admit the tapes. The appeal failed. The Court of Appeals upheld the findings of the medical tribunal that Dr. Edelsten was not of good character.

Guilty of Misconduct in a Professional Respect—Overservicing

"Between 1978 and 1984 Geoffrey Edelsten attempted to and did induce medical practitioners to whom he offered work as consultants or employees 'to over-service their patients by offering to enter into agreements with the said medical practitioner whereby they would be paid commissions for referring patients to specialist medical practitioners and/or companies associated with Geoffrey Edelsten.'"[7,8]

Pathology Referrals

The mechanism for overservicing is perhaps best explained using the pathology referral service. The doctors who were either employed by or were consultants to Dr. Edelsten's practice were paid by a company named Mediservices Proprietary Limited, which was controlled by Dr. Edelsten. He was one of two shareholders in a company named Omniman. The other shareholder was Trutza Investments P/L in which Edelsten and Monthaven P/L were the shareholders. Doctors working in Edelsten's surgeries were provided with pathology referral forms at various times in the name of OmniMed, Omniman, Alpha Pathology, or Macquarie Pathology. These medical practitioners referred pathology tests to Omniman, which, in turn, would send the pathology specimen to Macquarie Professional Services (MPS) or another specified pathology practice to carry out the relevant tests. Once MPS had completed its services, it sent accounts to the Federal Department of Health (the insurer); and when it received the money for the service, it was paid into a bank account that had been opened in the name of Omniman Trust Account. In accordance with an agreement that operated between them, Omniman received 67 percent of the value of the tests less ten dollars per patient and MPS received the ten dollars and the remaining 33 percent. The doctors who referred the specimens received regular commissions paid from OmniMed as inducements to overservice patients.[9] It could be argued that the scheme was designed to conceal the overservicing that was occurring, which, of course, it was.

According to the New South Wales Court of Criminal Appeal, the Medical Tribunal found that Dr. Edelsten had offered employment to a doctor whose terms of work were that she would receive a commission on everything referred within the building, meaning to any specialist service associated with

Dr. Edelsten and including all other services or tests such as pathology and x-ray.

In another example, Dr. Edelsten also offered employment to another doctor whose annual remuneration would be based on an annual base salary plus 10 percent of the gross fees on work performed or investigations ordered by her or 35 percent of gross fees. He told her that if she referred patients to in-house specialists, she would earn 10 percent of fees generated by those referrals.[10]

Other examples of overservicing were given in the evidence considered by the Court of Appeals. Another doctor said that on three occasions, Dr. Edelsten had telephoned him saying that he had not ordered as much pathology as Dr. Edelsten wished. Dr. Edelsten told him that "there are a lot of tests we can do and you really should be making full use of them." Dr. Edelsten then suggested that specific tests can be ordered routinely on pregnant women. When the employed doctor complained that not all the tests were justified, Dr. Edelsten replied that he wanted the tests done on everyone.[11]

Finally, a doctor who was employed at the Baulkham Hills Medical Centre said that she was paid a salary based on 35 percent of gross fees written by her. She gave evidence to the tribunal that on one occasion, Dr. Edelsten said to her, "I make very little money out of this practice. When I make money, it's out of pathology. I want you to order as much as you can."

On another occasion in 1984, a doctor commented to Dr. Edelsten, "I am not happy about being paid for doing pathology because I have found that it is illegal." Dr. Edelsten replied, "You are a fool; nobody will ever find out. The computers get confused when they are overloaded when your volume is high, and there is a large amount of money involved for you. Also, I pay you out of different companies so that nobody will ever know what is going on or where the cheques come from." The appeal against overservicing failed.[12,13]

Guilty of Misconduct in a Professional Respect—Fee Splitting

Until 1983, the patient's rebate for an ultrasonic cross-sectional examination was seventy-eight dollars, regardless of which practice provided the service. In 1978, however, the medical benefits insurance rebate was changed so that when the procedure was carried out within the one practice, the refund was reduced from $78.00 to $20.50. The distinction was known as a referred ultrasound, attracting a refund of $78.00, and a self-referred ultrasound, attracting a refund of $20.50. There was, at the time, no requirement for a referred ultrasound to be carried out by a specialist.

The tribunal alleged that Dr. Edelsten had entered into a fee-sharing arrangement with a radiologist so that patients who were referred for ultrasonic cross-sectional echography were charged by the radiologist at the higher rebate despite the fact that he shared the income received in respect of those services with Dr. Edelsten.[14]

There was a general (family) practice at Liverpool and an x-ray department next door. The x-ray department serviced the general practice and various other general surgeries in the region under Edelsten's control. Dr. Edelsten's practice manager arranged with the radiologist that he would carry out ultrasounds for the practice on the same basis that he provided x-ray services, that is, he would do the reporting on ultrasound tests and the same percentage for the use of facilities and services provided for him. This applied to a mobile ultrasound service in which an ultrasonographer would carry an ultrasound machine with a camera in her car to various addresses to carry out ultrasound examinations. She would then prepare reports by dictating into an audiotape that she would then leave with the film at the Liverpool x-ray premises. The radiologist would later drop by and sign the reports after a typist had completed them. The scans were then delivered back to the various original surgeries.

The court found that "an elaborate arrangement was devised in order to present the appearance" that the radiologist "was an independent medical practitioner whereas the fact was that he shared the receipts of the ultrasound services" with Dr. Edelsten and his partners.[14] "The essence of the complaint was that the appellant had received, by means of a fraudulent device, portion of the proceeds of ultrasonic treatment" given by the radiologist, which was charged at a higher rate.[14]

Apart from fee splitting with the radiologist, Dr. Edelsten also attempted to arrange fee splitting with doctors who worked for him. In one case, a doctor said that instead of paying her a salary, Edelsten told her that he would give her 50 percent of what was paid by the Health Insurance Commission if she agreed that she would collect the money and pay him a rental and give him half the money. On the day following the offer, she declined to be involved, saying that she did not know anything about ultrasound. This statement was met with the response from Edelsten that "he would show her how to do a couple and watch her do a couple and everything will be fine," although Dr. Edelsten had no training in ultrasound himself.

A similar arrangement was made with another doctor who also said that he had no experience in ultrasound but he entered into an agreement where he signed the headers and the assignment forms after checking that they tallied with the number of scans and then left them in his electricity box where they were collected later by a courier and returned to Edelsten's practices. The doctor said that he signed the reports and related ultrasound tests with respect to patients he had never seen, and he had ultrasound films and reports he had never examined. By this mechanism, the appearance presented to the Health Insurance Commission was that the ultrasound examinations had been carried out by a referred arm's-length practitioner and therefore qualified for the higher rebate.[15,16] Dr. Edelsten appealed, but the appeal on fee splitting failed.

Employment of an Unqualified Person to Remove Tattoos

Tattoo removal involves burning the superficial layers of skin containing the dye with a laser. The depth of the burn is critical to the final result. If the burn is too deep, it can result in an ugly scar. After the laser treatment, the laser site is allowed to heal, and the subsequent dead tissue falls off after a few days or is to be removed physically with forceps. In the case of Dr. Edelsten's patients, the final dressing for the resulting laser burn was Glad wrap, a plastic sheet sealant more commonly used in the kitchen.

A nursing sister was employed in Edelsten's Bankstown (a Sydney suburb) practice during 1980 and 1981. During that time, she was given training in tattoo removals by an employed doctor. She was transferred in 1983 to the George's Hall surgery nearby. She gave evidence to the tribunal that she received about twenty minutes' training from Dr. Edelsten and then assisted with several hundred laser tattoo removals after the doctor (either Dr. Edelsten or one of the other doctors) would give the local anesthetic and decide which areas were to be treated. Eventually, it was common for her to perform half or most of the removal, and she occasionally performed laser removals without a doctor being present in the room but never without a doctor being present in the building. Several patients gave corroborating evidence.[17]

Dr. Edelsten's appeal was dismissed with costs.[18]

Corporate Medicine

There is no doubt that Dr. Edelsten's thinking outside the square brought about a signal change; as clinics were open twenty-four hours a day, patients were bulk billed (direct billed to the Health Insurance Commission), and physicians could take rostered time off for their families and themselves. This was innovative and efficient for doctor and patient alike. One disadvantage of these corporate clinics was, however, that it became challenging to find a doctor who would do a home visit.

The Edelsten medical centers were gaudily decorated, incorporating variously a white grand piano, disco lights, and video machines. In 1977, Sydneysiders eagerly anticipated the opening of a half-million-dollar clinic that would cover six thousand square feet and employ nine doctors. Doors to consulting rooms opened automatically; waiting rooms were adorned with plush carpet for the comfort and pleasure of patients as they waited in snug armchairs, enjoying their choice of music via inbuilt stereo systems as they were served hors d'oeuvres and coffee from silver trays by receptionists in matching silver jumpsuits.[19]

Two years later, Dr. Edelsten was reportedly operating ten clinics, which employed sixteen doctors.[20] It was said that he located his medical centers close to a McDonald's restaurant, as "they had done all the marketing work." The older type of medical practice, of the *Dr. Finlay's Casebook* style, could still exist for those who wanted it. Dr. Edelsten himself worked in some of these clinics, although the pace must have been frenetic to fit in all that he had to do in a day as well as deliver one thousand babies a year for twenty years.[3]

Dr. Edelsten's Life outside Clinical Medicine

Dr. Edelsten was struck off the NSW Medical Register for ten years in 1988 for professional misconduct. He spent twelve months in prison in 1990, six months for soliciting Christopher Dale Flannery to "get a patient off his back" and six months for perverting the course of justice. Sentences to be served consecutively. He was a model prisoner by all accounts but received no remission of sentence. Mr. Edelsten presented powerful arguments on his websites in favor of his innocence, but the courts were unimpressed and did not reduce his sentence, and when he reapplied for admission to the medical register in 2001, he also failed. Again in 2003, he reapplied for admission, insisting that he was a changed man and of a changed character. He admitted to lying at previous attendances at court but said that he could now see the error of his ways. Despite that, he again failed to be reregistered.[21]

Mr. Geoffrey Edelsten's personal life outside medicine and commerce has been well chronicled in the printed and electronic media such that there is nothing to be gained by covering it again here. We have all seen him on bended knee in a bright-yellow silk suit proposing marriage to Gabi Grecko. Geoffrey and Gabi are seen in the image at the beginning of the chapter, attending a prominent race meeting in Sydney some years ago. His flamboyant and extroverted character is well known. It is worth recording Geoffrey's contribution to the Cronulla Sharks and to the Sydney Swans, however.

Cronulla Sharks

It was announced in the *6pm News* on July 22, 1986, that Dr. Edelsten discussed buying the Cronulla Sharks rugby league team with club officials. A week later, on July 29, the deal was announced all for $2.5 million! He and his then wife, Leanne, were seen outside the Regent Hotel, and although they attended one league game, the deal eventually fell through. The Cronulla Sharks were in financial difficulty when some of their sponsorship deals did not eventuate. The Cronulla rugby league club eventually came to the rescue, and the club continues to this day, even having won a Premiership.[22,23]

The Sydney Swans

The Swans Australian football league (AFL) team moved from Melbourne to Sydney in the early 1980s. They were called the Swans because they had many players who had moved from Western Australia, where the swan is the state emblem. After a short period of success, their future became somewhat tenuous. However, in a deal said to be worth $6.5 million over five years, Dr. Geoffrey Edelsten bought the Swans in 1985. This may have saved the Swans, as it was followed by a period of success on the field. However, financial security did not follow, nor was there an increase in membership. Dr. Edelsten resigned as chairman after less than twelve months, but the Swans remain in Sydney to this day.

A Brilliant Career

There are few individuals who have achieved so much and overcome so many obstacles as Dr. Geoffrey Edelsten. Having graduated in medicine in Melbourne, he was struck by a brain tumor that required surgery and then cardiac bypass surgery. Geoffrey then spent his time fruitfully, mostly between 1993 and 2004, by studying for seven master's degrees, a PhD in health care administration from the Pacific Western University, and law degrees from the University of New England and Monash University. He organized locum services and all-night medical services, which have reorganized the way we practice medical services in Australia. Some of these have been controversial, as they often result in the loss of the patient-doctor contact and make home visits difficult.

Unfortunately, Dr. Edelsten ran into a difficult period when it seemed that his judgment was clouded (as he admitted himself later) when he was found guilty of fraud by overservicing, fee splitting, employing an unqualified person to carry out professional services, and soliciting a known criminal to "get someone off his back." He was found to be "not of good character." As a result of this, Geoffrey was struck off the medical register and spent twelve months as a guest in Her Majesty's prison.

Dr. Edelsten continued his business interests after his spell in prison and has been variously described as a multimillionaire or a bankrupt. One cannot help wondering whether survivor resilience from the brain gave him the extraordinary strength to carry on regardless. He has always protested his innocence, but the Medical Tribunal never relented, and he was not reregistered.

Described as being "addicted to ostentatious displays of wealth," the *Weekend Australian* newspaper reported that Edelsten was found dead in his St. Kilda Road apartment in Melbourne on a Friday afternoon, June 11, 2021. He was aged seventy-eight.[24] Reports suggested no suspicious circumstances surrounding the death.[25]

Former Sydney Swans player Greg Williams said he was shocked by the news. "He was a great guy, he had a great heart, and he loved the Swans," Williams said. "People had an opinion of him, but he was a lot different than the actual opinion." This sentiment is supported in the respect and affection reflected in public comment following the announcement of the death.

By his own account, he has had a brilliant career.

Notes

1. Edelsten, G. W., T. R. Wenkart. "Use of Computers in a New Approach to General Practice." *Med. J. Aust.* July 25, 1970; 2(4): 203–4.
2. Edelsten, G. W. "Legislate against Tattoos?" *Med. J. Aust.* January 8, 1983; 1(1): 11.
3. geoffedelsten.com.au.
4. *Edelsten v Richmond Supreme Court of Appeal, NSW*; p. 4, lines 15–29. Available from https://www.caselaw.nsw.gov.au/decision/549f4fc830042624639fabba.
5. Ibid. p. 4, lines 35–50.
6. Ibid. p. 5, lines 5–50.
7. Ibid. p. 7, lines 35–40.
8. Ibid. p. 7, lines 40–50.
9. Ibid. p. 8, lines 15–50.
10. Ibid. p. 9, lines 13–24.
11. Ibid. p. 10, lines 15–25.
12. Ibid. p. 10 lines 30–44.
13. Ibid. p. 11, lines 17–24.
14. Ibid. p. 12, lines 8–15.
15. Ibid. p. 12, lines 15–24.
16. Ibid. p. 14, lines 35–50; p. 15, lines 1–29.
17. Ibid. p. 16, lines 21–51; p. 17, lines 1–36.
18. Ibid. p. 22, line 10.
19. Donnelly, B. "Doctors Lay on Silver-Suited Service." *Sydney Morning Herald.* August 28, 1977: p. 8.
20. Birnbauer, B. "Scheme Is No Sick Joke as Far as This Good Doctor Is Concerned." *The Age.* August 7, 1979: p. 4.
21. Staff. "Edelsten Tries to Re-Enter the Ranks of Doctors." *The Age.* November 25, 2003.
22. Abouchar, Dom. "Edelsten and the Sharks." Rugby League World. August 1986.

23. Staff. "Geoffrey Edelsten 'Buys' the Sharks, 1986." Sharks Forever. November 9, 2004.
24. Howe, Alan. "Eccentric Edelsten's Final Chapter at an End." *The Weekend Australian.* June 12, 2021: p. 1.
25. Dibb, A., J. Pierik, S. Spits. "Geoffrey Edelsten Found Dead in Melbourne Apartment." *The Sydney Morning Herald.* June 11, 2021.

Suggested Further Reading

http://www.sydneyswans.com.au/club/History/overview.

"The Crazy World of Dr. Geoffrey Edelsten and Gabi Grecko."

https://www.news.com.au/finance/business/inside-the-crazy-world-of-geoffrey-edelsten-and-gabi-grecko/news-story/ef9119cb4d7bb6903166a2d1ec83cbe0.

DR. ANDREW J. WAKEFIELD—PROFIT FROM MEASLES

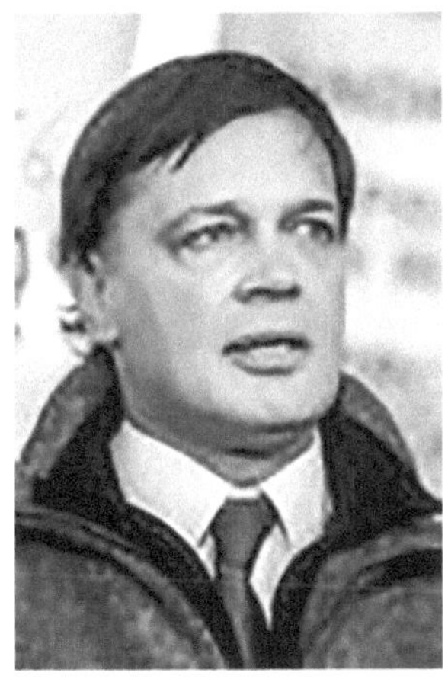

Photo: Peter Macdiarmid / Getty Images

It was still quite warm in Scotland in the middle of September 1940 when Margaret Lee came into labor. She knew it was coming, of course, but she was glad because her husband had just received his call-up papers. He was a pharmacist in town and in a protected occupation. He could have joined the medical corps but had chosen to volunteer with the rest, so now he had to present himself to his artillery unit in Kent. Margaret was happy that the baby would be born before he left. It did not matter to

Margaret that the Battle of Britain was in full flight over the English Channel. That was a long way away although Scotland had already taken its share of the wrath of the Luftwaffe. The baby was born at home, of course, because the hospitals were full. The baby was six pounds and twelve ounces and healthy.

The baby, called John, put on weight and progressed well until he was about sixteen months of age when he became febrile, alternatively lethargic and irritable, and his eyes became red, and he had a runny nose. His temperature rose to 40.1°, and he developed a rash that started around his neck. John became quite unwell, but his mother, Margaret, looked after him as well as she could. She cooled him down with wet blankets and kept him hydrated. It took over a week for the storm to pass and John's temperature to settle. The infection that John had was measles. He had survived it without vaccination because there was none.

How do I know all this?

Because that boy was me.

Prologue

When one reads about measles, mumps, and rubella (MMR) vaccine and its alleged link to autism, one gets the feeling that it is going to be one of those jokes: "Did you hear the one about the three people in a boat—one was a doctor, one was a journalist, and one was a lawyer …?" They are usually funny, but in this case, there was nothing funny about it. The doctor was *Dr. Andrew Wakefield*; the journalist, *Mr. Brian Deer*; and the lawyer, *Mr. Richard Barr*. There were other hapless passengers—some honest, some dishonest, some selfish, some selfless, and many irrational. The media, both printed and electronic, also carry a large part of the blame because of irresponsible reporting in the interests of anything that would increase sales. This case stretched for years over the United Kingdom, the United States, and Europe. Separating fact from fiction was almost impossible, as there were claims and counterclaims. But in this case, it was Mr. Brian Deer, neither a doctor nor a scientist, who exposed the fraud that underlies this story. As it was, unlike some other chapters in this book, the motive behind the deceitful findings was not academic fame or personal glory; it was simple criminal fraud and monetary greed on the part of Dr. Andrew Wakefield and numerous passengers in this boat, without a care for those who were harmed and who died in its aftermath. The effects reverberate to this day.

Dr. Andrew Wakefield was born in 1957 in Eton, Berkshire, England. His parents were both doctors, his mother being a general practitioner and his father a neurologist. His schooling was at the King Edward's School in Bath, and later he studied medicine at St. Mary's Hospital Medical School, now known as Imperial College School of Medicine, where he graduated in 1981. Further study resulted in him qualifying as a specialist surgeon in 1985. The following year, Dr. Wakefield moved to Toronto, Canada, where he took an interest in small bowel transplantation and rejection problems. Dr. Wakefield returned to the UK in 1990 as a senior lecturer in the departments of medicine and histopathology at the Royal Free Hospital and—from May 1, 1997—became a reader and honorary consultant in experimental gastroenterology with a stipulation in his contract that he was not involved in the clinical management of patients.[1]

Publications

Dr. Wakefield's first publication in a medical journal was in 1987, and it was related to mercury poisoning after swallowing a battery. This may have sparked an interest in the effects of ethylmercury, a related substance known as thimerosal, which was later used as a preservative for vaccines (other than MMR).[2] In 1989, he published twice, and one of these was related to Crohn's disease. From that time on, the number of his publications increased steadily to reach a maximum of eighteen per annum in 1995. Between 1987 and 2000, his name appeared related to ninety-six scientific articles, forty-eight as last author and eleven as first author. The articles as last author appear later in his career and probably reflect rising seniority. Of the ninety-six articles, thirty-one are specifically about Crohn's disease, and most of the remainder relate to other forms of inflammatory bowel disease (IBD). Several of the articles mention MMR or the wild measles virus connected to Crohn's disease, but in later years, reference is made to the measles and its possible relationship with encephalitis (inflammation of the brain).[3,4,5,6,7] There is no doubt that Andrew Wakefield was an authority on his subject, and it was this background that made him a credible witness in his area of expertise.

However, Dr. Andrew Wakefield also developed an interest in *autism*. There is no blood test or x-ray that can diagnose autism. It is a developmental and behavioral disorder that starts in childhood and lasts, in almost all cases, all of the child's life and can have a devastating effect on family and friends in severe cases. The diagnosis is made by observation of the child's behavior and a description from the parents. The signs include social ineptitude, lack of communication skills, repetitive behavior, and loss of learned skills such as walking and talking. Other features are often present; some are seen in healthy individuals but are not necessary to make the diagnosis. Some individuals have characteristics that are superior to those in the average person. The spread of unusual behavior is extensive, varying from reasonable to the extreme. The cause is unknown, but numerous factors can be associated with it, such as maternal infections, alcohol or drug consumption, and some inherited or genetic abnormalities. In 2013, the American Psychiatric

Association recognized four distinct autism diagnoses under one umbrella of autism spectrum disorder (ASD). In 1998, however, when this story started, the diagnosis most commonly used was autism. At that time, autism was reported in only about one to two cases in one thousand children, but it is reported many more times frequently nowadays, perhaps due to increased reporting rather than increased prevalence.[8] According to Dr. Andrew Wakefield, speaking on TV in May 2018, "By 2032 one child in two in the USA will be autistic. Eighty per cent of boys will be autistic."[8] The reporting of autism increased between 1996 and 2007. In 1996, the incidence was about 1:1,000; and by 2007, it was about 5:1,000. Whether this was due to an increase in the condition or an increase in reporting is not known.[9] Autism usually is described as having an onset in early childhood, but there are now reports in the press that the incidence in adults is increasing.

It has a long way to go before it reaches five hundred in one thousand, but in any case, when severe, the condition has difficult, sometimes devastating, implications for the family. Its onset is from about twelve months to two to three years of age, following the time that children have usually been vaccinated. It would be easy then to assume that if the condition commenced after the vaccination was given, the one might have caused the other. An example of the fallacy post hoc, ergo propter hoc (one thing happens because of another).

Inflammatory Bowel Disease

The bowel extends from the esophagus to the anus, but generally, when doctors talk about bowel disease, they mean the small bowel or the large bowel. The small bowel extends from the stomach to the large bowel. The distal end of the small bowel is called the ilium, and it terminates where it enters the cecum, being the first part of the large bowel or colon. This is called the ileocecal junction. There are various forms of inflammatory bowel disease (IBD), among them Crohn's disease and ulcerative colitis. These disorders and their cause are not fully understood, but there are several associated risk factors. In either case, they can cause unpleasant symptoms such as diarrhea, bloating, abdominal pain, constipation; and in some cases, they can be severely debilitating. Dr. Andrew Wakefield had a particular interest in the investigation of the causes, diagnosis, and treatment of people affected by IBD. He became a noted authority on IBD because of the extensive research work that he had put into it over several years. It made it very difficult to ignore him.[3,7,10,11]

Mumps, Measles, and German Measles

Mumps is a viral infection that attacks the salivary glands and, in some cases, other glands or organs, in rare cases, with dangerous side effects. Rubella (German measles) is a viral infection that can cause miscarriages in infected pregnant women or abnormalities in their unborn baby. Both can be prevented by vaccination.

Measles is a highly infective virus that usually strikes at an early age. It is the most serious of the three but can also be prevented by vaccination. In the absence of vaccination, it might be an epidemic in a nonimmune population and would usually cause a severe infective illness involving many of the body's systems. The mortality rate is 0.2–5 percent, depending on the resistance of the individual and the part of the world in which they are born. World Health Organization (WHO) records show that in 2016, there were 89,780 deaths from measles around the world, mostly among young children.[12] The year 2018 saw more than 140,000 deaths from measles, mostly in children under the age of five years. In 2019, 207,000 people died of measles as cases hit a twenty-three-year high.

The WHO had hoped to eliminate the disease by 2020 by achieving high vaccination rates. This goal was not achieved, partly due to the COVID-19 pandemic that stalled coverage due to a strained health system, which continues to this day. The year 2019 also saw explosive outbreaks of measles in countries where coverage was inadequate. Vaccine hesitancy remains yet another obstacle, as fewer parents vaccinate their children because of pronouncements by ignorant people like Donald Trump and Andrew Wakefield.[8,12,13,14] If enough people in the world were vaccinated, the virus (indeed, all three) would be eliminated, as it was for smallpox and has almost been for polio. The combined MMR vaccine has been in use in the US since the mid-1970s and was introduced in the UK in 1988. Previously, since 1968, the vaccines in the UK were given as three separate injections but were withdrawn in 1988 and replaced with single-dose MMR vaccine.[15,16]

Epidemics occurred, and in 1940 and 1941, for instance, there were over four hundred thousand cases in each year with a mortality rate of 0.2 and 0.3 percent respectively.[17] WHO figures show that for parents of children born in the UK in 1980, for instance, measles was still a real problem with almost 150,000 cases reported. As there is no specific treatment for measles, only systemic support can be offered, but the mortality rate in the UK has improved over the years so that by 2000 it was down to 0.04 percent.[17] Since then, the incidence of measles in the UK has been recorded in the hundreds.

Since the introduction of vaccination in the UK in 1968, the incidence of measles has steadily fallen. By 1998, measles was almost unknown because of immunization. Many younger doctors (and some older ones) have never seen a case.

At its peak in 1963, almost eight hundred thousand cases of measles were notified in England and Wales; but five years later, when the vaccination program started, the rate of notification dropped dramatically year by year so that within twenty years, the notifications were down to the hundreds.[18]

The number of cases vary depending on which part of the country is reporting, how effective the reporting is, whether the diagnosis was confirmed by a laboratory, and other factors; but there is little doubt that if a child was born in the 1950s or 1960s, its parents would be well aware of the presence of measles. The parents of a child born after 1990, however, might think that measles is irrelevant because they had never seen a case. *What then*, they might think, *is the point of vaccination against measles, a disease that does not exist?* The vaccine had been so efficient that it was a case of "In its efficiency may lie the seeds of its own destruction."

The World Health Organization Plans to Vaccinate Every Child in the World

Vaccination against mumps, measles, and rubella is recommended in children in two doses, at age twelve to fifteen months and then at four to six years. The vaccine is in the form of an attenuated virus, which means that the wild virus is weakened in the laboratory but still may cause a minor infection, which the body can fight off quickly, but allows the immune system to develop and repel any future attack by the wild severe virus. This principle is the same for all three viruses. The vaccination is highly effective, conferring protection on over 90 percent in most populations. Between 2012 and 2016, the Health Assembly's global push resulted in an increase in uptake of vaccination from 72 percent to 85 percent and resulted in an 84 percent reduction in deaths, estimated at 20.4 million.[14]

On June 13, 2017, the WHO announced that measles had been eliminated from Bhutan and the Maldives, a great triumph for a disadvantaged part of the world, especially since it is spreading again in parts of the USA and Europe.[16,19] Thirty deaths from measles were recorded in Romania in the fifteen months to June 2017. The WHO announced on October 24, 2018, that German measles had been eliminated from Australia due to the record-high rates of vaccination of 94.62 percent.[19]

The WHO and all the countries of the world intend to continue their vigil against measles, or it could return in epidemic proportions, and it is the policy of the WHO that measles is eliminated. To do this, they aim to vaccinate every single child in the world against measles twice, at one and four years of age, if possible. The vaccine to be used is MMR, of course, to protect against mumps and German measles as well as measles. Immunization is usually in the form of a combined single injection containing all three attenuated viruses but can be offered in three separate injections at intervals. There is no advantage in immunizing against the three viruses separately, and there may be a disadvantage, as vaccinations may be missed. There are, therefore, good reasons for immunization of all three viruses.[14]

Dr. Andrew Wakefield planned to benefit from this by discrediting MMR and having it replaced with his own patented single vaccine against measles. What a market! Wakefield's mouth must have watered. He had other plans.

Business Acumen

Dr. Andrew Wakefield had a considerable interest in business matters, and he was keen on promoting that business on the back of his medical and scientific knowledge of IBD. As early as 1995, he applied for a patent for a test to detect Crohn's disease by demonstrating the measles virus in the bowel or other body fluids.

In the months and years before the controversial journal article was published in *The Lancet* in February 1998, Mr. Richard Barr, a solicitor of the firm Dawbarns of King's Lynn, Norfolk, had been in touch with Wakefield; and in 1996, he approached Wakefield and asked if he would be prepared to act as an expert witness in upcoming legal suits in which parents wanted to sue the manufacturers of MMR vaccine for damage to their children caused by the vaccine.[20]

Mr. Barr was acting for an anti-vaccination action group known as JABS (Justice, Awareness and Basic Support) launched in Wigan, England. Dr. Andrew Wakefield was well known as an authority on bowel disease and the MMR vaccine and would make a valuable witness. The trouble was that all he had at that time to link MMR with bowel disease and autism was the yet-to-be-finished and unpublished paper in *The Lancet* in 1998. Mr. Barr organized the funding of £55,000 for Wakefield from the Legal Aid Board.[21] That meant that Wakefield would be taking money to gather evidence for lawsuits that were yet to come and that would depend on his evidence. It was an attractive proposition for Wakefield. He went on to promote his (business) point of view regardless. "The evidence is undeniably in favour of vaccine-induced bowel disease," he said.[22,23]

In July 1996, when the first child, in what was later to become known as one of the *Lancet 12*, was admitted to the Royal Free, Wakefield accepted the £55,000 from the UK Legal Board but did not declare it. Subsequently, he and *Professor Roy Pounder*, professor of gastroenterology, met with business administrators of the Royal Free Hospital to discuss their promising business venture. In June 1997, Wakefield applied for a patent in his name for a single measles vaccine. Mr. Brian Deer later reported the details of this business plan in the *British Medical Journal* in 2011. Venture capitalists would invest £2.1 million, which would be used for the detection and treatment of Crohn's disease and the diagnosis and treatment of autism. Income was estimated to be £3.3 million by the end of year three, rising to £28 million as the whole business came online. The name of the business would be Carmel Healthcare after Wakefield's wife, and there would be a laboratory called Unigenetics Inc. in Dublin, Ireland, to handle the pathology, including that from the USA. The laboratory received £800,000 in legal aid. It was also shown in later years that the laboratory used to test tissue samples for the lawsuits was the for-profit laboratory in Dublin, established explicitly for the purpose.[24] The laboratory was later shown to be incapable of processing a procedure called polymerase chain reaction (PCR), an incredibly technical procedure that required a high degree of quality control. Details of how the PCR was done were not given, making it impossible for others to test.[24,25,26,27,28]

A prospectus that came into the hands of Mr. Deer revealed that Wakefield would get 37 percent; the father of one child who was an investor would get 22.2 percent; the venture capitalist, 18 percent; Pounder, 11.7 percent; and the Irish pathologist, Professor O'Leary, 11.1 percent. Wakefield was also to be remunerated £40,000 per annum plus a travel allowance of £50,000. In the meantime, Wakefield was paid £150 per hour as a consultant, eventually amounting to £435,643 plus expenses from legal sources.[26]

Dr. Andrew Wakefield was well prepared for the replacement of the combined MMR vaccine with his single measles vaccine before the announced connection between MMR vaccine and autism.

The Lancet 12

It was with this background that Wakefield and others prepared to publish an article on February 28, 1998, in *The Lancet* mentioning nonspecific colitis (inflammation of the colon of no particular type) and pervasive development disorders (autism) in children who had been immunized by MMR recently. There were twelve children in the group described, and their parents claimed to have observed a behavioral change following the MMR vaccination. The twelve children were said to represent a consecutive series with chronic enterocolitis (prolonged standing inflammation of the bowel) and regressive developmental disorder (autism). They were subjected to numerous investigations, including colonoscopy, biopsy, electroencephalogram (EEG), magnetic resonance imaging (MRI), lumbar puncture, barium follow-through (bowel x-ray), and blood tests. These were done under the care and recommendation of Professor J. Walker-Smith, as Dr. Wakefield had no clinical rights. Of the twelve children, eight had been previously immunized with the MMR vaccine, and one had previously had measles. The parents suspected that the MMR vaccine was responsible for bowel disease.

The Press Release

Although the article was not going to say so in so many words, Wakefield knew that the concept that MMR vaccine might be the cause of autism would cause a furore, so he preceded the printed publication by calling a press release. In front of television cameras, under lights, five doctors—including the dean of the medical school, *Professor Arie Zuckerman*—made their breathless announcement. "For the first time, the MMR vaccine had been linked to a bowel disorder and the onset of autism in children."[15] Wakefield went on to announce that for the first time, he had found the measles vaccine in the bowel of IBD patients. This claim had already been shown to be untrue and had been directly contradicted by *Nicholas Chadwick*, a researcher in Wakefield's team,[24] but Wakefield did not seem to care. He carried on with some theory of his own to explain how the virus got from the gut into the bloodstream and across the blood-brain barrier into the brain, thereby causing autism.

The theory had already, long since, been discredited,[29] but Wakefield went on, "My concerns are that one more case of this is too many and that we put children at no greater risk if we dissociated those vaccines into three, but we may be averting the possibility of this problem." It was remarkable to call a press release before a publication in a scientific journal, but Wakefield was unrepentant. "It is a moral issue for me, and I cannot support the continued use of these three vaccines given in combination until this issue has been resolved," he said.[21,30] (What was not known at the time was that Wakefield had filed a patent nine months previously for a single-use vaccine for measles, from which he would profit greatly when parents and the WHO switched the immunization of their children from the triple vaccine MMR to the single vaccine that Wakefield had patented.)[31] Professor Zuckerman, who did not know of Wakefield's plans, became agitated at the reaction of the audience and, in fear of losing control of the horde, started banging the lectern and raised his voice, saying, "It is essential that public confidence in MMR is not damaged by the publication of this study. If this precipitates a scare that reduces the rate of immunization, children will start dying from the measles." He warned desperately, "Eight children, after all, do not provide proof of a link between MMR and autism."[15,32]

Professor Zuckerman must have been dreaming. To make an announcement like that and then expect parents not to worry is the stuff of fantasyland.

Dawbarns—Solicitors

In the weeks following the publication in *The Lancet*, its correspondence columns were filled with critical analysis from scientists and analysts. The popular press, however, showed no restraint in raucous headlines—such as "Ban Three-in-One Jab," "Doctors Link MMR Vaccine with Autism," etc.—but an interesting comment came in a letter from *Dr. Andrew Rouse* of the Wiltshire Health Authority only a few days after the publication in *The Lancet*. Dr. Rouse had found an organization called the *Society for the Autistically Handicapped* on the internet, and within their website was a fact sheet from a firm called Dawbarns inviting interested parents to contact them. The fact sheet invited parents "who believed that their child had been damaged, should seek proper compensation in the courts." It went on, "We are working with Dr. Andrew Wakefield of the Royal Free Hospital in London."[33]

Dr. Rouse also noted that in 1996, Rosemary Kessick had approached Dr. Wakefield because she was frantically worried about her son William, aged eight years. She reported that William had developed generally as a bright and active toddler until he had his MMR vaccination and then regressed developmentally, becoming unable to feed himself, to talk, and "lived in a world of his own." He had Crohn's disease, which sometimes left him screaming in pain. Rosemary thought that Dr. Wakefield might help when others could not.[33] William became one of the *Lancet 12* and one of more than three hundred children Dawbarns had assembled for litigation.[31] Dr. Rouse pointed out that contacts made in this way were likely to be "litigation biased."[31,32] Any conclusions from their study were, therefore, likely to be unreliable. Not that it seemed to bother Andy Wakefield. His business plan was all set to go.

Vaccination Rates

When Dr. Andrew Wakefield came along and suggested that there was a risk from the MMR vaccine, it was expected that many parents would decide not to immunize their children. Considering the dreadful implications of this press release, therefore, it is not surprising that it attracted national and international attention; indeed, it caused a tide of anxiety, which resulted in a substantial drop in vaccination rates in the UK and later in the USA.[16] Parents were aghast. Vaccination rates in the UK dropped from 92 percent to below 80 percent after the publication of the paper. For a population to have herd immunity requires a vaccination rate of 95 percent. Official figures showed that in 1998, there were fifty-six cases of measles in England and Wales, but this had increased to 1,348 cases by 2008. In April 2006, the first death in fourteen years from acute measles was recorded in England. Two children died from acute measles in 2008.[12,13] It was a sad reflection on the damage that can be done by a few words from people with their motives and, in this case, who did not care.

By 1998, measles was almost unknown in the UK because of immunization. However, after the publication of *The Lancet* paper in 1998, many parents were afraid to immunize their children. The effect was evident with the increased incidence of measles, which started rising again and reached a few hundred in 2002 (four years after *The Lancet* paper was published), reaching a peak of about two thousand in the year 2012 and again in 2013. There is no doubt that the incidence of measles is related to the vaccination rate in the community.[16]

When MMR vaccine was first introduced in the UK in 1988, it coincided with an increase observed in the incidence of autism. At first, parents of autistic children wondered why their children had been affected; and quite naturally, they looked around for causes. Many parents turned to their doctor for an explanation, but nobody had one. Around the same time, it was noticed that vaccinations for measles had increased with the intention of eradicating measles from the world. There is no doubt that the increased rate of vaccination resulted in a decrease in the incidence of measles and the consequent reduction in deaths due to the virus. Some parents thought that the increase in measles vaccinations might be linked to the increased incidence of autism. The incidence of autism continued to increase; however, as did the increase in the rate of MMR vaccination in line with WHO policy. Quite naturally, some parents started to wonder whether the two were related, perhaps due to the presence of the thimerosal in the vaccine. Thimerosal had not been used in vaccines for years, however, and it had never been used in the MMR vaccine.

Some other agent might be to blame. Dr. Andrew Wakefield was known to have published widely on Crohn's disease and a possible relationship with a virus. Because of this knowledge, he was approached in the mid-1990s by the firm of solicitors, Dawbarns, led by Mr. Richard Barr who was acting for a group of parents associated with an action group known as JABS, whose children were allegedly autistic. Mr. Barr was hoping that Dr. Wakefield could give evidence in subsequent legal suits brought by the parents against the manufacturers of the MMR vaccine. Dr. Wakefield, for his part, saw an opportunity here. He applied for a patent for a single measles vaccine and then set about discrediting the MMR vaccine. His business plan was detailed and would be built around the sale of his patented single measles vaccine when parents and doctors stopped using the MMR vaccine. He established a laboratory in Dublin, Ireland, that would handle all aspects of pathology and other tests connected with ileocecal bowel disease, viral studies, and autism, including those from the USA.

Thus, the scene was set for the commencement of his business venture when Wakefield held a press conference two days before an article was published in *The Lancet* on February 28, 1998. The article would describe twelve children who were alleged to have become autistic after receiving the MMR vaccine.

"The best laid plans of mice and men gang aft astray." When Robbie Burns, the Scottish poet laureate of the eighteenth century, said these words, he was talking to a field mouse whose den had been knocked over by a tractor. In this case, Dr. Andrew Wakefield was about to face a gale in the form of *Professor Mark Pepys*, FRS, who had just been appointed as head of medicine at the Royal Free Hospital in 1999. He had no belief in Wakefield or respect for him or his theories. He had told the Royal Free that he would not have come "if Wakefield was there," and he went on, "Do you know what they did? They promoted him"! He soon confronted Wakefield and demanded that his work be repeated to confirm it. Wakefield agreed but did nothing about it for two years. Wakefield then replied that he would do the work when he was ready. That was a bridge too far and marked the beginning of the end for Dr. Andrew Wakefield at the Royal Free Hospital. In October 2001, Wakefield's employment with the Royal Free Hospital was terminated, and he was told to pack his bags. Mr. Brian Deer reports that he received two years' salary and a statement clearing him of misconduct.

In December 2001, Wakefield departed finally from Royal Free Hospital "by mutual consent because they did not like my research" he said and moved to Austin, Texas, USA, in 2004 where he helped to start up Thoughtful House for the treatment of autism.[34]

The fuss was not confined to Britain. The increased prevalence of autism was worldwide, and in the USA, parents were looking for answers too. Wakefield's work did not go unnoticed there. At first, thimerosal (the preservative) was suspected, and numerous support groups sprang up hoping to find a link between thimerosal and Crohn's disease but, later, Crohn's disease and MMR and then MMR and autism.

Barnard Rimland, who had a son with autism and whose work at the Autism Research Institute had helped to redefine the disorder, had started a path for subsequent generations of would-be parent researchers. Rimland started an organization called Defeat Autism Now (DAN) that would collaborate with medical professionals who preferred to turn their back on the establishment (the DAN approach). Now that the internet made communications infinitely more accessible and more informative, other groups sprang up all over.

The National Alliance for Autism Research (NAAR) was launched by Eric and Karen London in Princeton, New Jersey, and the Cure Autism Now (CAN) was started by Jonathan and Portia Shestack in San Diego, California. These organizations and numerous others like them soon had followers all over the country and the support group Chapters Autism Speaks held regular meetings all over the USA to discuss their policies and strategies. It was easy to gather new members because all they had to say on their websites was "Do you have a child like ours? If so, you should consider joining us." Of course, lots of parents had a child like theirs, and membership increased exponentially. A fund was set up by the federal government whereby judgments could be awarded to parents without the manufacturer having to defend the case; otherwise, it would be so expensive for the manufacturer to pay damages that they would have to stop manufacturing the vaccine. A maximum of $250,000 was set for individual cases. There were three trial cases, all lost, with five thousand cases waiting to be tried.[35]

In 1993, *Albert and Sally Enayati* had a son who was diagnosed with autism. They met through CAN, and with Tommy Redwood, they founded an organization called the Coalition for Sensible Action for Ending Mercury-Induced Neurological Disorders (SafeMinds). This group and its subsequent behavior seemed intent to obstruct all rational thought that might deny a connection between the MMR vaccine and autism. Numerous scientific articles and media articles were published showing that MMR vaccines do not increase the chance of developing autism, but SafeMinds seemed to have a contradiction for them all.[27,34,35,36,37,38,39,40,41,42,43,44,45,46,47,48] As far as SafeMinds was concerned, the studies were too big, too small, rigged by government agencies, influenced by drug companies, anything but be right. Then in 2002, a report from Denmark seemed above reproach. For two years, it had tracked each one of more than 530,000 children born from the beginning of 1991 to the end of 1998, making it the most extensive MMR-autism study to date; after analyzing the children for a total of 2,129,864 person-years, the study concluded that MMR vaccination did not cause autism.[49]

Still, SafeMinds would not have it. They rubbished the authors in spite of their qualifications, saying, "It is a sad day in America when injured children are denied their due process." They went on, "It appears to support a thimerosal role in the increases in autism being reported in the study in Denmark." This was an extraordinary statement, as thimerosal (ethylmercury) had never been used in the MMR vaccine and had not been mentioned in the Danish study.[49]

Things began to heat up when in 2004, Mr. Brian Deer, a journalist writing in the *Sunday Times* who had taken an interest in the case some years before, now reported that Wakefield had failed to disclose that he was being funded by solicitors who were planning to use the evidence against vaccine manufacturers. The solicitors had been advertising on the internet, "If your child suffered from any or all of these symptoms, please contact us, and it may be appropriate to put you in touch with Dr. Andrew Wakefield."[25] That was terrible news for the Wakefield group because only Andrew Wakefield knew that he had been collaborating with solicitors. Ten of the paper's authors withdrew their names from *The Lancet* article, and in February 2004, *The Lancet* issued a "Retraction of an Interpretation."[50]

But Mr. Brian Deer was not done yet. In November 2004, *Channel 4* broadcast a one-hour *Dispatches* investigation by

Brian Deer who said "that he had documentary evidence that Wakefield had applied for a patent on a single measles vaccine before his campaign against the MMR, raising questions about his motives." Not only that but Mr. Deer also produced a copy of the patent itself, which explicitly stated that the use of MMR vaccine causes autism. Mr. Deer also revealed that Nicholas Chadwick, working under Wakefield's supervision, had failed to find the measles virus in the children reported in *The Lancet*.[51] Later, it came to light that Wakefield had taken blood from children at a birthday party in return for money, a fact to which he admitted.[52,53] It is a wonder that Walker-Smith and Murch did not withdraw their names from the paper then. Even then, *The Lancet* still did not retract the paper.

Having this information in the public domain was devastating for Wakefield, and he initiated libel proceedings against *Channel 4*, Mr. Brian Deer, and the *Sunday Times*. Within weeks, Wakefield applied to have the proceedings stayed because the General Medical Council (GMC) were proceeding against him contemporaneously. Mr. Justice Eady ruled against a stay of proceedings principally because the allegations of Mr. Deer were so serious and there would be no advantage to delay them.[54]

Mr. Deer's allegations are reproduced here:

(i) Wakefield spread fear that the MMR vaccine might lead to autism, even though he knew that his own laboratory had carried out tests whose results dramatically contradicted his claims in that the measles virus had not been found in a single one of the children concerned in his study and he knew or ought to have known that there was absolutely no basis at all for his belief that the MMR should be broken up into single vaccines

(ii) In spreading such fear, acted dishonestly and for mercenary motives in that, although he improperly failed to disclose the fact, he planned a rival vaccine and products (such as a diagnostic kit based on his theory) that could have made his fortune

(iii) Gravely abused the children under his care by unethically carrying out extensive invasive procedures (on occasions requiring three people to hold a child down), thereby driving nurses to leave and causing his medical colleagues serious concern and unhappiness

(iv) Improperly and/or dishonestly failed to disclose to his colleagues and the public that his research on autistic children had begun with a contract with solicitors who were trying to sue the manufacturers of the MMR vaccine

(v) Improperly or dishonestly lent his reputation to the International Child Development Resource Centre, which promoted to very vulnerable parents' expensive products for whose efficacy (as he knew or should have known) there was no scientific evidence.

Mr. Justice Eady's ruling states that "the views or conclusions of the GMC disciplinary body would not, so far as I can tell, be relevant or admissible," that *Channel 4*'s allegations "go to undermine fundamentally the Claimant's professional integrity and honesty," and that "it cannot seriously be suggested that priority should be given to GMC proceedings for the resolution of issues."

That was a temporary setback to Brian Deer. However, in December 2006, Mr. Deer released records obtained from the Legal Services Commission, showing that it had paid £435,643 in undisclosed fees to Wakefield to build a case against the MMR vaccine. Those payments, the *Sunday Times* reported, had begun two years before the publication of Wakefield's paper in *The Lancet*. Within days of Deer's report, Wakefield dropped all his libel actions and was ordered to pay all defendants' legal costs.

Life could not have been much fun for Andy Wakefield because he was (along with Professor J. Walker-Smith and Dr.

S. Murch) soon pulled up before the General Medical Council who had been following these events for some years now. The hearings lasted for 217 days, the longest in British history, even longer than McBride's 180 days in Australia. The charges were that he

- was being paid to conduct the study by solicitors representing parents who believed their children had been harmed by MMR;
- ordered investigations "without the requisite paediatric qualifications"— including colonoscopies, colon biopsies, and lumbar punctures (spinal taps)— on his research subjects without the approval of his department's ethics board and contrary to the children's clinical interests,[89] when these diagnostic tests were not indicated by the children's symptoms or medical history;
- acted "dishonestly and irresponsibly" in failing to disclose … how patients were recruited for the study as well as in his descriptions in The Lancet papers and in questions after the paper published, about what ailments the children had, and when those ailments were observed relative to their getting vaccinated;
- conducted the study on a basis not approved by the hospital's ethics committee
- purchased blood samples—for £5 each—from children present at his son's birthday party, which Wakefield joked about in a later presentation;
- showed callous disregard for any distress or pain the children might suffer.

It was all pretty damning stuff, and Wakefield denied the charges; but on January 28, 2010, the GMC ruled against him on all issues, stating that he had "failed in his duties as a responsible consultant" and acted against the interests of his patients and "dishonestly and irresponsibly in his controversial research." On May 24, 2010, he was struck off the United Kingdom medical register. It was the harshest sanction that the GMC could impose, and it ended his career as a physician. In announcing the ruling, the GMC said that Wakefield (along with Walker-Smith and Murch) had "brought the medical profession into disrepute," and no sanction short of erasing their names from the register was appropriate for the "serious and wide-ranging findings" of misconduct.[1] Wakefield argued that he had been unfairly treated by the medical and scientific establishment.[55] Murch's penalty was reduced on appeal from "serious professional misconduct" to "professional misconduct."

In February 2010, *The Lancet* finally retracted the whole article, twelve years after its initial publication.[56,57] Mr. Brian Deer had exposed the whole sordid story, starting with the faulty science and then moving to the fabrication of the facts Wakefield had made to suit the law cases and finally to show how the whole business plan was created to benefit Wakefield and others from the sale of a vaccine from which they would profit because they held a patent. In a piece published in the *British Medical Journal*, in 2011, Mr. Deer progressively demolished, one by one, each of the cases described in the *Lancet 12*, ensuring that the lawsuits would never succeed. He went on to say, "So that is *The Lancet 12*; the foundation of the vaccine scare. No case was free of misreporting or alteration. Taken together, NHS records cannot be reconciled with what was published, to such devastating effect in the journal."[15,25,26,27] "Wakefield, nevertheless, now apparently self-employed and professionally ruined, remains championed by 'a sad rump of disciples.'"

"Dr. Wakefield is a hero," says one mother. "I do not know where we would be without him." [27,39]

"To our community, Andrew Wakefield is Nelson Mandela, and Jesus Christ rolled up into one," says JB Handley, cofounder of Generation Rescue, a group that disputes vaccine safety, "and is a symbol of hope all of us feel."[58,59] These supporters were determined to be blind to the facts as shown by logic and science.[60] It is a mystery how they can defy the science that has shown us how to eliminate smallpox and, almost, poliomyelitis.

Everyone in this book has rusted-on supporters and seeing that the incidence of autism is rising along with the incidence of any variable, many would wonder whether autism is related to that variable. But this is only a case of post hoc, ergo propter hoc (just because one follows the other, it does not mean that one was caused by the other). Action groups such as AutismOne are still turning their attention to other causes of autism. For example, Snopes.com provides figures that show that the incidence of autism has been rising contemporaneously with the use of the weed killer glyphosate since 1990.[61] Citing this, the "senior scientist" reporting in the Snopes.com website claims that one child in two will be autistic by 2025 due to the use of glyphosate and refers the anxious parent to the contemporaneous increase of glyphosate and autism. It is only natural that parents should continue in desperation to search for a cause of autism, but at what cost when it is clear that there is no connection with measles?

Andrew Wakefield supporters are few and far between nowadays.

Except for the provision of safe drinking water, worldwide vaccination against infectious diseases has probably been the most successful community health project ever.[14] At the same time, due to Andrew Wakefield, there is little doubt that vaccination with MMR vaccine has caused more controversy than almost any other public health issue in history.

Few prospective parents, aged twenty-five in 2015, would have seen a case of measles, and little might have been said about it, as they would have been vaccinated over twenty years before. They may well have seen a few cases of autism in their friends' families, and if the individual was severely affected, the prospective parents might well want to consider whether to vaccinate their child if there was a risk that their child could be autistic as a result.

To this day, Andrew Wakefield is promoting the idea that MMR causes autism. In May 2018, he said on TV, "By 2032 half of all the children and 80 percent of all the boys in the USA will be autistic."[8,23]

- The *New York Times* noted, "Andrew Wakefield has become one of the most reviled doctors of his generation, blamed directly or indirectly, depending on the accuser, for irresponsibly starting a panic with tragic repercussions: vaccination rates so low that childhood diseases once all but eradicated here—such as whooping cough and measles among them—have reemerged, endangering young lives."[36]
- In 2010, the James Randi Educational Foundation awarded Wakefield the Pigasus Award for "Refusal to Face Reality." [62]
- In 2011, the journal *Annals of Pharmacotherapy* called it "the most damaging medical hoax of the last 100 years."[63]
- In January 2012, *Time Magazine* named Wakefield in a list of "Great Scientific Frauds."[64]
- In 2012, he was awarded the Lifetime Achievement in Quackery by the Good Thinking Society.[64]
- Perhaps most damaging of all was *Medscape* listing him as the "Worst Physician of the Year" in 2011.[65]

The saddest of all is that he was not charged with a criminal offense, as Deer called for in a CNN broadcast in 2011.[4]

Immunization is a community responsibility. Having one's child vaccinated contributes to herd immunity and makes it safer for all. To do otherwise makes it more dangerous for all.

Notes

1. General Medical Council. Re Wakefield Walker-Smith and Murch (internet). London: General Medical Council. January 28, 2010. Available from http://www.casewatch.org/foreign/wakefield/gmc_findings.pdf.
2. Mant, T., J. Lewis, T. Mattoo, S. Rigden, G. Volans, I. House, et al. "Mercury Poisoning after Disc-Battery Ingestion." *Human Toxicology*. 1987; 6(2): 179–181.
3. Smith M, Wakefield A. "Crohn's disease: ancient and modern." *Postgrad Med J*. 1994; 70(821): 149–153.
4. Lewin, J, A. Dhillon, R. Sim, G. Mazure, R. Pounder, A. Wakefield. "Persistent Measles Virus Infection of the Intestine: Confirmation by Immunogold Electron Microscopy." *Gut*. 1995; 36(4): 564–569.
5. Wakefield, A., R. Pittilo, R. Sim, S. Cosby, J. Stephenson, A. Dhillon, et al. "Evidence of Persistent Measles Virus Infection in Crohn's Disease." *Journal of Medical Virology*. 1993; 39(4): 345–353.
6. Wakefield, A., S. Montgomery, R. Pounder. "Crohn's Disease: The Case for Measles Virus." *Ital. J. Gastroenterology and Hepatology*. 1999; 3(April): 247–254.
7. Thompson, N., R. Pounder, A. Wakefield, S. Montgomery. "Is Measles Vaccination a Risk Factor for Inflammatory Bowel Disease?" *The Lancet*. 1995; 345(8957): 1,071–1,074.
8. (Internet). 2018 (cited October 22, 2018). Available from https://www.independent.co.uk/news/world/americas/andrew-wakefield-anti-vaxxer-trump-us-mmr-autism-link-lancet-fake-a8331826.html.
9. Newschaffer, C. J., L. A. Croen, J. Daniels, E. Giarelli, J. K. Grether, S. E. Levy, D. S. Mandell, L. A. Miller, J. Pinto-Martin, J. Reaven, A. M. Reynolds,

C. E. Rice, D. Schendel, G. C. Windham (2007). "The Epidemiology of Autism Spectrum Disorders." *Annual Review of Public Health*. 28: 235–258. Available from https://www.annualreviews.org/doi/full/10.1146/annurev.publhealth.28.021406.144007.

10. Wakefield, A., A. Dhillon, P. Rowles, A. Sawyerr, R. Pittilo, A. Lewis, et al. "Pathogenesis of Crohn's Disease: Multifocal Gastrointestinal Infarction." *The Lancet*. 1989; 334(8671): 1,057–1,062.

11. Wakefield, A. "MMR Vaccination and Autism." *The Lancet*. 1999; 354(9182): 949–950.

12. "Measles." World Health Organization (internet). 2018 (cited October 5, 2018). Available from http://www.who.int/news-room/fact-sheets/detail/measles.

13. Bosley, S. "Resurgence of Deadly Measles Blamed on Low MMR Vaccination Rates." *The Guardian* (internet). 2018 (cited October 5, 2018). Available from https://www.theguardian.com/society/2018/aug/20/low-mmr-uptake-blamed-for-surge-in-measles-cases-across-europe.

14. Sanitas, M. "Why Is Measles Making an Unpleasant Comeback?" Huffington Post–Life (internet). 2017 (cited November 16, 2018); Available from https://www.huffpost.com/entry/why-is-measles-making-an-unpleasant-comeback_b_595bbddfe4b0326c0a8d1333.

15. Deer, B. "MMR: The Truth Behind the Crisis." *The Sunday Times*. 2004.

16. World Health Organization. "Number of Reported Measles Cases in the United Kingdom of Great Britain and Northern Ireland." WHO. 2018. http://apps.who.int/immunization_monitoring/globalsummary/countries?countrycriteria%5Bcountry%5D%5B%5D=GBR&commit=OK#.

17. Gov. UK. "Measles Notifications in England and Wales 1940–2016." London: Public Health, England. 2017 https://www.gov.uk/government/publications/measles-deaths-by-age-group-from-1980-to-2013-ons-data/measles-notifications-and-deaths-in-england-and-wales-1940-to-2013.

18. Oxford Vaccine Group. "Measles: Annual Number of Notified Cases in England and Wales since Vaccination Was Introduced in 1968." Oxford. 2018 http://vk.ovg.ox.ac.uk/measles.

19. Dow, A. "Infection Every Expectant Mother Feared 'Eradicated' in Australia." *Sydney Morning Herald*. 2018.

20. Wakefield, A. "Vaxxed: from Cover Up to Catastrophe." Vimeo: Cinema Libre Studio. 2016. https://itunes.apple.com/us/movie/vaxxed-from-cover-up-to-catastrophe/id1162913858?ct=t():.

21. Deer, B. "Revealed: MMR Research Scandal." *The Times*. February 22, 2014.

22. Stott, C., M. Blaxill, A. Wakefield. "MMR and Autism in Perspective: The Denmark Story." *Journal of American Physicians and Surgeons*. 2004; 9(3): 89–91.

23. Wakefield, A. "Why I Owe It to Parents to Question Triple Vaccine." *Sunday Herald*. 2002: 2–10.

24. Mnookin, S. *The Panic Virus: Fear, Myth and the Vaccination Debate*. 1st ed. Collingwood, Vic.: Simon and Schuster. 2011. p. 161.

25. Deer, B. "*The Lancet*'s Two Days to Bury Bad News." *BMJ*. 2011; 342(Jan. 18 2): c7,001.

26. Deer, B. "How the Vaccine Crisis Was Meant to Make Money." *BMJ*. 2011; 342(Jan. 11 4): c5,258.

27. Deer, B. "How the Case against the MMR Vaccine Was Fixed." *BMJ*. 2011; 342(Jan. 5 1): c5,347.

28. Deer, B. "Wakefield's 'Autistic Enterocolitis' under the Microscope." *BMJ*. 2010; 340(Apr. 15 2): c1,127.

29. Mnookin, S. op. cit. p. 107.

30. Deer, B. "Royal Free MMR Video News Release, 1998." Briandeer.com (internet). 1998 (cited October 20, 2018). Available from https://briandeer.com/wakefield/royal-video.htm.

31. Mnookin, S. op. cit. p. 116.

32. Mnookin, S. op. cit. p. 108.

33. Rouse, A. "Autism, Inflammatory Bowel Disease, and MMR Vaccine." *The Lancet*. 1998; 351(9112): 1,356.

34. Sathyanarayana, Rao T., C. Andrade. "Ethical Issues in Research: Study Design and Publication-Worthiness as a Case in Point." *Indian Journal of Psychiatry*. 2015; 57(1): 1.

35. Samson, K. "Federal Vaccine Court Opens Controversial Autism Proceedings." *Neurology Today*. 2007; 7(13): 1.

36. Associated Press. "Journal: Study Linking Autism and MMR Was a Fraud." *Democrat and Chronicle*. 2011.

37. Dominus, S. "The Crash and Burn of an Autism Guru." *The New York Times*. 2011.

38. Halsey, N., S. Hyman. "Measles-Mumps-Rubella Vaccine and Autistic Spectrum Disorder: Report from the New Challenges in Childhood Immunizations Conference Convened in Oak Brook, Illinois, June 12–13, 2000." PEDIATRICS. 2001; 107(5): e84.

39. Freckelton, I. *Scholarly Misconduct*. 1st ed. Oxford, UK: Oxford University Press. 2016.

40. Macrae, F., D. Wilkes. "Damning Verdict on MMR Doctor: Anger as GMC Attacks 'Callous Disregard' for Sick Children." *Daily Mail*. 2010.

41. Godlee, F., J. Smith, H. Marcovitch. "Wakefield's Article Linking MMR Vaccine and Autism Was Fraudulent." *BMJ*. 2011; 342(Jan. 5 1): c7,452.

42. Smeeth, L., C. Cook, E. Fombonne, L. Heavey, L. Rodrigues, P. Smith, et al. "MMR Vaccination

and Pervasive Developmental Disorders: A Case-Control Study." *The Lancet*. 2004; 364(9438): 963.

43. Mughal, S., A. Saadabadi. "Autism Spectrum Disorder (Regressive Autism, Child Disintegrative Disorder)." StatPearls Publishing (internet). 2018 (cited October 1, 2018); NCBI Bookshelf. Available from https://www.ncbi.nlm.nih.gov/books/NKB525976/?report+printable.

44. Center for Diseases Control and Prevention. Atlanta, Ga.: US Department of Health and Human Services. 2015. https://www.cdc.gov/vaccinesafety/concerns/thimerosal/index.html.

45. Sabra, A., J. Bellanti, A. Colón. "Ileal-Lymphoid-Nodular Hyperplasia, Non-Specific Colitis, and Pervasive Developmental Disorder in Children." *The Lancet*. 1998; 352(9123): 234–235.

46. Deer, B. Briandeer.com—Brian Deer (internet). Briandeer.com. 2018 (cited October 21, 2018). Available from http://briandeer.com/.

47. Langdon-Down, G. "Law: A Shot in the Dark; the Complications from Vaccine Damage Seem to Multiply in the Courtroom." *The Independent*. 1996; 25.

48. "Medical Journal: Study Linking Autism, Vaccines Is 'Elaborate Fraud.'" CNN. 2011.

49. Madsen, K., A. Hviid, M. Vestergaard, D. Schendel, J. Wohlfahrt, P. Thorsen, et al. "A Population-Based Study of Measles, Mumps, and Rubella Vaccination and Autism." *New England Journal of Medicine*. 2002; 347(19): 1,477–1,482.

50. Murch, S., A. Anthony, D. Casson, M. Malik, M. Berelowitz, A. Dhillon, et al. "Retraction of an Interpretation." *The Lancet*. 2004; 363(9411): 750.

51. Deer, B. "Molecular Testing in Wakefield's Own Lab Rebutted the Basis for His Attack on MMR."

Briandeer.com (internet). 2007 (cited November 13, 2018). Available from https://briandeer.com/.

52. Dyer, O. "Andrew Wakefield Is Accused of Paying Children for Blood Samples." *BMJ.* 2007; 335(7611): 118.2–119.

53. Dyer, O. "Wakefield Admits Fabricating Events When He Took Children's Blood Samples." *BMJ.* 2008; 336(7649): 850.1–850.

54. Deer, B. "MMR Doctor Andrew Wakefield Fixed Data on Autism." *The Sunday Times.* 2009.

55. British and Irish Legal Information Institute. Approved Judgement. London: British and Irish Legal Information Institute; Nov 2005.

56. Wakefield, A., S. Murch, A. Anthony, J. Linnell, D. Casson, M. Malik, et al. "RETRACTED: Ileal-Lymphoid-Nodular Hyperplasia, Non-Specific Colitis, and Pervasive Developmental Disorder in Children." *The Lancet.* 1998; 351(9103): 637–641.

57. The Editors of *The Lancet.* "Retraction—Ileal-Lymphoid-Nodular Hyperplasia, Non-Specific Colitis, and Pervasive Developmental Disorder in Children." *The Lancet.* 2010; 375(9713): 445.

58. Rayner, J. "My Child First." *The Observer* (London, Greater London, England). 2000; 31.

59. Alison, R. "Defiant Parents Stand by Decision: No Regrets despite Their Children Catching Measles." *The Guardian* (London, Greater London, England). 2002; 3.

60. Harrison, J. "Wrong about Vaccine Safety: A Review of Andrew Wakefield's 'Callous Disregard.'" *The Open Vaccine Journal* (internet). 2013; 6(1): 9–25. Available from https://www.autism-watch.org/books/callous_disregard.pdf.

61. Mikkelson, D. "Fact Check: Glyphosate Herbicide Will Cause Half of All Children to Have Autism

by 2025?". Snopes.com (internet). 2018 (cited November 17, 2018). Available from https://www.snopes.com/fact-check/glyphosatan/.

62. James Randi Educational Foundation. "The 5 Worst Promoters of Nonsense." 2010.

63. Flaherty, D. "The Vaccine-Autism Connection: A Public Health Crisis Caused by Unethical Medical Practices and Fraudulent Science." *Annals of Pharmacotherapy*. 2011; 45(10): 1,302–1,304.

64. Park, A. "Great Science Frauds." *Time* magazine (internet). 2012 (cited November 18, 2018). Available from http://healthland.time.com/2012/01/13/great-science-frauds/slide/andrew-wakefield/.

65. "Physicians of the Year: Best and Worst." Medscape. 2011.

Suggested Further Reading

Deer, Brian. *The Doctor Who Fooled the World*. John Hopkins University Press. 2020.

Editor's Note

MMR vaccine, autism, and other possible precipitating agents caused so much controversy that it swamped the printed, broadcast, and internet media that almost all the citations above can be found in four or five places. In many cases, arguments were printed in the press or medical journals and broadcast on television, radio, and the internet as well as being discussed at conferences and special interest groups. It has clearly not been possible to reference everything related to the events that occurred. The reader will have no trouble following any thread desired to satisfy their curiosity about Andrew Wakefield and the MMR scam, however.

CHAPTER EIGHT

DR. WILLIAM G. MCBRIDE— THE DEBENDOX DEBACLE

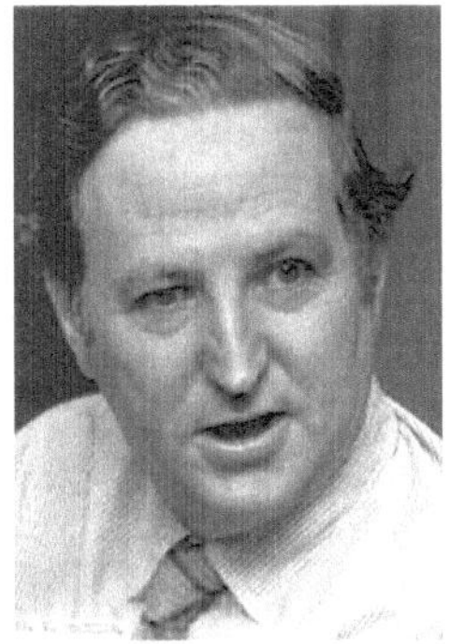

Photo: Alamy

Prologue

Every now and again, something comes along that changes the course of medicine. The discovery that thalidomide causes fetal abnormalities if taken by women in the early stages of pregnancy was such an event. It fell to *Dr. William Griffith McBride* to announce this discovery to the world. Dr. McBride had the opportunity to be remembered as the Father of Modern Teratology, but sadly, he contaminated his place in history because he did not have the humility to handle such an enormous responsibility. He set himself aside, above his peers, making his own rules, thereby bringing about his own downfall, ending his career in controversy.

Dr. William Griffith McBride was born in Sydney on May 25, 1927. He attended Canterbury Boys' High School, a selective school in Sydney at the time.

His medical training was at the University of Sydney Medical School, where he graduated in 1949. After resident hospital appointments at St. George Hospital in Sydney and Launceston Hospital in Tasmania, Dr. McBride applied for and fortuitously was successful in being appointed to the Women's Hospital, Crown Street in Sydney. The resident position there only became available when a successful candidate took leave to get married.[1] In those days, to become a specialist obstetrician and gynecologist in Australia, one had to complete two years' training before going to London to be examined by specialists there to qualify for Membership of the Royal College of Obstetricians and Gynaecologists (MRCOG). (Nowadays, Australia and New Zealand have their own Royal Australian and New Zealand College of Obstetricians and Gynaecologists—Ed.) After spending 1952 and 1953 at the Women's Hospital, Dr. McBride traveled to London as a ship's surgeon on the RMS *Orontes*.[2] He waited five months to sit his examinations during which he studied for the exams and enjoyed the pleasures of England. Surprisingly, because Australian graduates were highly prized among the English aristocracy, he was not employed at any hospital as a registrar as most Australians were to advance their surgical skills (by practicing on NHS patients[!]—Ed).

Back in Sydney, McBride was successful in his application for medical superintendent at the Women's Hospital, a position that he held until 1957. During that time, he exhibited perhaps the first evidence of the flaw in his character. McBride did not mind using other people's data to promote his selfish desire to achieve his ambitions. In this case, he used the data from the fertility clinic at Crown Street to apply for the prestigious degree of Doctor of Medicine (MD), a degree awarded by the University of Sydney only to original research of the highest standard.[3] The only trouble was that the data accessed for the thesis entitled *Some Aetiological Factors in Spontaneous Recurrent Abortion* came from the fertility clinic's records without the consent or knowledge of the director of that unit, *Dr. Allan Grant*, who was overseas during 1958–1959.[4] Additionally, the bylaws of the university state that the work will be "a record of the original research undertaken by the candidate who shall state the sources from which his information was derived, the extent to which he availed himself of the work of others and the portion of the work he claims as his original."[5] Dr. Allan Grant had founded the clinic in 1938, and in the intervening twenty years, a mass of data had been collected from thousands of patients. When Dr. Grant returned and found what McBride had done, he was "irritated" and said, "We had been working on it for years, filling out tables, adding them up." He continued, "Then McBride came along and summarised it all. His thesis was written when I was in America. I did not know anything about it until I saw it in a journal that he had been awarded an MD." He went on, "It was not the right thing to do, to descend on the figures while I was away."

Nevertheless, Grant was a gentleman and conceded that McBride's thesis was "good work" and that he had carried out "at least part of the research" and remained friendly with McBride after that.[6]

In 1957–58, Dr. McBride was appointed to the visiting (specialist) staff at the Women's Hospital, St. George, Bankstown and South Sydney Hospitals and entered private practice. In 1957, he also had to complete his obligation as medical superintendent at the Women's Hospital, so it was no surprise that he quickly became swamped.

I first met Dr. William McBride in 1964 when I was a medical student at the Women's Hospital, Crown Street in Sydney. I was rostered there with another student as part of our undergraduate training in obstetrics and gynecology. One morning, we were instructed by our supervisor to meet with Dr. McBride for a tutorial in the surgeon's room just outside the operating theater. We attended as required and took a seat. In due course, Dr. McBride came out of the operating theater and sat on a couch in the surgeon's room. He stretched out and asked us a question about ectopic pregnancies, and then he promptly fell asleep! The other student and I raised our eyebrows at each other but were reluctant to awaken the great man. After ten minutes or so, the anesthetist came out of the theater, wakened Dr. McBride, and told him that the next case was ready. Dr. McBride got up and entered the theater, and that was the last that I saw of him for three years. During those three years, I occupied myself graduating in medicine and with other hospital appointments.

I returned to the Women's Hospital in 1968 and remained there, training in obstetrics and gynecology, except for a two-year break in 1972 and 1973 when I went to the UK for further training. I returned to the Women's Hospital in 1974 and remained there until the hospital closed in 1983. From 1977 until 1983, I was on the visiting staff as an obstetrician and gynecologist on the same team as Dr. McBride.

Thalidomide

Thalidomide is a miserable drug. It is a true teratogen in that it can damage the embryo in the absence of toxicity in the mother. It is mostly harmless to humans, although it is known that it can cause peripheral neuritis (nerve damage) in some. It is now known that it can damage the unborn baby when given to its mother between thirty-four and fifty days after the last menstrual period. Even then, the mother shows no evidence of toxicity.[7] It was probably the first true teratogen to be recognized. Before thalidomide, it was not realized that there was such a drug. What made thalidomide so treacherous is that the dreadful manifestations it had on the unborn were not seen for seven or eight months after it had wrought its malicious effects. The damage was, therefore, not easy to identify.

Thalidomide was first marketed in Australia in 1960 under the brand name *Distaval*, although it had already been marketed in the UK under that name and in Germany, where it was developed, as *Contergan*. In New South Wales, thalidomide was marketed by the Distillers Company, until then perhaps better known for selling Scotch whisky. The NSW representative for Distillers, *Mr. William Hodgetts*, visited *Dr. Reg Hamlin* at the Women's Hospital, Crown Street on August 18, 1960, and, afterward, Dr. William McBride as well as others to promote Distaval as a sedative during labor.

Shortly after thalidomide was included in the pharmacy, a patient was admitted in early pregnancy with intractable vomiting, known as hyperemesis gravidarum. In spite of all efforts, the vomiting would not stop. McBride, having run out of ideas, commenced the woman on Distaval, and the vomiting stopped within two days. He was most impressed by this and started to prescribe the drug more frequently. It must be remembered that at that time, thalidomide was regarded as a harmless wonder drug.[8] Dr. McBride must be given credit for his use of the drug under the circumstances.

Other obstetricians in the hospital were using phenobarbitone or Debendox, which had already been on the market for several years, but they did not embrace thalidomide as did McBride.[9] And so it was that Dr. McBride was the only obstetrician at the Women's Hospital who was using thalidomide in routine practice.

By this time, McBride's practice was increasing. There was a ward in the Women's Hospital where women who were miscarrying or threatening to miscarry were accommodated. It was noticed by the nursing staff that an unusually high proportion of these women were patients of Dr. McBride. Then in late 1960, several miscarriages of abnormal fetuses occurred, and three children with abnormalities were born to patients of Dr. McBride. The nursing staff pointed out to Dr. McBride that the patients all seemed to be his.

Sister Sarah Bird (not her real name), the nursing unit manager on the night labor ward, drew his attention to this but does not claim to have made the connection with thalidomide. That was left to others. Dr. Reg Hamlin, the medical superintendent (later of fistula fame in Ethiopia), kept a map in his office and stuck a pin in it wherever the mother lived. For a time, the nuclear reactor at Lucas Heights came under suspicion, but that was soon discounted. Lucas Heights is not far from Hurstville where McBride had his consulting rooms. After the third child was born with abnormalities, it was apparent that this was not just a simple case of bad luck. McBride studied the records of the women who had abnormal children and noticed that the one thing that they had in common was that their mother took thalidomide in early pregnancy.

He saw Dr. Hamlin on Tuesday—June 13, 1961—and told him of his suspicions. Hamlin rang the hospital pharmacy and had thalidomide removed from its shelves, becoming the first hospital in the world to do so.[10] In doing this, Dr. McBride saved many lives and children from being born with abnormalities in Australia alone.

Then began a period in which McBride had to do everything he could to stop the sale of thalidomide in Australia and preferably the rest of the world until more was known about it. He called Mr. William Hodgetts—the representative of the distributors, Distillers Company Biochemical (Australia) Limited (DCBCAL)—to his office in Macquarie Street on July 6, 1961. He told him of his anxieties regarding the safety of thalidomide because he had delivered three children with abnormalities. Mr. Hodgetts notified London immediately, but it is said that they did not receive notification until November 21, 1961. Distillers pointed out that thalidomide had been on sale in the United Kingdom for two years and four years in Germany (where it was manufactured) by Chemie Grünenthal. In the meantime, McBride says that he wrote to *The Lancet* on July 30, 1961, but that the letter was rejected and returned by surface mail reaching him in November that year. Neither the letter to *The Lancet* nor the letter of rejection from *The Lancet* has ever been located.[11] Dr. McBride later stated in a letter to *The Lancet* that he had copies of the relevant letters lodged with the National Library of Australia, which would prove that his first paper existed and had been rejected. A search of McBride's documents in the library, however, has not been successful in finding the letter.[12] What is certain is that Dr. McBride wrote a letter to *The Lancet*, which was published on December 16, 1961.[13]

In that letter to *The Lancet*, McBride said, "In recent months I have observed that the incidence of multiple severe abnormalities in babies delivered of women who were given the drug thalidomide (Distaval) during pregnancy, as an antiemetic or as a sedative, to be almost 20 percent."[14] That letter proved to be a signal event, as it was the first time that a connection had been made between the ingestion of thalidomide in pregnancy and congenital abnormalities in the unborn child and had been published in a medical journal in the English language.

McBride himself reports in 1967 that after a scientific meeting in Dusseldorf on November 18, 1961, when thirty-four newborns with defects of the long bones were reported, *Professor Widukind Lenz* of Hamburg raised the prospect of whether thalidomide might be to blame.[15] It has been reported that Lenz had published a paper on the topic in the *German Medical Journal* on November 22, 1961.[16,17] Controversy has raged among scientific circles about who was the first to warn the world about the dangers of thalidomide. Lenz himself has credited McBride as the first. McBride, on the other hand, in a paper in the journal *Teratology*, says that "thalidomide was withdrawn from the market because of Lenz and McBride's independent observations."[18] The truth would seem to be academic, as the essential thing was that thalidomide was withdrawn from world markets, preventing it from causing further abnormalities.

William McBride was now famous. He was recognized as the man who had warned the world about a terrible toxin. He lectured around the world, traveling frequently. He was awarded Commander of the British Empire in June 1969[19] and the Order of Merit from L'Institut de la Vie in France on June 22, 1971.[20] He was Father of the Year and Man of the Year in 1972 and made an Officer of the Order of Australia in 1977[21] and was on the TV show *This Is Your Life* in 1978.[22] Life was undoubtedly on the up-and-up for Dr. William McBride. Those were the halcyon years. McBride continued to study thalidomide. Others study it to this day, and it is now much more widely understood.[23,24,25,26,27,28]

Patients came from far and wide to see the great man, regardless of their problem, whether it was infertility, cancer, or pregnancy. His practice grew so much that he was almost unable to cope. Not that that was difficult to do when his caesarean section rates, reported by a private health fund, went up to 88 percent in 1979[29], and he simply abandoned patients when he was going overseas, leaving them to others without asking them and without making arrangement for their care, an offense of which he was later found guilty by the Medical Tribunal.[30] That was not an isolated incident, as suggested by the court. Many other events occurred. For example, he was suspended for a month by St. George Hospital in January 1988 because he failed to show up for an operation, and that was a common occurrence at the Women's Hospital, Crown Street before it closed in 1983.[31]

The Rise of Foundation 41

The award of the Order of Merit from L'Institut de la Vie carried with it a monetary prize of F100,000, about $40,000. Within months of his arrival back in Australia, McBride announced that he would donate the $40,000 to establish a foundation dedicated to researching the forty weeks of pregnancy plus the first year in life, provided he could find twenty-four other benefactors who would donate a similar amount, making a total of $1 million. The foundation would be called Foundation 41.

After some initial resistance from other donors, Apex, a charitable organization, stepped into the breach and made a large donation.[32] Two prominent Apexians, *Mr. Stuart Hudson* and *Mr. Peter Richard*, became founding directors and governors. They worked tremendously hard, launching an appeal throughout Sydney for $500,000. *Mr. John Darling*, chairman of BP Australia, was appointed as chairman of the board of management of Foundation 41. Foundation 41 was soon up and running with contributions coming from Lions, Rotary, Westpac Bank, schools from all over New South Wales, and numerous others. Foundation 41 was incorporated in New South Wales and became a registered charity on March 29, 1972.[33] It was only a matter of months before the Australian commissioner of taxation allowed a donation to be tax-deductible, provided that the foundation adopted a more appropriate form of scientific accountability. To satisfy the commissioner, Foundation 41 was obliged to form a Research Advisory Committee (RAC). The RAC consisted of four outside professors experienced in scientific research and one other, who was, not surprisingly, Dr. William McBride. McBride presided over this committee and was also the medical director on the board of management of Foundation 41. This put him in a critical and unique position of power within the organization. There was no Peer Review

Committee and no Ethics Committee. Now that he had his own personal, private research unit, he had to do something with it. He had unfettered right to do anything he wanted, and that is just what he did. And it finally led to his downfall.

Not surprisingly, now that Foundation 41 was up and running, McBride was keen to continue his research on thalidomide. He was often asked his opinion on whether a child's abnormalities were due to thalidomide, and even twelve years later, it was not known how thalidomide caused these abnormalities. Until that time, it was thought that defects of the limbs were due to developmental failures in the mesoderm (bones, muscles, vessels). To solve the puzzle, Dr. McBride sent x-rays of five children whose mothers were known to have taken thalidomide during pregnancy to *Dr. Janet McCredie*, a senior staff radiologist at the Royal Prince Alfred Hospital, and asked her opinion. Could Dr. McCredie tell from the x-rays whether the abnormalities had been caused by thalidomide? Dr. McCredie was at first reluctant to help, as she was not experienced in this area; however, she agreed to study the films out of curiosity. Later, Dr. McCredie laid the films out side by side and categorized the abnormalities. She noticed that the malformations were similar to others that she had seen in adults with leprosy, diabetes, and syphilis, in which the cause of the defects was attributable to nerve damage. As thalidomide was known to cause nerve damage in adults, it occurred to Dr. McCredie that she might be viewing cases of nerve damage in the fetus. Dr. McCredie explained her theory to Dr. McBride who disagreed with her, but she continued to have discussions with him in early 1972 when he consulted her about other abnormalities in children who were born showing the effects of thalidomide. During this time, McBride changed his view and agreed that the mechanism of damage caused by thalidomide was likely to be derived from the nerves and not the muscles.

Later in 1972, Dr. McCredie traveled to England, where she consulted a friend, *Professor Howard Middlemiss*, at the University of Bristol who had extensive experience in the radiology of sensory nerve damage. He soon agreed with McCredie that the radiological signs were consistent with nerve damage and suggested that she write an MD thesis on the subject but, in the meantime, submit a manuscript to the journal *Clinical Radiology*, which she did using the five cases of McBride, with his permission, and fifty others from Britain.[34,35] She spent many hours in the library in Britain researching her theory and preparing a paper for publication. The journal *Clinical Radiology* is a quarterly publication, and the article did not appear in print until April 1973, six months after it had been submitted. It carried both names, with McBride as the junior author. He had insisted that his name should appear in the article, although he had done none of the work. He had only asked Dr. McCredie for her opinion on x-rays of five thalidomide-affected children. He offered research help to Dr. McCredie from Foundation 41 but only if his name appeared on the article.[36,37,38]

Within two months, McBride published an article on the neural crest theory of McCredie in his name alone in an obscure journal called *International Research Communications System (IRCS)* in June 1973. He later attended a meeting on birth defects in Vienna where he read a paper on the neuropathology theory of McCredie without acknowledging her. It was not the only example of McBride's use of her work to further his own ambitions. Dr. McBride later presented papers on Janet McCredie's neuropathology theory at scientific meetings and made press announcements without asking or acknowledging her. Despite other attempts by McBride to plagiarize Dr. Janet McCredie, she was awarded the 1977 Twining Medal of Britain's Royal College of Radiologists and, in 1979, the Peter Bancroft Prize for postgraduate medical research at the University of Sydney. She is now recognized for her development of the theory of neuropathology.[39] Dr. McCredie was awarded the degree of Doctor of Medicine by the University of Sydney in 1979 for her thesis on the subject.[40] This would seem to be another example of how McBride cared little for how he plagiarized the work of others.

To quote *Bill Nicol*, the author of *McBride: Behind the Myth*, "There is little doubt that McBride did Dr. McCredie a grave disservice in the way he sought to establish ownership of the neural-crest theory. He did so almost entirely through Foundation 41." As the foundation prospered, so too did its research on the subject.

Few could have foreseen the consequences.[41]

Imipramine

On one of his visits to the Royal Prince Alfred Hospital to discuss the x-ray findings of thalidomide with Dr. McCredie, McBride thought that he saw some similarities to those seen in abnormal children born to mothers who had been on imipramine during pregnancy. Imipramine is a tricyclic antidepressant and was widely and commonly prescribed throughout the world. It was marketed by *Ciba-Geigy* under the trade name *Tofranil*. It was estimated that in 1972 alone, 1.6 million women in Britain had taken the drug and doctors were writing about fifteen million scripts per annum. McBride wrote to the *Medical Journal of Australia* (MJA). The letter to the MJA was published on March 4, 1972 and warned that he had seen a child with the absence of arms or legs and was aware of two others. The mothers, he said, "had taken imipramine in their pregnancy." McBride immediately announced his anxieties in the popular press.[42]

The afternoon tabloids the *Mirror* and *Sun* boomed that "its effects are at least as devastating as thalidomide." Shaun McIlraith in the *Sydney Morning Herald* published a piece on

March 4, 1974, with a sobering photograph of a two-year-old girl with no arms.[43] In later interviews that day, the number of abnormal children increased. He had not only three confirmed cases of his own but also another "possible four cases" that he had heard about. These four cases were more difficult to prove because it was not possible to confirm that their mothers had taken imipramine. He claimed in a statement to the *Mirror* that "our research has shown conclusively that this antidepressant has its effect on the nervous system and can cause babies to be born without arms or with short stumps instead of arms." It seems that he was now claiming that drugs that affect the nervous system can cause abnormalities in the fetal neural crest, a theory that he had previously denied in conversations with Dr. Janet McCredie. Nonetheless, his fame and standing were such that he could not be ignored, and the news spread like wildfire around the world.

The Australian Drug Evaluation Committee (DEC) had been formed after the thalidomide disaster about ten years previously. Under the chairmanship of *Sir William Morrow*, it had been the watchdog of adverse drug reactions. Information was gathered from numerous sources, including doctors and nurses, hospitals, and pharmacists. The committee had not been sitting on its hands. For eighteen months, it had been surveying births at five major hospitals in Sydney and Melbourne and had collected information on over 43,000 births, detecting no increase in congenital abnormalities in women who had taken imipramine. Now it needed to stand and be counted. In a statement on behalf of the committee, while being careful with his words, Sir William contradicted McBride. He said, "The Committee is not aware of any definite cause and effect relationship between imipramine and congenital abnormalities."

Over the next two weeks, there was uproar. McBride took calls from around the world day and night. There were calls from government agencies, doctors, radio, television and printed press, and others wanting to report more cases of congenital abnormalities. The press complained that the government had taken no action to prevent further congenital abnormalities. After three or four days, however, McBride changed his attitude, saying, "I admit that the evidence is circumstantial, but it's circumstantial evidence that they cannot ignore." Amidst all the fuss and DEC's refusal to ban the drug without further evidence, McBride softened his attitude. He offered to provide evidence to DEC that the affected children's mothers had taken imipramine. He could provide only one x-ray to the DEC, however, that of Michelle, the two-year-old who had no arms. The other two children were still to be x-rayed. Later, McBride would admit that only one woman out of the three had taken imipramine, the other two having taken another drug, amitriptyline.

When taken in context with the other four supposed victims whose mothers were not known for sure to have taken imipramine, McBride's warning was becoming shaky, at best. He admitted to the committee that his original statements about imipramine were incorrect. The committee reaffirmed its previous decision.[44,45,46,47]

Bill McBride was not one to be cowed by the odd committee or two. He was defiant and is reported to have said, "By God, I will fight for these babies. I think that if I can save just one child from the effects of these tricyclic drugs, I will have done my job." McBride was dissatisfied that the Department of Health had not withdrawn imipramine from the market. It did not seem to have occurred to him that many women would have already withdrawn themselves from the drug due to the publicity and therefore have deprived themselves of its benefit. Later reports suggested that abortions were carried out needlessly due to anxiety. Dr. McBride was quoted saying, "I personally feel that if a woman needs antidepressants, she shouldn't be pregnant and is better off having an abortion." He went on, "If you cannot cope with life before a child arrives you will be much worse off afterwards."[48] This statement is extraordinary coming from a person who claimed to be so caring about children. It may reflect the pressure he felt at the time.

As the media frenzy passed, the imipramine controversy was concluded by a statement from the DEC that "McBride had corrected certain details in his original letter to the *Medical Journal of Australia* and that in conclusion, the committee would reiterate that, although the absolute safety of imipramine during pregnancy has not been established, current assessment proves no causal relationship with congenital abnormalities of the limb." One would have thought that McBride might now get back to his medical practice and his farm in Dungog. But it was not so.

Amniocentesis means passing a needle through the abdominal and uterine wall into the gestation sac to collect amniotic fluid. In the late 1970s, amniocentesis for the detection of chromosome abnormalities became more frequent, as it was realized that as maternal age increased, so did the risk of a chromosome abnormality. The only cytogenetics laboratory in NSW at the time was at the Prince of Wales Hospital–Randwick, which had a limited capacity to diagnose chromosome abnormalities from amniotic fluid.

The New South Wales Health Commission, therefore, placed a limit on the age at which amniocentesis could be performed. At the time, the age limit was thirty-nine years. Dr. McBride did not like to be told when he could or could not send amniotic fluid anywhere, so he established a cytogenetic laboratory in Foundation 41 and collected the amniotic fluid from patients himself without ultrasound guidance, sending the fluid to his own laboratory in Foundation 41. A member of the cytogenetic unit in Foundation 41 reports, "His collections are perfect. I believe he is an excellent technician and that he collects amniotic fluid very quickly and he does it very well because his amniotic fluid is clear."[49]

This was entirely incorrect, as that member was not aware that when McBride failed to collect amniotic fluid, he merely sent the patient across the lane from Foundation 41 to have the procedure carried out properly under ultrasound control in the hospital. The fluid was then usually bloodstained due to the previous failed attempts. McBride did what he liked in Foundation 41.

The ILZRO Project

McBride and Foundation 41 had close links with British Petroleum (BP). The prize of $40,000 that he had won from the L'Institut de la Vie in France had been funded by the French branch of British Petroleum, and the chairman of the board of Foundation 41, Mr. John Darling, was also the chairman of the board of BP Australia. The purpose of the International Lead Zinc Research Organization (ILZRO) project was to study the effects of lead levels on the intelligence and behavior of affected children. The psychologist involved was *Ms. Barbara Black*. McBride submitted two applications for funding to the National Health and Medical Research Council (NHMRC). Both were rejected, so his application was sent to the Australian Lead Development Association and ILZRO. This was successful. Insisting that his name be first on the application, the paper was submitted to the *Medical Journal of Australia*.[50] Breaking with tradition, McBride preempted the findings and announced to the public at Foundation 41's Open Day on May 28, 1982, "We did not find any risk in Sydney children. I think it is futile and a waste of the nation's resources to completely remove lead from petrol at a time when the world's reserves of fossil fuels are being rapidly depleted. I stress our blood levels indicate no cause for alarm." The editor of the MJA was furious when this was reported in the *Sydney Morning Herald* six weeks before publication in the MJA. He added a lengthy editorial at the end of the article identifying the source of funding and indicating that "it had been written without the knowledge or approval of all of the authors."[51]

Agent Orange

During the Vietnam War, the United States used Agent Orange as a defoliant. It consisted of 2,4,5-T and 2,4-D weedicides in a fifty-fifty combination and was sprayed over vast tracts of forests from bomber aircraft to eradicate most broad-leaved and woody plants. 2,4,5-T is a synthetic chemical whose temperature must be tightly controlled during manufacture, as the process contaminates the chemical with traces of dioxin, a highly toxic contaminant that is known to be teratogenic. In the context of war, the damage done by Agent Orange was of no great concern if it landed on enemy troops. What was of more interest was that some of the sprays might have fallen on friendly troops, including the Australian military. By 1966, 2.3 million gallons of Agent Orange had been sprayed over about one-seventh of Vietnam. Its military use was stopped in 1970, and it was banned from most domestic consumption in 1972. The production of 2,4,5-T was ceased entirely in 1982.[52,53]

McBride was interested in 2,4,5-T, having used it himself on his farm in Dungog. He told a young research scientist in Foundation 41's Developmental Biology Department, *Mr. Phil Vardy*, to prepare a study on the effects of 2,4,5-T. He told Mr. Vardy to spray some 2,4,5-T on the rabbits' food, which he did, but they would not eat it, so he told Mr. Vardy to put it in their water, but they would not drink it. Some died, some became sick, and some became dehydrated. The experiment had been ill-planned, and Mr. Vardy had not been given time to prepare it correctly. It was a complete failure, but it did not stop McBride from announcing that 2,4,5-T was safe, which we now know not to be true.

In 1981, a researcher named *Ms. Kerry Fagan* joined Foundation 41. Ms. Fagan had extensive experience, in particular, with the transmission of chromosome abnormalities from parent to child. McBride seemed to be hoping for funding from the Vietnam Veterans Association, and Ms. Fagan prepared a proposal for funding to the Department of Veterans Affairs. McBride altered the application by canceling the requirement for the father's chromosomes. The application failed, and the number of Vietnam veterans willing to contribute decreased to a trickle. The study evaporated.[54] This interference by McBride was typical of his mismanagement of research projects. During its life, Foundation 41 applied for twelve National Health and Medical Research Council (NHMRC) grants, and it never received one. Not one.[55]

Elective Induction of Labor

In 1974, *Dr. Jack Lyle*, a psychologist, was seconded to Foundation 41. His task, with the assistance of Ms. Barbara Black, was to organize several studies into what effect induced labor might have had on intelligence and physical ability of children whose mother's labor had been induced. Dr. Lyle left Australia in 1976 on sabbatical leave, and when he returned, he found that his work had been published without his name on the paper. After he protested, his name was added to the paper, but the same work was published in the *Medical Journal of Australia* two years later without Dr. Lyle's name. This was another example of plagiarism, in this case, of Dr. Jack Lyle and Ms. Barbara Black. [56]

Around this time, McBride published several articles suggesting that elective induction of labor before term resulted in children who might have higher intelligence than those who were allowed to labor spontaneously.[57,58] One might assume, reasonably, that these were efforts to justify his enormously high elective cesarean section rates.[59]

Debendox/Bendectin

Dicyclomine, doxylamine, and vitamin B6 were marketed from 1956 as a single pill under the brand name Debendox in Australia and the UK and Bendectin in the USA. It was useful for the treatment of morning sickness in pregnancy.[60,61] Dicyclomine was removed from the combination in the USA in 1976 as it was ineffective as an antiemetic (anti-nausea medication). It remained as a combination of the three substances elsewhere in the world. Debendox had been extensively studied, and by 1977, its use was widespread, as it was one of the few drugs that might help morning sickness.

There is some evidence that women who have nausea and vomiting in pregnancy may be less likely to spontaneously miscarry.[62,63,64] This would be cold comfort to those women who become very distressed by the condition. At any rate, Debendox was the only drug on the market that helped morning sickness that was approved by the Food and Drug Administration in the USA. The national drug agencies of the United Kingdom, Australia, Switzerland, and Germany found no evidence of teratogenicity.[65] Because it was officially approved and had been shown to be efficacious and safe, it was widely used.[66,67,68,69,70,71,72,73,74,75,76,77] By 1977, it was estimated that twenty million women had used it;[78] and in 1978, one million prescriptions had been issued in the USA alone.[79] In one case, a correction was published after thirty years, altering a decimal point and therefore changing the incidence of abnormalities after taking Debendox from 13 percent to 1.3 percent due to a typographical error![80] It seems that nobody took any notice of the error in the first place, or they recognized it for what it was.[81]

So there was convincing evidence that Debendox was safe to take in pregnancy. That did not deter McBride though. He was after Debendox.

The Mekdeci Case

By his own account, Dr. McBride's interest in Debendox was triggered in 1978 when he received a letter from *Mrs. Betty Mekdeci* of Orlando, Florida. Mrs. Mekdeci inquired whether McBride thought that her son's abnormalities might have been caused by Debendox. McBride thought that his general knowledge of the composition of the Debendox was adequate to say that it could cause malformations of this type. This was only an opinion, however, so he requested funds from Merrell in Australia to study the effects of Debendox, but this request was declined. McBride then asked the company for a supply of pure doxylamine and dicyclomine, but he was again rejected. Dr. McBride still had no concrete evidence that Debendox could cause congenital abnormalities and he was due to travel to Florida to give evidence for Mrs. Mekdeci, so he bought commercial Debendox, crushed the tablets, and fed them in large doses to fourteen pregnant rabbits. None produced an abnormal litter.[82] (It is not recorded whether they got morning sickness—Ed.)

McBride flew to Orlando, Florida, to give evidence for the Mekdecis at the trial, only to find Professor Widukind Lenz providing evidence for Richardson-Merrell Inc. There was no ill will between them. Indeed, they were friends, but the Mekdecis lost the case.[83,84] They received nothing, not even costs, having claimed $10 million. Regardless of this, hundreds of other cases were being lined up to claim damages against Richardson-Merrell!

McBride suspected, perhaps quite reasonably, that the reason that Richardson-Merrell would not supply dicyclomine was that they had a sizeable commercial stake in the sale of the drug. In support of this theory, *Admiral G. Crabb*, retired from the Royal Australian Navy and working for a security organization, warned McBride that the pharmaceutical company was searching for dirt on McBride, possibly to be used in court. The admiral also advised Dr. McBride to be careful crossing the road and not to travel on trains in the United States.[85,86]

Back in Australia and not being able to get his hands on pure doxylamine or dicyclomine, McBride decided to test scopolamine, also known as hyoscine, a related anticholinergic drug. This alone should have cast doubt over the research, as scopolamine is not an ingredient of Debendox. "A horse in the same stable," McBride would say. He tested six New Zealand white rabbits by adding scopolamine to their drinking water. The water came from a bottle with a rubber bung in it. Leakage from the bottle was inevitable and ended up forming a wet patch in the sawdust at the bottom of the cage, so the amount of scopolamine ingested was calculated using the amount of water estimated to be in the wet patch and the water remaining in the bottle.[87] McBride, crediting Mr. Vardy and Ms. French, submitted the findings in a paper to the *Journal of Toxicology and Applied Pharmacology*. Not surprisingly, the article was rejected, having been criticized on scientific grounds.

McBride then made several modifications to the paper that he thought might satisfy the peer reviewers, and it was finally accepted for publication by the *Australian Journal of Biological Sciences*.[88] While McBride was overseas, a packet of reprints arrived at Foundation 41 addressed to McBride, Vardy, and French. Phil Vardy opened this packet and found that many of the facts had been altered from the original submission, and there were two more rabbits than were in the study. Vardy confronted McBride with this when he returned from overseas. This was the beginning of a period of acrimonious accusations and counteraccusations, threats and counterthreats, dismissals, reappointments, and resignations. The Research Advisory Committee insisted that McBride write to the *Australian Journal of Biological Sciences* and publish a correction, but he only published a "Note" in 1983 saying that the experiment would be repeated.[89] The journal noted that Mr. Vardy and Ms. French had withdrawn their names from the paper.[90]

In the meantime, the Women's Hospital, Crown Street—adjacent to the Foundation 41 building—closed in 1983, and the staff was transferred elsewhere, McBride to the Royal Hospital for Women in Paddington. But Merrell Dow (as it was now called) stopped producing the drug in 1983 although it was still approved by the FDA, therefore denying women its benefits from then on. Although there was no evidence that Debendox was harmful, indeed it was the preferred drug by the FDA for the treatment of morning sickness. *Mr. David Sharrock*, the managing director of Merrell Dow, announced that the drug would no longer be produced and was being withdrawn from the market. This was because, in spite of the continuing failure of legal cases to show that Debendox was harmful, the cost of defending each case and the associated insurance premiums were so high that it was becoming a financial burden on the company. There were said to be hundreds of cases waiting to be defended.[91] Life went on, but the women of the world were denied the relief from morning sickness that had been available from one of the most tested and safest drugs ever.

It is interesting to note that in 1962, so recently after his observations on thalidomide, McBride was not above warning others about the risks of drawing premature conclusions. He said, "Let us be on the alert by all means and report our observations, but we must be critical, as many pregnant women and their husbands are unnecessarily upset by uncritical accusations of drugs as being the cause of all congenital abnormalities."[92] It is advice that McBride would have done well to take himself.

The *Science Show* with Norman Swan

On December 12, 1987, Dr. Norman Swan, a Scottish-born pediatrician turned journalist, broadcast on the ABC, national radio's *Science Show*—a program focused on fraud and dishonesty among the medical fraternity. Dr. William McBride was overseas at the time but arrived back the next day, walking into a veritable storm.[93,94,95] He was accused of fraudulently altering the data of a scientific experiment that he claimed was evidence of Debendox causing abnormalities in unborn babies in a similar way to thalidomide. The board of Foundation 41 met the next day and decided to tough it out, but this was going to prove difficult because hard evidence of the fraud was provided by Mr. Phil Vardy.[96] McBride denied many of the statements of Mr. Vardy and Ms. Jill French but at the same time tried to back off from his own accusations about Debendox by pointing out that scopolamine was not an ingredient of Debendox. McBride claimed that his findings about scopolamine did not relate to Debendox. This was a bit bizarre, as he had already given evidence against Debendox on two occasions in the USA.[97] It was also a bit late, as Debendox had been withdrawn years before.

The furore would not die away. Eventually, after five months, the board held an inquiry under the chairmanship of Sir Harry Gibbs, recently retired from the Supreme Court. The other members of the inquiry would be Professor Robert Walker and Professor Roger Short. The committee commenced its hearings on July 25 and completed them on November 2, 1988. Their findings were devastating. The committee found McBride guilty of scientific fraud.[98,99,100,101]

McBride resigned the next day but was reappointed later after a dispute among the board.[102,103]

The Fall of Foundation 41

From the beginning, McBride ran Foundation 41 as his personal fiefdom. He hired and fired as he chose. He chaired the Research Advisory Committee (RAC) as his own reporting session rather than as a serious research planning forum. *Professor Michael Bennett* arrived from England to take up the position of professor of obstetrics and gynecology at the Royal Hospital for Women in Paddington and found himself on the RAC but was unable to obtain any agenda papers before the meeting. He resigned from the committee after one meeting. *Professor Rodney Shearman* at the University of Sydney found that his name was being used on advertising material without his consent and demanded that it be removed, which it was without apology or recognition. Although the NHMRC supports about one thousand research projects at any one time, Foundation 41 never qualified for a single grant. Ever.[104]

According to Mr. Peter Richards and Mr. Stuart Hudson, life governors and founding directors of Foundation 41, Dr. McBride did not contribute all his $40,000 prize money to Foundation 41. They say that he put in only two payments of $8,000 each. Mr. Richards and Mr. Hudson were both former Apex leaders, who had motivated their members to raise more than $500,000 for Foundation 41 and say that McBride had spent the balance of the $40,000.[105] As the news of the fraud spread, charitable donations dried up, and the foundation had to consider amalgamating with others or selling its real estate.[106,107,108]

Controversy followed him all his life.[109,110]

The next year, McBride faced a complaint from *Merrilyn Walton* on behalf of the Health Care Complaints Unit of the New South Wales Department of Health. There were nine charges relating to his patients' clinical management and six in relation to his research. The subsequent Medical Tribunal was perhaps the longest in medico-legal history at that time. It sat for 180 days, of which McBride gave evidence on forty-six. It took almost four years for the tribunal to hand down its decision, and when it did, it pulled no punches. He was found guilty of only one of the clinical cases, that of abandoning a patient in hospital, but among other criticisms, regarding the scientific fraud, the Tribunal said, "McBride's acts were not made in haste; they were not made by a man in poor physical or mental health. His acts demonstrated a course of conduct of premeditated deception in the field of medical research and indicated a serious flaw or defect in his character, a trait of dishonesty."

The Tribunal concluded that the appropriate order was for the removal of Dr. McBride's name from the medical register.[111,112,113] McBride repeatedly appealed the decision and, in 1995, applied to be reregistered on the basis that he had "identified the defect in my character and realised the error of my ways." The Medical Tribunal rejected the application, saying that McBride had "continued absence of insight."

Stephen Lock, once the editor of the *British Medical Journal*, said of McBride, "The most astounding feature of Dr. William McBride's eventual admission that he had published false and misleading data was the excuse that he gave: that the ends justify the means."[114]

An application in 1998 to the Tribunal, however, was successful, and McBride was allowed to return to medicine, having admitted dishonesty and undertaken to refrain from medical research and be supervised in his practice. Having regained his registration, he no longer practiced in New South Wales but worked in American Samoa and then lived quietly with his family back in Sydney.[115,116]

Epilogue

The greatest tragedy in this story is the withdrawal of Debendox/Bendectin from the market and, therefore, its unavailability to women who might benefit. Nausea and vomiting in pregnancy is a sickening disease, and Debendox is the one drug that can help it. It is now unavailable for all the wrong reasons.

The next tragedy is that Dr. William Griffith McBride had to do no more than he had already done in unveiling the harmful effects of thalidomide, and he would have been remembered as the Father of Teratology. He went off on his own crusades, targeting one thing after another, whether right or wrong. One of his greatest problems was that he was not a team player. He listened to nobody. Sadly, he also damaged the image of scientific research.

Dr. W. G. McBride died in Sydney on June 27, 2018. His send-off was enormous, fit for a state funeral.

As Mr. Stuart Hudson had once said, "You either loved him or hated him. There is no in-between with Bill McBride."

Notes

1. McBride, W. *Killing the Messenger*. 1st ed. Cremorne, NSW, Australia: Eldorado; 1994. p. 30.
2. Ibid. pp. 36–38.

3. McBride, W. *Some Aetiological Factors of Recurrent Abortions*. Sydney: MD thesis submitted to the University of Sydney; 1960.

4. Nicol, B. *McBride: Behind the Myth*. 1st ed. Crow's Nest, NSW: ABC Enterprises for the Australian Broadcasting Corp.; 1989. pp. 5–6.

5. Bylaw XII.8 (1) of the University of Sydney.

6. Nicol, B. op. cit. p. 6.

7. Kennedy, D. "Thalidomide: a Byword for Tragedy. *O&G Magazine* (internet). 2016 (cited August 17, 2018); vol. 18, no. 1. Available from https://www.ogmagazine.org.au/18/118/thalidomide-byword-tragedy/.

8. Nicol, B. op. cit. p. 15.

9. Ibid. p. 13.

10. Ibid. pp. 16–17.

11. Ibid. p. 20.

12. O'Neill, J., B Lagan. "McBride Thalidomide Discovery Papers Elude Search." *Sydney Morning Herald*. November 19, 1988: 3.

13. McBride, W. G. "Thalidomide and Congenital Abnormalities." *The Lancet*. December 16, 1961; 2(7216): 1,358.

14. Ibid.

15. McBride, W. "Thalidomide Embryopathy." *Teratology*. 1977; 16(1): 79–82.

16. O'Neill, J., B. Lagan. op. cit. *Sydney Morning Herald*.

17. Lenz, W., K. Knapp. "Thalidomide Embryopathy." *Archives of Environmental Health: An International Journal*. 1962; 14–19.

18. McBride, W. "Thalidomide Embryopathy." *Teratology*.

19. McBride, W. *Killing the Messenger*. 1st ed. Cremorne, NSW, Australia: Eldorado; 1994. p. 91.

20. Ibid. p. 93.

21. Nicol, B. *McBride: Behind the Myth*. p. 174.

22. Ibid.
23. McBride, W. "Teratogenic Action of Thalidomide." *The Lancet.* 1978; 311(8078): 1,362.
24. McBride, W. "Thalidomide May Be a Mutagen." *BMJ.* 1994; 308(6944): 1,635–1,636.
25. "Is Thalidomide a Mutagen?" *InPharma Weekly.* 1994; (944): 21.
26. Smithells, R. "Thalidomide May Be a Mutagen." *BMJ.* 1994; 309(6952): 477.
27. Kida, M. "Thalidomide May Not Be a Mutagen." *BMJ.* 1994; 309(6956): 741.
28. Ashby, J. "Thalidomide Is Not a Mutagen." *Nature.* 1997; 389(6647): 118.
29. Nicol, B. *McBride: Behind the Myth.* p. 174.
30. McBride, W. *Killing the Messenger.* p. 216, complaint 6.
31. Hogarth, M., B. Lagan, J. O'Neill. "The Foundation and Fall." *Sydney Morning Herald.* November 19, 1988; pp. 81, 88.
32. Nicol, B. *McBride: Behind the Myth.* pp. 75–76.
33. Ibid. p. 80.
34. Ibid. p. 101.
35. McCredie, J., W. McBride. "Some Congenital Abnormalities: Possibly Due to Embryonic Peripheral Neuropathy." *Clinical Radiology.* 1973; 24(2): 204–211.
36. Ibid.
37. McCredie, J., J. Cameron, R. Shoobridge. "Congenital Malformations and the Neural Crest." *The Lancet.* 1978; 312(8093): 761–763.
38. McCredie, J. "The Action of Thalidomide on the Peripheral Nervous System of the Embryo." Proceedings of the Australian Association of Neurologists. 1975; 12: 135–140.
39. Nicol, B. *McBride: Behind the Myth.* p. 112.
40. Ibid. p. 113.

41. Ibid. p. 113.

42. Ibid. p. 30.

43. McIlraith, S. "Deformity Fear; No Drug Action." *Sydney Morning Herald*. March 4, 1972: 2.

44. Nicol, B. *McBride: Behind the Myth*. p. 42.

45. Staff. "Imipramine Check by Makers." *Sydney Morning Herald*. March 8, 1972: 3.

46. McIlraith, S. "Deformity Fear; No Drug Action." *Sydney Morning Herald*. March 4, 1972: 2.

47. Jacobs, D. "Imipramine (Tofranil)." *South African Medical Journal*. 1972: 1,023.

48. Nicol, B. *McBride: Behind the Myth*. pp. 44–45.

49. Nicol, B. *McBride: Behind the Myth*. p. 87.

50. McBride, W., B. Black, B. English. "Blood Lead Levels and Behaviour of 400 Preschool Children." *Medical Journal of Australia*. 1982; 2(1): 26–29.

51. Nicol, B. *McBride: Behind the Myth*. p. 88.

52. Zimdahl, R. "A History of Weed Science in the United States." Amsterdam: Elsevier; 2010.

53. Hall, W., D. MacPhee. "The Agent Orange Controversy in Australia: A Contribution to the Debate." *Australian and New Zealand Journal of Public Health*. 1985; 9(2): 109–119.

54. Nicol, B. *McBride: Behind the Myth*. p. 94.

55. Hogarth, M., B. Lagan, J. O'Neill. "McBride Projects Failed to Win Government Funds." *Sydney Morning Herald*. November 22, 1988: 12.

56. Ibid.

57. McBride, W., J. Lyle, B. Black, C. Brown, D. Thomas. "A Study of Five Year Old Children Born after Elective Induction of Labour." *Medical Journal of Australia*. 1977; 2(14): 456–459.

58. Black, B., W. McBride. "Children Born after Elective Induction of Labour." *Medical Journal of Australia*. 1979; 2(7): 362–363.

59. McBride, W. G., B. P. Black, C. J. Brown, R. M. Dolby, A. D. Murray, D. B. Thomas. "Method of Delivery and Developmental Outcome at Five Years of Age." *The Medical Journal of Australia*. April 21, 1979; 1(8): 301–4. doi: 10.5694/j.1326-5377.1979.tb112116.x. PMID: 449802.

60. Hays, D. "Bendectin: A Case of Mourning Sickness." *Drug Intelligence & Clinical Pharmacy*. 1983; 17(11): 826–827.

61. Henderson, I. "Congenital Deformities Associated with Bendectin." *Can. Med. Assoc. J.* 1977; 117(7): 721–2.

62. Milkovich, L., B. van den Berg. "An Evaluation of the Teratogenicity of Certain Antinauseant Drugs." *American Journal of Obstetrics and Gynecology*. 1976; 125(2): 244–248.

63. Kullander, S., B. Källén. "A Prospective Study of Drugs and Pregnancy: II. Anti-Emetic Drugs." *Acta Obstetricia et Gynecologica Scandinavica*. 1976; 55(2): 105–111.

64. Collins, F. "Morning Sickness Associated with Lower Miscarriage Risk." NIH Directors Blog. October 4, 2016. Available from https://directors-blog.nih.gov/2016/10/04/nausea-in-pregnancy-is-associated-with-lower-miscarriage-risk/.

65. Korcok, M. "The Bendectin Debate." *Can. Med. Assoc. J.* 1980; 123: 992–8.

66. Check, W. "CDC Study: No Evidence for Teratogenicity of Bendectin." JAMA: *The Journal of the American Medical Association*. 1979; 242(23): 2,518.

67. Food and Drug Administration Advisory Committee. "The Bendectin Peer Group Report." Washington, DC: US Department of Health, Education and Welfare. 1975.

68. Paterson, D. "Congenital Deformities." *Can. Med. Assoc. J.* 1969; 101(3): 175–6.

69. Shiono, P., M. Klebanoff. "Bendectin and Human Congenital Malformations." *Teratology.* 1989; 40(2): 151–155.

70. Henderson, I. "Congenital Deformities Associated with Bendectin." *Can. Med. Assoc. J.* 1977; 117(7): 721–2.

71. Harron, D., K. Griffiths, R. Shanks. "Debendox and Congenital Malformations in Northern Ireland." *BMJ.* 1980; 281(6252): 1,379–1,381.

72. Smithells, R., S. Sheppard. "Teratogenicity Testing in Humans: A Method Demonstrating Safety of Bendectin." *Teratology.* 1978; 17(1): 31–35.

73. "The 'Bendectin' Debate: Teratogenic Potential Unlikely." *InPharma Weekly.* 1980; 266(1): 5–6.

74. Paterson, D. "Congenital Abnormalities Associated with Bendectin." *Can. Med. Assoc. J.* 1977; 116(12): 1,348.

75. Korcok, M. "The Bendectin Debate." *Can. Med. Assoc. J.* 1980; 123(9): 992–8.

76. Therapeutic Goods A. "Fifty Years of Independent Expert Advice on Prescription Medicines." Australian Government Department of Health (internet). 2014 (cited August 20, 2018). Available from https://www.tga.gov.au/book/fifty-years-independent-expert-advice-prescription-medicines-02.

77. Holmes, L. "Teratogen Update: Bendectin." *Teratology.* 1983; 27(2): 277–281.

78. Henderson, I. "Congenital Deformities Associated with Bendectin."

79. Check, W. "CDC Study."

80. Fleming, D., J. Knox, D. Crombie. "Debendox in Early Pregnancy and Fetal Malformation." *BMJ.* 1981; 283(6284): 99–101.

81. "Correction. Debendox in Early Pregnancy and Fetal Malformation." *BMJ*. 2010; 340(May 2010): c2,196.

82. McBride, W. *Killing the Messenger*. pp. 119–120.

83. Kolata, G. "Jury Exonerates Bendectin in Mekdeci Case." *Science*. 1981; 212(4495): 647.

84. Kolata, G. "Jury Clears Bendectin." *Science*. 1985; 227(4694): 1,559.

85. Synnot, J. "Ex-Admiral Backs McBride's Claim." *Sydney Morning Herald*. January 19, 1999: 27.

86. McBride, W. *Killing the Messenger*. pp. 124–126.

87. Ibid. p. 127.

88. McBride, W., P. Vardy, J. French. "Effects of Scopolamine Hydrobromide on the Development of the Chick and Rabbit Embryo." *Australian Journal of Biological Sciences*. 1982; 35(2): 173.

89. McBride, W. "Note on the Paper 'Effects of Scopolamine Hydrobromide on the Development of the Chick and Rabbit Embryo' by W. G. McBride, P. H. Vardy and J. French." *Australian Journal of Biological Sciences*. 1983; 36(2): 171.

90. McBride, W., P. Vardy, J. French. "Effects of Scopolamine Hydrobromide on the Development of the Chick and Rabbit Embryo." *Australian Journal of Biological Sciences*. 1988; 41(4): 589.

91. Hays, D. "Bendectin: A Case of Mourning Sickness."

92. McBride, W. "Drugs and Foetal Abnormalities." *BMJ*. 1962; 2(5320): 1,681.

93. Scott, L., A. Conway. "Doctor Flies into Trouble." *Sydney Morning Herald*. December 13, 1987: 5.

94. Lagan, B. "McBride: Storm over Cheating Claims." *Sydney Morning Herald*. December 14, 1987: 1.

95. O'Neill, G. "Changes Said to Be in McBride's Hand." *Sydney Morning Herald*. December 14, 1987: 4.

96. Lagan, B. "McBride Rejects Allegations of Fraud." *Sydney Morning Herald*. December 15, 1987: 1.

97. Beale, B. "Tests Not Debendox Connected." *Sydney Morning Herald*. December 15, 1987: 6.

98. Nicol, B. *McBride: Behind the Myth*. p. 161.

99. Humphrey, G. "Scientific Fraud: The McBride Case—Judgment." (Internet). Journals.sagepub.com. *Med. Sci. Law* vol. 34, no. 4: pp. 299–306. 1994 (cited August 16, 2018]. Available from http://journals.sagepub.com/doi/abs/10.1177/002580249403400405?journalCode=msla.

100. Lawson, M. "McBride Found Guilty of Fraud." *Nature*. 1993; 361(6414): 673.

101. Dayton, L. "Thalidomide Hero Found Guilty of Scientific Fraud." *New Scientist* (internet). 1993 (cite August 16, 2018); (1862). Available from https://www.newscientist.com/article/mg13718620-800-thalidomide-hero-found-guilty-of-scientific-fraud/.

102. Dempster, Q. *Whistleblower*. 1st ed. Sydney: ABC Books; 1997.

103. Lock, S. "Misconduct in Medical Research: Does It Exist in Britain?" *BMJ*. 1988; 297(6662): 1,531–1,535.

104. Hogarth, M., B. Lagan, J. O'Neill. "McBride Projects Failed to Win Government Funds." *Sydney Morning Herald*. November 22, 1988: 12.

105. Hogarth, M., B. Lagan, J. O'Neill. "The Foundation and Fall." *Sydney Morning Herald*. November 19, 1988: pp. 81, 88.

106. Hogarth, M. "Foundation 41 Seeks Merger." *Sydney Morning Herald*. November 21, 1988: 5.

107. Hogarth, M., B. Lagan, J. O'Neill. "The Skeleton in Foundation 41's Cupboard." *Sydney Morning Herald*. November 21, 1988: 12.

108. Staff. "Foundation 41 Moves to Halt Fund-Raising Crisis." *The Age*. November 21, 1988: 20.

109. McLaren, M. "Family of Renowned Doctor Forced to Defend His Name Just days after His Death." 2018 [cited 16 August 2018]. 2GB: *Ray Hadley Morning Show* (internet). Available from https://www.2gb.com/family-of-renowned-doctor-forced-to-defend-his-name-just-days-after- his-death/.

110. Ripley, A., E. Fitzgerald. "Doctor Warned World of Thalidomide." *SMH*. July 18, 2018: Obituaries.

111. Humphrey, G. "Scientific Fraud: The McBride Case—Judgment." (Internet). Journals.sagepub.com: *Med. Sci. Law* vol. 34, no. 4: pp. 299–306. 1994 (cited August 16, 2018). Available from http://journals.sagepub.com/doi/abs/10.1177/002580249403400405?journalCode=msla.

112. Lawson, M. "McBride Found Guilty of Fraud." *Nature*. 1993; 361(6414): 673.

113. Dayton, L. "Thalidomide Hero Found Guilty of Scientific Fraud." *New Scientist* (internet). 1993 (cited August 16, 2018); (1862). Available from https://www.newscientist.com/article/mg13718620-800-thalidomide-hero-found-guilty-of-scientific-fraud/.

114. Lock, S., F. Wells. *Fraud and Misconduct in Medical Research*. 1st ed. London: BMJ Publishing Group; 1993.

115. Freckelton, I. *Scholarly Misconduct Law, Regulation, and Practice*. 1st ed. Oxford: Oxford University Press; 2016. pp. 142–146.

116. Ripley, A., E. Fitzgerald. "Doctor Warned World of Thalidomide." *Sydney Morning Herald*. 2018.

Suggested Further Reading

Nicol, Bill. *McBride: Behind the Myth*. 1st ed. Crow's Nest, NSW: ABC Enterprises for the Australian Broadcasting Corp.; 1989.

McBride, William. *Killing the Messenger*. 1st ed. Cremorne, NSW, Australia: Eldorado; 1994.

Dempster, Quentin. *Whistleblowers*. Australian Broadcasting Corporation. Sydney: 1997.

Freckelton, Ian. *Scholarly Misconduct; Law, Regulation, and Practice*. Oxford University Press. Oxford UK. 1st edition, 2016.

Lock, Stephen, Frank Wells. *Fraud and Misconduct in Medical Research*. BMJ Publishing Group, London; 1993.

Walton, Merrilyn. *The Trouble with Medicine: Preserving the Trust between Patients and Doctors*. Allen and Unwin; 1998.

Martin, Brian. *Scientific Fraud and the Power Structure of Science*. Published in *Prometheus*. 1992; vol. 10, no. 1: pp. 83–98.

CHAPTER NINE

DRS. PEARCE AND CHAMBERLAIN—ECTOPIC MAGICIANS

Prologue

This is a tale of two men, both of whom were highly intelligent and successful, but one of whom was stupid in the extreme and the other was naive in the extreme. The stupidity of one and the naivety of the other would bring them both down.

Ectopic Pregnancy

An ectopic pregnancy is one that occurs outside the uterine cavity. Fertilization of the ovum by the spermatozoon occurs in one fallopian tube or the other, usually on the side of ovulation. Once the ovum is fertilized, it is called a zygote, and it usually takes as many as four days to make its way down the tube into the uterus, under the influence of the wave-like movement of the tube itself. The zygote divides as it develops and may drift in the uterine cavity for a day or so until it implants into the uterine wall, which is lined with decidua—the lining of the uterus that has been specially prepared to receive it. Pregnancy hormones start to be detectable soon after this.

If the progress of the zygote is delayed for any reason, it may die, or it may implant in the fallopian tube itself, as the lining of the tube is similar to the lining of the uterus. In this case, it is called an ectopic pregnancy. The fallopian tube, however, is not designed to accommodate a developing pregnancy (the zygote is called an embryo after five weeks), and eventually it may rupture the fallopian tube, sometimes with resultant disastrous bleeding, often around eight to ten weeks of pregnancy. In this case, there are symptoms, such as pain and bleeding, that give a clue to the diagnosis. Treatment such as surgery or chemical treatments are indicated, and the pregnancy and often the tube is lost for further reproductive purposes.

Since the advent of diagnostic ultrasound, it has been possible to diagnose most cases of tubal pregnancy before pain and symptoms appear. High-frequency transvaginal ultrasound allows a close examination of the pelvic contents, including the fallopian tubes. If there is a pregnancy in the uterus, it is usually easily visualized as early as six weeks after the last menstrual period. Also, a pregnancy in the fallopian tube and fetal heartbeats (meaning fetal circulation and life) can usually be seen at this stage.

Before the development of diagnostic ultrasound, ectopic pregnancies were not diagnosed early in the pregnancy and had to be dealt with surgically when they bled or caused pain. One case described in 1915 was of a woman who was undergoing an open abdominal operation to remove a fibroid when the surgeon found an ectopic, which he judged to be alive. Having the uterus open where he had removed the fibroid, he decided to use the surgical incision in the uterus to transfer the ectopic pregnancy, which he had discovered serendipitously, to the uterus. The operative findings described the fallopian tube as "soft and healthy, enlarged to the size of a walnut but not distended."[1] This seems like a contradiction in terms, and the surgeon's description of how he transplanted the pregnancy to the uterine cavity and secured it there with two sutures suggests an extraordinary degree of skill and a lot of luck. It seems entirely possible that there was an undiagnosed and undetected pregnancy already in the uterus and that it was the one that survived the removal of the fibroid.

Another transplant of an ectopic from the tube to the uterus was described in 1990 from Randolph, Vermont, USA, although the case occurred clinically in 1980. The reason for the ten-year delay in reporting the case was not explained.[2] The patient was a twenty-seven-year-old woman who presented with "severe pain elicited with palpation in the tubal area." On this basis, the patient underwent open abdominal surgery at which a normal corpus luteum (evidence of ovulation and probably the cause of the pain—JA) was noted on the left side and a 4–5 mm tubal mass (probably too small to cause pain—JA). The surgeon then fashioned an infusion tube with a rubber bulb on one end and punctured the uterine wall with the tube. The chorionic sac with enclosed fetus was aspirated up the tube and expelled into the lining of the uterine cavity with gentle pressure. The tube must have been quite wide in diameter to accommodate a 4 mm sac without damage to the sac. Puncturing the uterine wall with such a large diameter instrument usually traumatizes the uterus and causes considerable bleeding. These cases and others indicate that there was interest in salvaging living ectopics, especially in infertile women.[3] Nobody had shown how to do it reliably, however.

John Malcolm Pearce

Mr. Malcolm Pearce was born in 1954. (The English cling to a quaint habit of calling senior surgeons "Mr.," a hangover from the days when surgeons were still members of the Barbers Union—Ed.) By the time he was forty years of age, he was a successful obstetrician and gynecologist, a senior consultant at St. George's Hospital in Tooting, South London, England, and on the editorial board of the *British Journal of Obstetrics and Gynaecology* and, basically, at the top of his profession. He was held in high regard as an expert in obstetric and gynecologic ultrasound and was well published with about thirty in the major journals, about half of which were as first author and the others evenly split between contributing and last author. Most of the publications were in the *British Journal of Obstetrics and Gynaecology*, where he was an assistant editor. Mr. Pearce was no junior doctor struggling to get up the ladder; he was already well up the ladder. His salary on the National Health Scheme was over £50,000 per annum, and this was supplemented by his private practice income.[4]

The Fraud

Then for some reason best known to himself, Mr. Pearce decided to publish a case that never happened. Through the *British Journal of Obstetrics and Gynaecology*, he announced to the world that a twenty-nine-year-old African woman (patient X) had presented for ultrasound examination just over five weeks after her last menstrual period.[5] Pearce reported that the woman had no symptoms but previously her right fallopian tube had been removed and the left tube had been repaired, in both cases because of a previous ectopic pregnancy. Mr. Pearce goes on to describe how he operated on the woman by opening her abdomen, dissecting the early gestation sac from the fallopian tube and placing it inside the uterine cavity by gently blowing it into the cavity using a tube inserted into the uterine cavity via a catheter through the cervix after removing a strip of uterine lining with a sharp instrument. The operation was completed, and the pregnancy checked by ultrasound two days later. The fetus was seen to be alive on ultrasound, and the patient was discharged home after four days. The pregnancy was checked by ultrasound at eight weeks, twelve weeks, and eighteen weeks when it was seen to be well if a little smaller than average. Further checks of fetal growth and well-being were carried out at twenty-eight weeks, thirty-two weeks, and thirty-six weeks when healthy growth was demonstrated, and all were well. The woman had a normal delivery at thirty-eight weeks of a healthy 2.7 kg female infant.[5]

Having described the progress of the pregnancy, Mr. Pearce then continued in the report to discuss in detail why he was successful. He mentioned that he had attempted this procedure previously on eight occasions between five- and eight-week gestation without success although on one occasion he claimed that fetal heart movement was detected on the day after the operation. The whole of this case report and the subsequent discussion seem extraordinary, as it was entirely a figment of his imagination. It is particularly surprising that the medical community did not question the veracity of this tale, as the woman who presented had only missed a period by a little over a week and had no symptoms whatsoever. So why did she present? The reason was not explained in the case report. As well as that, it defies the imagination to believe that a gestation sac at five or six weeks, whose circulation is entirely dependent on the fetus, could be surgically transplanted into a uterus whose circulation is entirely dependent on the mother.

Professor Geoffrey Chamberlain Is Sucked In

Nonetheless, Pearce went to press. Mr. T. Manyonda, a senior registrar, coauthored the paper and probably wrote most of it on Malcolm Pearce's instructions. An investigation by the St. George's Hospital found that he had no knowledge of the fraud.[6] *Professor Geoffrey Chamberlain*, however, had cosigned the original report in a custom known as gift authorship, which means that his name was last on the publication although he had no real knowledge of the details. This provided legitimacy to the report, but unwittingly, it brought him down with Mr. Pearce.[7]

Professor Chamberlain was sixty-four years of age when the report on the successful transfer of an ectopic pregnancy was published in the *British Journal of Obstetrics and Gynaecology*. He was editor in chief of that journal and president of the Royal College of Obstetricians and Gynaecologists, who were the owners of the journal. Chamberlain was head of the Department of Obstetrics and Gynaecology at the St. George's Hospital and was at the peak of his career. He would have been looking forward to retirement and probably a knighthood.

When the news broke that an ectopic pregnancy had been successfully transferred to the uterus, it created great interest in the medical community and the public. Dr. Gedis Grudzinskas at the London Hospital reported that he had so far been unsuccessful with three cases but "would now try again with renewed vigor."[3,8] The *Guardian* newspaper shrieked that "Britain has pioneered an operation to rescue ectopic pregnancies."[9]

All would probably have been well and the fraud never noticed except that Dr. Pearce also published an article in the same issue of the same journal claiming he could reduce the incidence of recurrent miscarriages in women with polycystic ovary syndrome (PCOS).[10] This study claimed to have 191 women with polycystic ovaries who have had three consecutive miscarriages. Half of these women were given human chorionic gonadotropin (HCG) from early in a subsequent pregnancy, and half were given a placebo (an inactive pill). Neither the patients nor the investigators knew which group the patients were in until twelve weeks' gestation, if the pregnancy got that far.

The polycystic ovarian syndrome is not an uncommon condition, occurring in about one woman in ten to twenty, but its diagnosis is not always obvious. It results in reduced fertility, however, and assembling 191 women with PCOS and three consecutive miscarriages would have been a formidable task, typically requiring many centers to be involved. In addition, Pearce claimed that he had followed these women twelve weeks into their next pregnancy to assess the effect of HCG. This article was also a figment of his imagination. He must have been dreaming if he thought that his colleagues would not notice. And he was dreaming. They did notice. They found it incomprehensible that such a large study had gone on over several years in their hospital without their knowledge. Mrs. Alison Peattie, a senior lecturer in gynecology at the medical school, remarked, "I was completely stunned and embarrassed; I kept thinking, why should I know nothing about this?"

The News Was Out

When this exciting news got out, Professor Chamberlain ordered an inquiry in the hospital. It was quickly discovered that Mr. Pearce's password had been used to change the records. It transpired that patient X had indeed miscarried and her records had been changed and replaced by another patient, patient Y, who—Mr. Pearce said—was not eligible for treatment under the NIIS. Mr. Pearce told Professor Chamberlain that he had changed the records to protect patient Y who was afraid that details of a previous miscarriage would come out. One patient whose details had been changed had been born in 1910 and was dead at the time of the alleged transfer. *Sir Robert Kilpatrick*, chairman of the disciplinary committee convened by the General Medical Council, later said, "Mr Pearce not only sought personally to mislead others but to implicate colleagues, including junior doctors, in a web of deceit that has had incalculable consequences for public confidence in the integrity of research."[11]

Professor Chamberlain and *Mr. Isaac Manyonda*, who coauthored the work on the ectopic pregnancy, and *Dr. Rosoel Hamid*, who coauthored the paper on the trial of HCG, were reported to have no first-hand knowledge of the fraudulent nature of the study but had unwittingly assisted in its summary and publications on Mr. Pearce's instructions; each received letters from the General Medical Council reminding them of their duty to check research before accepting responsibility for it. Mr. Pearce resigned from St. George's Hospital in December 1994 and was struck off the General Medical Register in June 1995.

The articles on ectopic pregnancies and polycystic ovarian disease were retracted along with twenty-three other scientific papers previously published by Mr. Pearce and various coauthors between January 1989 and December 1994.[6] The news of the fraud was quick to spread outside medical circles, and the newspapers had a field day. The *Guardian* headlined an "Inquiry on Fake Gynaecology Research" and again "Doctor Lied on Pregnancy Treatment," and in June 1995, the *Observer* recommended "Watching the Researchers."[12,13,14] News of the fraud spread around the world.

Professor Chamberlain said later, after the General Medical Council hearing, that in hindsight accepting gift authorship was "Not a good idea. I rubber stamped this paper out of politeness and because Mr Pearce asked me, as Head of Department. It never occurred to me that it might be a lie. It was refereed twice before publication, and the referees did not suspect that it was false either." He went on, "Obviously Malcolm has been extremely silly on this occasion, but in the past, he has done a lot of good."[14] Professor Chamberlain observed that gift authorship was a bad idea, and it is no longer practiced.

Professor Chamberlain resigned as editor of the *British Journal of Obstetrics and Gynaecology* and president of the Royal College of Obstetrics and Gynaecology. He remained as head of staff at the hospital until his retirement and was held in high esteem. When he retired, after leaving St. George's Hospital, he became Apothecaries' Lecturer in the History of Medicine at Swansea University from 2000 to 2008. He died in 2014 aged eighty-four, and the Royal College of Obstetricians and Gynaecologists established the Professor Geoffrey Chamberlain Award in his memory. It was a sad end to a proud and genuine career.[1]

Epilogue

Mr. Pearce's motivation to publish a case reporting that an ectopic gestation had been transplanted into the uterus is unclear. He must have known that the case was going to attract worldwide attention and that he would have to answer questions about it. Further, his publication of 191 patients in a randomized double-blind series was bound to attract widespread attention from his own hospital and the medical community in general. It was so ridiculous that it was implausible. It almost seems that he expected to be discovered. If his motivation was to attract attention, he certainly did that; but in the process, he exposed himself to scientific ridicule, which saw him undone. Sir Robert Kilpatrick, chairman of the disciplinary committee, said, "Scientific fraud is dangerous. Medical knowledge worldwide is developed in part on the published results of previous research."[15]

Unfortunately, Mr. Pearce's reputation was not the only reputation that was tarnished. As has been the case in several other fraudulent incidents in this book, findings of a few have resulted not only in loss of trust in the work of those authors but also the honest work of others. Sadly, in this case, Professor Geoffrey Chamberlain's worthy career also came to grief.

Notes

1. Wallace, C. "Transplantations of Ectopic Pregnancy from Fallopian Tube to Cavity of Uterus." *Surgery, Gynecology and Obstetrics*. 1917; 24: 578–579.
2. Shettles, L. "Tubal Embryo Successfully Transferred in Utero." *American Journal of Obstetrics and Gynecology*. 1990; 163(6): 2,026–2,027.
3. Grudzinskas, J. "Treatment of Ectopic Pregnancy: Ablate or Relocate—the Newest Dilemma?" *Human Reproduction*. 1994; 9(8): 1,584.
4. Jones, J. "Watching the Researchers." *The Observer* (London, Greater London, England). June 11, 1995: 12.
5. Pearce, J., I. Manyonda, G. Chamberlain. "Term Delivery after Intrauterine Relocation of an Ectopic Pregnancy" (this article has been retracted). *Brit. J. Obstet. Gynaecol.*: An International Journal of Obstetrics and Gynaecology. 1994; 101(8): 716–717.
6. "Retraction of articles." *Brit. J. Obstet. Gynaecol.*: An International Journal of Obstetrics and Gynaecology. 1995; 102(11): 853. Royal College of Surgeons. Chamberlain, Geoffrey Victor Price (internet).
7. Royal College of Surgeons; 2014. Available from https://livesonline.rcseng.ac.uk/biogs/E006425b.htm.
8. Grudzinskas, J., M. Palomino, P. Armstrong, A. Lower. "Relocation of Ectopic Pregnancy to the Uterine Cavity: A Dream or a Reality?" *Brit J. Obstet.*

Gynaecol.: An International Journal of Obstetrics and Gynaecology. 1994; 101(8): 651–653.

9. Fursland, E. "Lifesaver in the Tube." *The Guardian.* August 2, 1994: 30.

10. Pearce, J. M., R. Hamid. "Randomised Controlled Trial of the Use of Human Chorionic Gonadotrophin in Recurrent Miscarriage Associated with Polycystic Ovaries" (this article has been retracted). *Brit. J. Obstet. Gynaecol.*: An International Journal of Obstetrics and Gynaecology. 1994; 101(8): 685–688.

11. Dobson, R. "Science: Doctoring the Evidence." *The Independent* (internet). August 9, 1998 (cited August 9, 2018). Available from https://www.independent.co.uk/artsentertainment/science-doctoring-the-evidence-1170688.html.

12. Pilkington, E. "Inquiry on 'Fake' Gynaecology Research." *The Guardian.* November 18, 1994: 3.

13. Millhill, C. "Doctor 'Lied on Pregnancy Treatment.'" *The Guardian.* June 6, 1995: 6.

14. Dyer, O. "Consultant Struck Off for Fraudulent Claims." *Brit. Med. J.* 1995; 310(6994): 1,554–1,555.

15. Webb, G. "J Malcolm Pearce—Obstetrician Whose Faked Research Ended Two Careers." Dr Geoff (internet). 2017 (cited August 9, 2018). Available from https://drgeoff-nutrition.wordpress.com/2017/11/28/j-malcolm-pearce-obstetrician-whose-faked-research-ended-two-careers/.

CHAPTER TEN

DR. MARK WEINBERGER— THE NOSE DOCTOR

Prologue

One of the most remarkable things about *Dr. Mark Weinberger* is that he accumulated over 350 malpractice cases and twenty-two counts of health-care fraud in such a short time, about three years. There is no way that a surgeon or a physician can generate such a record merely by being careless. He had to work at it, deliberately and uncaringly damaging patients without regard for their well-being at the same time feeding his financial greed. When he realized that he was in trouble, he disappeared for almost five years, leaving behind massive debts, before being found camped on the side of Mont Blanc in the Italian Alps.

Dr. Mark Weinberger

Mark Weinberger's paternal grandparents, *Silvia* and *Irving*, were Hungarian refugees who arrived in the United States in 1937 with their two young sons, Richard and Frederick. In 1944, Silvia and Irving bought a luncheonette on the Grand Concourse in the Bronx, New York. Sylvia made chopped liver to sell in the luncheonette, but initially, it was out of favor because most respectable Jewish women thought that it was beneath them not to make their own. It eventually found favor and became a $2 million business. The name was abbreviated from Mrs. Weinberger's Food Products to Mrs. Weinberg's Food Products because it was too long to fit on the label, according to Mrs. Weinberger.[1] The manufacturing part of the food business was sold in 1989, but Irving continued to have an interest in the marketing side for a time.

Robert McGill Thomas Jr., then a well-known journalist with the *New York Times*, was born and grew up in Shelbyville, Tennessee, where chopped liver was rare and schmaltz was not part of the vernacular. In his obituary on Sylvia Weinberger who died in 1995 at the age of eighty-nine, he wrote, "There was something mythic, too, about Sylvia Weinberger, who used a sprinkling of matzoh meal, a pinch of salt and a dollop of schmaltzmanship to turn chopped liver into a commercial success."[1]

Frederick, who was to become Mark's father, was also involved in the chopped liver business for a time before he was hired as a government physicist in Washington. Fred married Fanny, and they had three sons, Jeff, Mark, and Neil. Mark Weinberger, the middle child, was born on May 22, 1963. They lived in Mamaroneck in Westchester County, New York, and all three attended Scarsdale High School. Later, Jeff studied at Columbia University, while Mark and Neil attended the University of Pennsylvania.[2]

Mark completed his undergraduate degree cum laude at the University of Pennsylvania and graduated at the David Geffen School of Medicine at the University of California in Los Angeles in 1989.[3,4] His specialist training in otorhinolaryngology (ear, nose, and throat abbreviated to ENT) and plastic surgery was completed in 1995 in Chicago while on a fellowship.

Dr. Mark Weinberger commenced practice in Merrillville in 1996. This was a blue-collar working town in the Midwest about thirty miles from Chicago. It seemed an excellent choice, as there were many chimneys belching smoke and the winters were cold, both conditions favoring sinus disease, assuring Weinberger of plenty of clients. It was not long when, in 1999, one of the earliest suspicions arose when *Mr. Rob Tepperman* of Münster sensed that something was wrong after Dr. Weinberger performed surgery on him to relieve sinusitis, but Tepperman's condition deteriorated. His wife had called Weinberger in his office to request details on follow-up after the surgery, but Weinberger did not meet her and only spoke on the phone and was "rather belligerent." Tepperman consulted a lawyer after he was advised by another ENT surgeon that his operation had probably been unnecessary, but he did nothing about it until he heard that Weinberger had fled.[5]

The Sinuses

The sinuses are paired air-filled spaces in the skull. There are two frontal sinuses above the eyes and two maxillary sinuses behind the cheek. Also, there are small (sphenoid) sinuses close to the back of the bridge of the nose, and there are small (ethmoid) sinuses behind the nose. The sinuses are lined with mucosa, which is continuous with the mucosa of the nose, and the secretion in the sinuses is swept slowly into the nose by tiny hairlike structures called cilia. This helps to keep the mucosa of the nasal passages moist. It is also postulated that the sinuses reduce the weight of the skull and increase the resonance of the voice. The sinuses communicate with the back of the nose through small orifices called ostia. Should these ostia become blocked for any reason—such as infection, trauma, allergy, or polyps—the mucous secretions in the sinus can become trapped and possibly infected. Blockage of the ostia can usually be helped by using decongestants or antibiotics, and surgery is seldom indicated. In days gone by, surgery to drain the sinuses was carried out either through the mouth or the cheek using a trocar and cannula. Nowadays, however, surgery of the sinuses has been revolutionized by fiber-optic endoscopy. With this technique, a thin tube with a fiber-optic endoscopy light is inserted in the nose so that the surgeon can visualize the anatomy and hopefully relieve any obstruction. This method of surgery on the sinuses is required only in a small fraction of patients, but Dr. Mark Weinberger recommended it to at least 90 percent of his patients, often at the first visit. Considering that on some days he saw as many as one hundred patients and in some months he took on 120 new patients, it is no wonder that he was busy. Mark soon leased a computed tomography machine. These machines cost $1–2 million, and the price was reflected in the lease. Computed tomography (CT) is the investigation of choice in most cases of chronic sinusitis compared with plain x-rays, MRI, or other forms of imaging; so Weinberger's CT machine would have been another good little earner. Unfortunately, when the patients and the scans stopped coming, the lease payments on the machine did not.

Michelle Kramer

Mark Weinberger was in a club called Glow in Chicago when he met *Michelle Kramer*, aged twenty-five. She was slim, blonde, and attractive. She was working toward a PhD in psychology in Chicago. They were instantly drawn to each other and fell in love. Mark promised to look after her as a "princess for the rest of your life,"[6] words that we know today were hollow. In spring 2001, Mark proposed on bended knee to Michelle Kramer in the Piazza Navona in Rome, one of the most romantic places in the world, surrounded by hired singers.[2] Later that year, on November 1, 2001, his young bride arrived in the Chicago Botanic Garden in a horse-drawn carriage, and they were formally married.[6] Michelle herself reported that the marriage was not exactly smooth. Her father died from lung cancer, and Michelle was overcome with grief, but Mark seemed oddly unsympathetic and irritated that her father's health had interfered with their life. They managed to carry on, however, and decided to rejuvenate their marriage with a second wedding in Ravello, Italy, in the spring of 2002 on a cliff overlooking the ocean. Weinberger flew in fifteen guests and accommodated them in Villa Cimbrone, a twelfth-century villa, which included Winston Churchill, D. H. Lawrence, and Greta Garbo on its guest list.[2]

The Nose and Sinus Center

By mid-2001, he was busy, advertising frequently and widely in the *Times* (Munster, Indiana) and elsewhere.[7] He was practicing in the Nose and Sinus Center from a suite at W. Eighty-Ninth Avenue, Merrillville, Indiana, where he claimed to specialize in nasal and sinus problems, having helped "thousands of patients to breathe easy." "Dr Mark Weinberger," he blared, "Founder and Medical Director of the Nose and Sinus Center combines his education and experience with the safest, most, advanced and most effective treatments to offer long-term relief from nasal and sinus problems."[8] He dedicated his clinic "exclusively to nose and sinus care, sinus headaches, nasal blockage, snoring, cosmetic re-sculpting, the most advanced technology, and optical imaging."[7]

The Weinberger Sinus Clinic

On November 20, 2002, Dr. Weinberger formally unveiled a beautiful new stand-alone brick building overlooked by a stone sculpture (featuring a huge nose), expressly built as a "one-stop shop" for the Weinberger Sinus Clinic at E. Ninth Drive, Merrillville. Members of the chamber of commerce, including the president, were there to help Mark at the ribbon-cutting ceremony, opening the center with a fanfare.[9]

Dr. Weinberger was not slow to promote his own perceived qualities. He said that he had set out to create a new standard of excellence in patient-friendly, high-tech, high-quality care and had, in so doing, been able to satisfy a great need for his patients. He cited a recent feature in the *US News and World Report* that called sinusitis the most common chronic illness in the country affecting thirty-seven million people. He said that "because of the location of the sinuses around the eyes and near the brain it is likely that when the sinuses are inflamed these structures are impaired too." He went on to relate this problem to the way he saw it affecting his patients and gave this as "an example of his inspiration to change the conventional practice of his particular specialty." "This is a real problem that affects people's lives, their work, their sleep, and their families. Now, why should someone with such a problem have to go to several different doctors and facilities and suffer through long waiting periods and mounds of paperwork to get a diagnosis? The obvious answer is they shouldn't, and no, they don't." Weinberger went on, "In most cases we can arrive at a diagnosis and treatment plan during the first visit. And I don't mean temporary relief from a few pills, I am talking about long-term relief."[10] Already he was having delusions of grandeur!

After the unveiling, guests were treated to a tour of the complete surgical and treatment facilities available, including a CT scan machine.[9] Dr Weinberger's father had lent him $1 million to purchase this machine in the belief that he was making an investment that his son would care for him for the rest of his life.[11] The whole concept of the clinic was one of complete diagnostic testing, including treatment, surgery, and follow-up all in the one location. Mark Weinberger was the only physician, so his behavior was unfettered. He could read his own CT scans, organize his own operating lists, and be as rude as he liked to anyone.

The capital cost of the facility was in the millions, not to mention the service costs and staff, and Mark Weinberger spared no expense. The operating tables themselves cost many thousands of dollars, and the equipment for endoscopic fiber-optic examination of the nasal passages and sinuses was also very costly. Television monitors and photographic material are required to visualize and record what the surgeon is doing, but in the case of Dr. Mark Weinberger, it might have been better not to know.

Dr. Mark Weinberger was well on his way to making those millions, and he was fond of flaunting it. He employed maids, cooks, a skipper for his yacht in the Mediterranean, and three drivers, one of whom drove him an hour to work each day and then always went to collect his lunch at his favorite Japanese restaurant and one of whom remained on duty outside. He took ten days off every month to go overseas, often in a private jet, usually to the Mediterranean where he and Michelle would chill out. They lived a life of luxury, bought a condominium in Chicago and property in the Bahamas. They flew by Concorde to London and went to the Cannes Film Festival and rubbed shoulders with celebrities. They bought an eighty-foot yacht, the *Corti-Seas,* for $4 million and shopped at Versace and Dior. Michelle Kramer (now Weinberger) thought that her husband was making about $200,000 per week, doing as many as fifteen operations a day.[6,13]

Trouble

But trouble was not far away. *Phyllis Barnes* had attended Weinberger's clinic on September 6, 2001, complaining of hoarseness and a sore throat. Weinberger ordered a CT scan at his office and recommended an endoscopic sinus operation, which he performed. Ms. Barnes later attended hospital on November 22, 2001, complaining of difficulty breathing. She was quickly diagnosed with throat cancer. Just before Weinberger's flamboyant opening of the Weinberger Sinus Clinic, a lawyer, Robert J. Allen, filed a complaint on behalf of the estate of the patient, Phyllis Barnes, who had died from cancer of the throat on September 16, 2004.[4,13,14] The attorney claimed that Weinberger had performed an unnecessary sinus operation upon her and had failed to diagnose the tumor. Other specialist surgeons who saw Phyllis Barnes after Weinberger said that the swelling in and around her neck was so apparent that one would have had to miss it deliberately. Another noted that Weinberger was the worst doctor it had been his misfortune to know. Subsequently, dozens of the Weinberger's former patients filed complaints with that lawyer, suspecting they, too, had unnecessary surgery, some being charged up to $40,000, paid by insurers. Another attorney, *Barry Booth*, filed similar claims on behalf of another twenty-five patients, some of whose children had surgery.[4,13,14] One patient, *Amy Verhoeve*, aged thirty-two, went to Weinberger's Merrillville offices suffering from a minor sinus complaint and was told that she needed surgery, according to *Leslie Dixon*, an Indianapolis attorney whose law firm represented several patients. After the operation, her condition did not improve, so she saw another specialist who examined her and said that nothing for which she had been billed had been performed. To make matters worse, she now had a hole in her sinus, which required treatment.[15] Another patient, *William Boyer* of Gary, one of the earliest patients to sue Weinberger for malpractice, testified in court that his vocal cords had been damaged during surgery by Weinberger. His testimony was given with a raspy voice. He later won damages for $300,000.[16] Another client, *Kayla Thomas*, was aged nine years. Weinberger prescribed the same sinus surgery that he did for all his patients. Kayla was later diagnosed with a pituitary tumor.[2]

Michelle, his wife, reported that Mark's behavior was becoming increasingly eccentric, even alarming. He kept a laptop computer and a mobile phone in every room, installed numerous security cameras throughout the house and a safe in every room, and became obsessed with staying fit, working out three times a day.[6] The employees also became concerned with Mark's behavior. He became withdrawn and short-tempered, often not replying when asked a question. Sometimes he came to work without shaving and occasionally walked around the office not fully dressed.[2] On one occasion, several men went to the office carrying briefcases and entered the clinic's conference room. It is now thought that they were Hasidic Jews from New York and they were trading diamonds for cash. About that time, Weinberger took over the clinic's bookkeeping and allegedly siphoned $2 million from the business. Numerous boxes were delivered to the office obviously containing camping gear. Michelle later found some of this still in a room in the house when she returned from Greece.

By summer 2004, malpractice claims against him were mounting, and he was feeling the pressure. Michelle was becoming worried about Mark. Then Mark planned an exceptional trip for Michelle and her mother and three other friends to get away from it all. Michelle thought that it might be a turning point. He flew them to Mykonos, an island in Greece, on September 18, 2004. He and Michelle flew first-class to Paris and all of them on to Mykonos by NetJets, his shared private jet company. When Michelle and Mark arrived in Mykonos, the motor yacht was not there, and Mark was frantic. She later found that he had sent the vessel to Greece and to Cannes to deliver shipments of survival gear. His eighty-foot motor yacht was a day late mooring in the marina in Mykonos. He and Michelle stayed on the vessel, while the others were accommodated in a hotel ashore. It was Michelle's thirtieth birthday soon, and she had recently suffered a late miscarriage from which she was still recovering. Mark bought her two costly diamonds as a gift.[11] But Mark Weinberger was planning much more than that.

The next morning, September 21, 2004, Michelle woke on the yacht to find that Mark was not there. At first, she thought he must have gone for a jog; but when he did not return, she became worried and started to search the island. The yacht's skipper, *Lupo Clerici*, reassured her, however, that Mark had only gone to Paris to have the diamonds set as earrings for her birthday and that he would be back later that day.[11]

Mark Weinberger never came back.

The Doctor Who Disappeared

Michelle called everyone who might know where Mark was, including the American Embassy in Greece, but no one had heard from him. Then the captain of the yacht gave Michelle a mobile phone number that Mark had left with him previously, and she called that number. Mark answered and sounded quite happy, but when she said to him softly, "Mark," he did not reply for a few seconds and then quietly hung up. Docking fees for the yacht amounted to $40,000, and Michelle needed to get back home. She flew back home commercially with the other friends on September 26 after six days in Greece, using borrowed money, and went to his office.[4] She found shredded documents there and pieced them together, finding the name of a hotel in Paris and a receipt for a plane ticket from Paris to Cannes. She called the FBI; being the last person to see him alive, she realized that she would come under suspicion. She found books on how to speak Italian and learned that he had been stockpiling survivalist gear such as compasses, water purification equipment, thermal underwear, a GPS, a satellite phone, flashlights, maps (of Greece, Italy, Western Europe, Paris), a book *How to Be Invisible,* sleeping bags, and a waterproof wallet and passport holder; Mark had been planning all along to live a life without her. Then she received a phone call from the private jet company that she and Mark had used to fly to Greece. Mark apparently had asked the company to tell her she could use his account to fly from Greece to Paris and then home. Mark had not realized that she was already back home. Michelle then flew to France and went to the hotel mentioned in the shredded papers, but the front desk clerk said that Mark had left the day before. She visited the clubs and cafés they had once loved, but no one had seen him. She searched for him in Cannes and Charles de Gaulle airport, but no one had seen him, and she never found him. His credit cards were still being used across Europe to buy clothes and for casinos, including Cannes, until they ran out of funds. Reports came in that he had been seen in China, Monte Carlo (south of France), and Israel,[11,17,18] but no one really knew where he was.[6] Mark Weinberger had vanished.

Back at home in Chicago, Michelle found that Mark had left her with $6 million in debt. She had no prospect of honoring the debt. She was unable to maintain the house, and the banks were after him for defaulting on the loan, and the malpractice suits were snowballing. He was being accused of performing bogus surgery on his sinus patients, including operating on children who were too young to even have sinuses. Michelle had no choice; having found that it was impossible to deal with the massive debt, she filed for bankruptcy. From that time on, she got on with life as best she could, but she never heard from Mark Weinberger again.

The Runaway Doctor

In an excellent piece called "The Runaway Doctor" in the magazine *Vanity Fair*, *Buzz Bissinger* says that "in the name of sheer greed he performed hundreds of sinus related surgeries that were not only completely unnecessary but also made some patients' conditions worse; he left behind accusations that he had scared patients into having surgery by showing them hideous but phony images of their supposed illnesses; he left behind alleged missed diagnoses in which he failed to detect throat cancer in a woman who subsequently died, and missed the tumor on the pituitary gland of an eight-year-old girl while operating on her sinuses with surgery she never should have had because her sinuses were not yet fully formed."[2] In other words, over a period of approximately three years, he racked up around one hundred malpractice cases per annum and one case of insurance fraud about every six weeks.

Many doctors do not get one malpractice suit in a lifetime. It was not just carelessness that generated so many malpractice suits; it was malignant deliberation. Not that it mattered much at the time because nobody could find Dr. Mark Weinberger to file the lawsuits against him.

Not only did Mark Weinberger fail to return on that morning of September 21, 2004, but he also deliberately disappeared, doing his best to make himself invisible. This was evident, as he answered the telephone when Michelle called and was still using his credit cards. He had not been kidnapped or murdered, his body thrown in the ocean.

Monica Specogna

Courmayeur is in Northwest Italy, in the Aosta Valley, 4,016 ft above sea level, on the southern side of Mont Blanc.

Mont Blanc is 15,781 ft, and the border with France, which is on the northern side, passes through the summit. Courmayeur is a picturesque, scenic alpine village with a population of around three thousand, popular with skiers and tourists. In Via Regionale, there is a small grocery store one level up from ground level, where Monica Specogna served at the counter. Monica loved the mountain, she loved to ski, to head off on a bicycle, and to trek to strange places. She was content in Courmayeur.

Mark Weinberger would change all that.

One day in the winter of 2007–8, Mark Weinberger came into her store. Buzz Bissinger, who interviewed her, says that she told him that "Mark was a client like any other." She went on, "He was pleasant and talkative. We spoke about music but not about anything else." Monica had worked in the music industry previously, playing bass and heavy metal guitar and doing the sound mixing for several small albums. Mark Weinberger, who also had an interest in music, had rented a tiny flat down a series of steps, below ground level at number 39 Via Regionale directly below the grocery store. Over the next year, they began to see each other more frequently when he came into the store. Gradually a relationship developed between them, and they went skiing together more often.[2]

Weinberger lied to Monica from the beginning. He told her that he was a retired Wall Street stockbroker and that he had made enough to live a peaceful life without having to work. He said to Monica that he had earned enough money to maintain the lifestyle that he had in the United States, with cars, diamonds, planes, and a yacht. "Now," she said, he "scorned money and the wealth and lifestyle that went with it and the money that was brought to Courmayeur by rich skiers." Weinberger said that he had been living in Monte Carlo and traveling around Europe by bicycle. His arrival in Courmayeur was by chance, according to Weinberger.

Camping on the Mountain

Then in late spring 2009, Mark and Monica decided to cycle 170 miles from Courmayeur to Grindelwald, Switzerland, at the foot of Mount Eiger. When they returned, Mark announced that he was going to camp on the mountain for the rest of the summer. He seemed to be drawn to the isolation because of its challenges. Mark settled there in a tent and visited from time to time for groceries and supplies. Later that year, he decided that he would camp at a higher altitude for a year and write a book about the experience, hoping to make enough money to settle with Monica in Grindelwald and perhaps adopt children. Monica had reservations about this plan because Mark had decided to camp two thousand feet above Courmayeur in the Val Ferret, where conditions could be deadly.

But there in the Val Ferret, Mark made his camp in late September. For whatever reason, whether he forgot or whether he thought that he could not be found, Dr. Mark Weinberger stopped paying the rent on his little flat in Courmayeur. By December, the agent was becoming annoyed about the outstanding rent, so he went to the Carabinieri, taking Mark's photograph, which Mark had given him when he rented the apartment. The photograph and the details on the passport showed Mark's identity. When the Carabinieri checked their database, they found that Mark was on an Interpol arrest warrant and on *America's Most Wanted*. Unfortunately, they did not know where he was.

The End Cometh

Mark came down from his tent in the Val Ferret on the tenth of December 2009, Monica's thirty-ninth birthday, and they went skiing together. The next day, a friend rang Monica and told her that Mark was not whom he said he was. The friend, probably a mountain guide, told Monica that Mark was wanted by the FBI. After Mark had returned to his tent, Monica went online to *America's Most Wanted* website. There she discovered who Mark really was and what he was accused of doing. She was aghast. All the happiness of the previous year had turned to custard. Monica was an honest and sincere person. No matter how difficult it would be, Monica had to turn Mark in, or she would be unable to live with herself. She printed a copy of the page from the website of *America's Most Wanted* and took it to the Carabinieri. Due to inclement weather, the Carabinieri were unable to fly by helicopter into the Val Ferret until December 14. They did not find the campsite that day, but they did see traces showing where he had been. The next day, using a snowmobile, they located him near the Elena Refuge, six thousand feet above sea level. When *Captain Giuseppe Ballistreri*, head of Carabinieri in that area, asked Weinberger what he was doing there, he replied, "I just want to live a quiet life." When he was unable to produce identification other than a ski pass, he was asked to accompany the Carabinieri back to barracks. Once there, he hungrily wolfed down a large bowl of pasta and posed for photographs. Shortly afterward, he went to the toilet where he produced a small carpet knife and attempted to cut his own throat. Although he caused some bleeding, he missed the major blood vessels despite being a head and neck surgeon and did little damage other than a superficial cut.[2] Mark Weinberger was extradited to the United States on February 25, 2010.

Prison and the Criminal Cases

On arrival in the United States, Weinberger was imprisoned without bond in the Federal Metropolitan Correctional Center in Chicago until he appeared in federal court in Hammond,

Indiana, on October 22, 2010, where he pleaded guilty to twenty-two charges of criminal fraud. His lawyers, in a plea deal with federal prosecutors, agreed to a prison term of four years, but there was an outcry from his victims and Michelle Kramer that the sentence was too lenient.[2] In October 2012, a federal court judge, Philip Simon, sentenced Weinberger to seven years in prison for insurance fraud, a federal crime.[19] At that stage, Weinberger had been in jail for almost three years and requested that he be allowed to spend the remainder of his term in a low-security prison in Florida close to where his father lived.[20]

The Clinic and the Civil Cases

After Dr. Mark Weinberger vanished on September 21, 2004, without leaving a forwarding address or a contact number, staff and patients back at the clinic began to wonder what was happening. At first, some work carried on, but there was no surgery. They contacted the company's lawyer who placed the company in receivership. *Mr. Robert Handler* was appointed as the receiver on October 5, 2004. It was his challenge to get the company up and running again in the absence of the proprietor. Handler put the patient invoices of the company in the hands of a debt collection agency in the hope of recovering some outstanding monies owed to the clinic. He soon received numerous calls from patients who complained that they had been receiving bills for consultations and surgery that they never had.[21] He established that debts were about $7 million, with only $7,000 in the bank. His plan was to employ other ENT specialists as soon as possible so that the clinic could carry on and honor its debts. Announcements were made in the local press that the clinic would open again,[22] but it soon became evident that no other surgeon was prepared to take over an undertaking, which depended on such unethical practices, and the clinic was put on the market as real estate.[23]

When it became public knowledge that Mark Weinberger had been found, numerous patients and their lawyers were delighted because they thought that now they had someone whom they could sue. Their delight was to be short-lived. Indiana law had been revised in the 1980s and allowed the banks and insurance companies access to the offender's estate before the victim. Attorney *Ken Allen*, acting for the estate of Phyllis Barnes, said that although she had won $1.25 million in damages, it would require further lengthy legal battles to ensure that she saw any of it.[13,24] Furthermore, Weinberger's medical indemnity company *Medical Assurance Company Inc.* referred to a clause in their policy that stated that the insured had to cooperate with the company in defense of any claim. Weinberger, of course, had been out of touch and anonymous for five years and was unable to assist the company. Even when he returned, he refused to work with the company, which therefore asked the court to declare that Weinberger had breached his responsibilities under the contract and therefore that *Medical Assurance* no longer had a duty to defend or indemnify him. The court found in favor of *Medical Assurance*.[25] This meant that there was no easy way to compensate for the 350 malpractice cases lined up against him. Under Indiana law, malpractice cases must be reviewed by an independent panel of three physicians before they go to trial. This meant a massive amount of preparation on the part of the court and the lawyers.

Several lawyers entered class actions on behalf of patients. In 2013, Lake County judge *John R. Pera* approved a $55 million settlement according to two legal firms acting on behalf of 282 former patients who had sued Mark Weinberger. On average, each patient would receive $250,000, ranging from $120,000 to $470,000. The maximum compensation under Indiana law was $1.25 million with the first $250,000 being paid by the doctor or his malpractice insurance company. It was not immediately clear how Mark Weinberger would pay the $250,000. Because Weinberger's insurance company, *Medical Assurance*, had been absolved of any liability, the compensation was to come from the *Patient's Compensation Fund*, which is paid for by doctors and other health-care providers. The Indiana Department of Insurance administers the fund, but the state does not contribute to the fund itself.[25] About seventy other cases, clients of the law firm Kenneth G. Allen and associates, remain to be finalized.

Epilogue

The reasons for Dr. Mark Weinberger's misbehavior do not seem complicated. He was not searching for academic glory because there is nothing in the scientific literature to suggest that he wanted to be remembered by inventing some revolutionary technique or procedure. He was not interested in finding a cure for deafness; indeed, he was not interested in the ear. Perhaps this was fortunate, as he may have caused more deafness than he cured. Weinberger seemed to be driven by pure greed. Later, he became the subject of an episode in the TV series *American Greed*.[26] The producers of that program seemed to have got it right. Perhaps he fell into a downward spiral of financial desperation, requiring more and more cash to feed his everlasting hungry lifestyle. In the end, his actions became simply criminal, as he held no regard or empathy for the well-being of his patients. He clearly knew that what he was doing was unethical and unlawful because when he realized that he was about to be exposed, he planned his disappearance meticulously and managed to disappear for five years. At the end of that time, he must have been wondering how long he could last without detection, and he may well have been hoping that he would be detected and bring it all to an end. Mark

Weinberger was a cruel doctor who hurt hundreds of patients to satisfy his greed.

He has fully earned a place in this book.

Notes

1. Kaufman, M. "Robert McG. Thomas, 60, Chronicler of Unsung Lives." *The New York Times*. January 8, 2000.
2. Bissinger, B. "The Runaway Doctor." *Vanity Fair*. December 21, 2010.
3. Healthgrades.com (internet). Dr. Mark Weinberger, MD—Merrillville, IN—Ear, Nose, and Throat & Plastic Surgery. Available from https://www.health-grades.com/physician/dr-mark-weinberger-w6hkc.
4. Staff reporter. "Wife Says Missing Medic Was Targeted." *The Chicago Tribune*. October 28, 2004.
5. Stafford, D. "Settlement Reached in Weinberger Medical Malpractice Suits." Theindianalawyer.com (internet). July 3, 2013. Available from https://www.theindianalawyer.com/articles/31829-settlement-reached-in-weinberger-medical-malpractice-suits.
6. Advertisement: *The Times* (Munster, Indiana). "Sinus Care in a Specialized Facility." March 15, 2002.
7. Pesta, A. "The Day My Husband Disappeared." *Marie Claire* (internet). March 16, 2011. Available from https://www.marieclaire.com/culture/news/a5872/con-artist-husband/.
8. Advertisement: *The Times* (Munster, Indiana). "Breathe Easy." May 3, 2001.
9. Advertisement: *The Times* (Munster, Indiana). "The Nose & Sinus Center." December 11, 2002.
10. Anonymous: The Doctor from Hell | Get into Medical School (internet). Dr Mark Weinberger Get-into-

medicalschool.com. May 23, 2011. Available from https://www.get-into-medicalschool.com/dr-mark-weinberger/.

11. Hooper, J. "Americas Most Wanted: Doctor Found Living in a Tent on Mont Blanc." *The Guardian.* December 11, 2009.

12. Laverty, D. "Nose Doctor's Day in Court Will Have to Wait." *The Times* (Munster, Indiana). June 23, 2005.

13. Laverty, D. "Where Is Dr. Mark Weinberger?" *The Times* (Munster, Indiana). October 17, 2004.

14. Wilson, C. "Fugitive Doctor Found in Italy." *Chicago Tribune* (Chicago, Illinois). December 20, 2009.

15. Grimm, A. "Surgeon Sentenced to 7 years." *Chicago Tribune* (Chicago, Illinois). October 13, 2012.

16. Staff reporter. "Sinus Doctor May Be in the South of France." *The Times* (Munster, Indiana). December 10, 2004.

17. Laverty, D. "Missing Doctor May Be in Israel." *The Times* (Munster, Indiana). October 20, 2004.

18. Daily News Wire Services. "Fugitive Doctor Gets Prison for Massive Patient Fraud." October 13, 2012.

19. Grimm, A. "Surgeon Sentenced to 7 Years." *Chicago Tribune* (Chicago, Illinois). October 14, 2012.

20. Staff reporter. "Agency Contacts Patients." *The Times* (Munster, Indiana). November 4, 2004.

21. Laverty, D. "M'ville Sinus Clinic Could Reopen in Coming Weeks." *The Times* (Munster, Indiana). November 8, 2004.

22. Laverty, D. "Controversial Merrillville Clinic Won't Reopen Doors." *The Times* (Munster, Indiana). January 12, 2005.

23. Kasarda, B. "Laws Dampen Malpractice Suit Victory." *The Times* (Munster, Indiana). March 4, 2009.

24. Pozgar, G. "Patient Care Case Law." Burlington, Mass.: Jones & Bartlett Learning; 2012.

25. Staff reporter. "Nose Doctor's Patients Settle Lawsuits for $55M." Associated Press: *USA Today*. June 25, 2013.
26. CNBC (a division of NBCUniversal). "Mark Weinberger: Nose No Bounds." May 2, 2011.

Suggested Further Reading

Bissinger, Buzz. "The Runaway Doctor." *Vanity Fair*. 2010.

Pesta, Abigail. "The Day My Husband Disappeared." *Marie Claire* (internet). 2011. Available

from https://www.marieclaire.com/culture/news/a5872/con-artist-husband/.

CHAPTER ELEVEN

DR. PAUL VOLKMAN—THE PILL MILL MAN

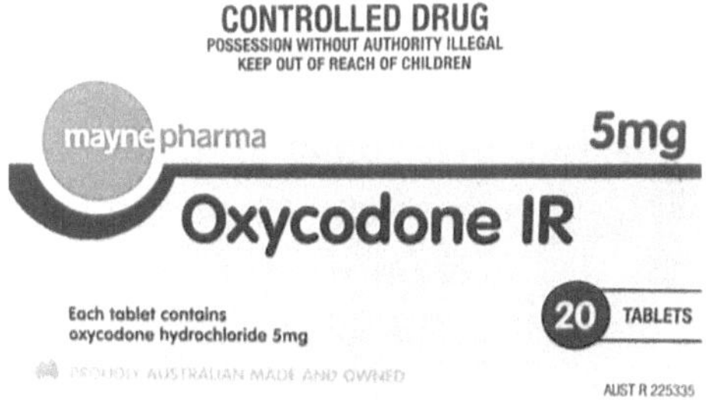

Photo: John Anderson

Prologue

Ohio, USA, lies to the south of the Great Lakes and is mostly forested and picturesque. Scioto County is a small county located to the south of the state on the northern bank of the Ohio River. About eighty thousand lived there at the 2010 census. The main town in Scioto County is Portsmouth, close to the north bank of the Ohio River near the confluence with the much smaller Scioto River to the west.

Portsmouth was home to about forty thousand people in 1940, reduced to twenty thousand by 2010 due to the slow demise of the steelworks and the shoe factory.[1] It is said that the method of manufacturing shoelaces originated there. It would soon be known as the Pill Mill Capital of America. About sixty-five kilometers (forty miles) north of Portsmouth is Chillicothe in Ross County. About eight hundred kilometers (420 miles) to the east of Portsmouth lies Chicago, Illinois, eight hours away by road. Kentucky is on the other side of the Ohio River to the southwest, and West Virginia is to the southeast of Portsmouth, also on the other side of the river. Deer roam in the woods of Scioto County.

That was not why it was famous though.

Opiates and Opioids

An opiate is a drug that comes from a specific species of the poppy plant. Opiates include morphine, codeine, and papaverine. They derive from the fluid, sometimes described as a latex, that oozes from incisions on the seed of the poppy. The poppy has been farmed all over the world, including China and India, from time immemorial, but in the case of the pill mills, it usually came from Latin America, particularly Mexico, where it was grown by farmers who once farmed sugarcane until they realized that there was more money in farming the poppy. The latex produced from the flower is not quality-controlled and therefore varies in concentration and purity. An opioid is a broader term, which includes related synthetic (i.e., manufactured) substances derived from, or independently produced, to be similar in chemical structure as the opiates. Opioids manufactured by pharmaceutical companies are subject to quality control and can be relied upon to have the correct dose in each tablet and be of reliable purity. Their desired effect is to relieve pain and induce a feeling of well-being, and they do this very well.[2]

Unfortunately, opiates, as well as relieving pain, can cause *tolerance*, *dependence*, and *addiction*. *Tolerance* results in an increasing dose being required to achieve the same effect. If a person becomes *dependent* on a drug, it means that although they regularly use the drug, it can be withdrawn by reducing the dose gradually, causing little discomfort. To be *addicted* means that they cannot do without the drug even when it causes inconvenience or uncomfortable side effects. When the drugs were first synthesized in the 1980s, these addictive effects were not fully appreciated. The combination of tolerance and addiction makes it difficult to withdraw from the opiates, and increasing doses are required to satisfy the feeling of euphoria that they induce.

Withdrawal from Opiates

When a drug-addicted person is unable to obtain supplies of the opiate to which they are addicted, they are likely to experience withdrawal symptoms. These can start as early as six hours, depending on the drug, the previous dosage, and how long they have been addicted. They can include joint, bone, and muscle aches and pain, anxiety, fever, diarrhea, nausea and vomiting, abdominal cramps, depression, goosebumps, chills, and intense drug cravings, lasting four to five days. The severity of these symptoms will vary from user to user and from drug to drug, but in general, they cause pains, insomnia, sweating, loss of appetite, racing heart, and runny nose. Effects will be similar regardless of the drug involved, although perhaps not as severe. There is evidence that some pharmaceuticals—such as naloxone, which is an antidote—can be lifesaving when given to an overdose victim by reversing the effects of the opioids.[3]

Withdrawal from the drug is an ugly sight, resulting in the addict becoming more and more desperate to satisfy their need. Some will rely on theft and violence to obtain more of the drug. The opioids, such as oxycodone, are a valuable medical resource when used for pain relief, but when used recreationally, with no need to relieve pain, they are poison. Pharmaceutical agencies have been engaged in a search for potent analgesics (pain relievers) that do not have addictive side effects. Several similar painkillers have been developed, but so far, all have an addictive character. The most commonly prescribed is oxycodone, but others are used, such as Vicodin, one of the most widely prescribed and frequently abused pain relievers in the US. It is a combination of two pain relievers; acetaminophen (commonly known by the trade name Tylenol) and hydrocodone (synthetic codeine). Vicodin is marketed under a number of proprietary brand names, including Vicodin, Lortab, Anexsia, Zydone, Lorcet, and Norco. Vicodin is considered an effective pain reliever when used as prescribed over the short term. Careless, inappropriate, or deliberate misuse can have severe consequences, including drug dependence and addiction. Other opiates that are available (not necessarily on prescription) are codeine, heroin, hydrocodone (Vicodin), hydromorphone (Dilaudid), methadone, meperidine (Demerol), morphine, oxycodone (Percocet or OxyContin), and fentanyl.

Opioid Overdose

Overdose of opioids is by far the most common way that deaths occur due to prescription drugs. Recent statistics show that in 2012, 259 million prescriptions were written for painkillers in the USA. Almost all of the world's hydrocodone supply is consumed by Americans, and 81 percent of oxycodone prescriptions are written in America.[4]

In Florida alone, there were over seven deaths per day due to overdoses of prescription drugs in 2010; and in the USA overall, deaths from overdoses of prescription drugs overtook deaths from motor vehicle accidents.[5,6] The deaths were not confined to Florida; in Ohio, for example, there were 4,149 deaths in 2016 alone. *Philip Eil* noted that Associated Press reported that in 2010, one baby in ten was born in Scioto County addicted to opiates.[7,8]

The Opioid Crisis

So how did this all come about? In 1996, the FDA approved the sale of the recently developed OxyContin by the pharmaceutical company Purdue. The approval was based on the assumption that because the preparation was slow-release, it would be nonaddictive. According to *Sam Quinones* in his book *Dreamland*, the belief that the opiates were not addictive started when the *New England Journal of Medicine* published a short letter on January 10, 2000, from Ms. Jane Parson and Dr. Hershel Jick from the Boston University School of Medicine. In the book, Quinones describes a crucial letter to the editor of the *New England Journal of Medicine* in 1980, in which the authors stated, "Although there were 11,882 patients who received at least one narcotic preparation, there were only four cases of reasonably well-documented addiction in patients who had a history of addiction. We conclude that despite widespread use of narcotic drugs in hospitals, the development of addiction is rare in medical patients with no history of addiction."[9]

What role did this letter play in how physicians justified the use of opioids to treat pain?

The letter explained that after the thalidomide disaster in the 1960s, the hospital had built a database containing details of three hundred thousand inpatients and the drugs that they had been given while hospitalized. Of these, twelve thousand patients had been given opioids, and only four had become addicted. This letter was later taken to be evidence that the risk of addiction to opioids was low. It was not mentioned that the subjects were all inpatients and that the amount of opioid dispensed was tightly controlled.[10] Numerous physicians accepted that OxyContin was not addictive although their training in medical school had left them in no doubt that opioids were addictive. Those doctors who were at the forefront of treating pain or specialized in pain management thought that the opiates were a gift from heaven. And a gift from heaven they were, but not in the way that you might think because this left a fertile background for Purdue Pharma to send their sales representatives to sow the seeds of the wonder drug. And that is what they did. One thousand salespeople descended on seventy thousand health practitioners to spread the gospel.[11]

There are numerous ways that an opiate overdose can occur. The vast majority are accidental and result from an opiate-dependent person taking a larger-than-usual dose when he or she meant to take a specific treatment. Sometimes the overdose is due to taking an unfamiliar combination of opiates, and sometimes it is due to taking an unexpectedly high amount of substance due to unavailability of the usual dose. Some opioid overdoses are deliberate suicides. Some opiates are from pharmaceutical companies, where the quality control of the drug is tight, but some are from other sources where there is little or no quality control and, therefore, the quantity of drug per dose is unknown. Hence the recent increase in Florida, where a clampdown on the so-called pill mills has resulted in drug addicts turning again to Mexico Mud, which is not so constant in quality. Mexican Mud is the crude form of heroin that is produced from the poppy farms in Mexico. According to the World Health Organization (WHO), due to the effect on the part of the brain that regulates breathing, opioids in high doses can cause respiratory depression and death. An opioid overdose can be identified by a combination of three signs referred to as the opioid overdose triad. The signs are pinpoint pupils, unconsciousness, and shallow breathing. The breathing can become so shallow that the heart stops and the unconsciousness becomes permanent.

Some Facts about the Opiate Epidemic

1. Almost all of the world's hydrocodone is consumed by Americans.
2. In 2012, 259 million prescriptions were written for painkillers in the USA, about one bottle for every adult.
3. Of the world's oxycodone prescriptions,
   81 percent are written in America.[4]
4. Over four hundred thousand Americans died
   from overdoses of prescription drugs or illegal opioids in the last twenty years.
5. For the first time since WWII, life expectancy has
   fallen in the USA because of opioid deaths.
6. In 2010, one baby in ten was born in
   Scioto County addicted to opiates.[7,8]
7. There were more than 117 deaths from drug overdoses from 2000 to 2008 in Scioto County alone.
8. Eleven million Americans are addicted to opioids.

Pill Mills

The desperation to obtain the drug and the willingness of the physicians to prescribe it, initially in the belief that it was not addictive, led to the rise of the pill mills, probably starting in Florida, USA.

In 1990, physicians in the USA began to use various opiates, which had been recently developed, for the treatment of pain. Synthetic opioids, such as oxycodone (which have a molecular structure similar to morphine), were effective at relieving postoperative pain, as well as for chronic pain, such as intractable back pain, cancer pain, and other pains that might have resulted from injuries sustained at work. They were a boon to legitimate health care.

In Florida, though, a new business model sprang up. Out the front, it was called a pain management center or similar, but its sole purpose was to make money for the proprietors by selling prescription opiates, such as oxycodone. It was called a pill mill. Instead of the physician who worked there being engaged in a family first–style health center—looking after the whole family and all their health needs, with medical records on-site and equipment to check the physical health of mother, father, and children—all that was there was a safe to secure the money and the drugs, prescription pads, and an attendant to see that the money was collected. There were no physical examinations, no medical records, limited or no medical equipment, and no counseling or plan put in place for recovery or rehabilitation. Pain was treated by pills alone; no other treatment was available. You could select your own medicines, which were dispensed in large volumes. Large crowds often gathered outside the clinic. Payment was by cash only, and no advice was given. There could even be a dispensary on-site. If a physician was there, he or she might have carried a gun. All that was needed was someone with a Drug Enforcement Administration (DEA) license. This business model became a pill mill.

Sam Quinones, writing in his highly acclaimed book *Dreamland*, says that around 1970–1980, in parts of America—like Portsmouth, Ohio—things were not so good. The industry started moving away to countries where labor was cheap. By 1980, the Detroit Steel mill had closed.[12] The housing market was sliding, leaving only a rental market, and unemployment had increased to an unhealthy level with people moving away to find work elsewhere, leaving only the skeleton of a town that had once been a bustling business center. At least 117 people died from drug overdoses between 2000 and 2008 in Scioto County alone. One grieving mother rented a shop in town as a memorial and filled it with photographs of those who had died.[13] Life was not so good for many folks. The pill mills flourished all over the country in this vacuum with astonishing speed.

Some examples of this follow.

Dr. John Lilly opened an office in Portsmouth (now described as the OxyContin Capital of the World). Lilly was charged with corrupt activity, unlawful possession of a dangerous weapon, and aggravated trafficking of drugs in 2001.[14] He got three years in prison for his trouble, but that did not seem to stop others.

Dr. Thomas J. Weed, one of Florida's best-known pill doctors, flagrantly advertised his clinic on television, bragging how easily patients could obtain supplies from him. He usually took less than five minutes per patient and was known to have "seen" seventy patients in a day. Medical and police reports say that nine patients died of an overdose in 2004 and 2005 after having taken drugs prescribed by Dr. Weed.[15] The average family doctor might see, listen to, or advise and reassure twenty to thirty people. One cannot provide proper medical care to seventy patients in a day.

The authorities were watching though. In 2005, there were said to be over 150 clinics in Broward County, Miami, alone; but by 2009, over one hundred had been closed down.[16] This clamping down on the availability of opioids probably contributed to opioid addicts switching to Mexico Mud, a crude latex-like substance derived from farmed poppy seeds. It is cheaper and inferior to opioids produced in pharmaceutical laboratories.

Dr. John Christensen

In 2013, officials charged Dr. John Christensen with two counts of murder and seventy-six other counts mostly related to drug or insurance fraud. His trial, in a Palm Beach County courtroom, began three years later, on October 25, 2016. The charges of murder were reduced to manslaughter, to which he pleaded guilty. And as a result of plea bargaining, he was sentenced to four years in prison on the manslaughter charges; and on the seventy-six other charges, he was fined $262,000 but imprisoned on those charges. He also agreed to repay $1.1 million to the federal government in Medicare fraud and not to reapply for his medical license. When he was sent to prison, he had served almost a year in custody, so he still had three years to go. He was aged sixty-five years.[17,18, 19]

Dr. Jasna Mrdjen

The epidemic was not confined to Florida, though. Dr. Jasna Mrdjen was prosecuted in Los Gatos in the San Francisco Bay Area in 2015 for inappropriately prescribing narcotics to an addict who later died. She was also facing twelve other charges, including feloniously dispensing a controlled substance to an addict. Evidence was also presented that she had prescribed an undercover officer, posing as a construction worker, 870 OxyContin and oxycodone tablets without ever having examined him or taken a history. She also directed him away from pharmacies that might refuse to fill his prescription and advised him how to pass a urine test.[20]

Dr. Gerald Klein

Also in the year 2015, *Dr. Gerald Klein* was charged with first-degree murder following the death of Joey Bartolucci due to an overdose of prescribed opiates. Dr. Klein was aged eighty and had been a specialist surgeon in earlier years. He had taken employment in 2008 with a Jeff George and his brother Chris who had operated pill mills valued at $40 million in Lake Worth, Boca Raton, and Broward County, Florida. The brothers were later jailed for running illegal clinics and the manslaughter of Joey Bartolucci, which occurred because of their clinics.[21] Chris was given a three-year reduction in his sentence for giving evidence in another case against two doctors, and Jeff was hoping for similar treatment for giving evidence against Dr. Klein. Ironically, Dr. Klein was found not guilty of the murder of Bartolucci but was found guilty of drug offenses.[18,19] Clearly, as they say, there is no honor among thieves.[22,23,24,25]

Dr. Shelinder Aggarwal was a pain management doctor who operated a pill mill, named Chronic Pain Care Services, in Huntsville, Alabama. In 2012, about eighty to 145 patients a day visited Aggarwal's clinic, with him seeing the majority of patients and writing all prescriptions. According to court documents, initial patient visits typically lasted five minutes or less, and follow-ups two minutes or less. Aggarwal did not obtain prior medical records for his patients, did not treat patients with anything other than controlled substances, often asked patients what medications they wanted and filled their requests, prescribed controlled substances to patients whom he knew were using illegal drugs, and did not take appropriate measures to ensure that patients did not divert or abuse controlled substances. His plea agreement summarizes an interaction with a patient, which was captured on video. In it, Aggarwal notes that the DEA viewed him as the "biggest pill-pusher in North Alabama" and that many of his patients were "dropping like flies, they are all dying."

According to the prescription drug monitoring program (PDMP), Alabama pharmacies filled about 110,013 of Aggarwal's prescriptions for controlled substances in 2012. That would equal about 423 prescriptions per day if he worked five days a week and resulted in approximately 12.3 million pills. The PDMP rated Aggarwal as the highest prescriber of controlled substances filled in Alabama in 2012, with the next highest prescriber writing a third as many prescriptions. There is no way that Aggarwal could handwrite 423 prescriptions in a day. He must have been using a printer to pump them out.

Medicare data shows Aggarwal was the highest prescriber in the United States of Schedule II controlled substances under Medicare in 2012. Schedule II substances include the opioid painkillers oxycodone, oxymorphone, hydromorphone, and morphine. He was the nation's highest Medicare prescriber of opioid painkillers at the height of his practice.

As to Aggarwal's health-care fraud scheme, he pleaded guilty to requiring patients to undergo unreasonable and unnecessary urine drug tests that he did not need or use in their treatment. Aggarwal acknowledged that the tests he ran depended not on patients' treatment but on how much he could bill for tests. He often ignored urine test results showing patients were using illegal drugs.

Between January 2011 and March 2013, urine drug tests accounted for about 80 percent of paid claims that Aggarwal submitted to Medicare and Blue Cross Blue Shield (BCBS) for a total reimbursement of $9.5 million. According to his plea agreement, "Aggarwal's primary motivation for testing patients' urine specimens, and submitting those claims for payment, was financial gain." Aggarwal pleaded guilty in October to one charge of distributing a controlled substance outside the scope of professional practice and not for a legitimate medical purpose in July 2012 and to one charge of conspiring to execute a health-care fraud scheme against Medicare and BCBS of Alabama between January 1, 2011, and March 31, 2013. Aggarwal earlier repaid $2.8 million to Medicare and $45,843 to BCBS of Alabama following audits.

The US Department of Justice–North Alabama District reports that on February 7, 2017, in Birmingham, Alabama, a federal judge sentenced Dr. Aggarwal, aged forty-eight, to fifteen years in prison for illegally prescribing controlled substances and committing health-care fraud involving $9.5 million in unneeded and unused urine tests. The judge also directed Aggarwal to forfeit $6.7 million and his former clinic on Turner Street Southwest, Huntsville, and ordered Aggarwal to pay $6.7 million in restitution to Medicare and Blue Cross Blue Shield of Alabama.[26]

Dr. David Proctor—Godfather of the Pill Mill

In his book *Dreamland*, Sam Quinones does not mention much about Dr. David Proctor, a Canadian, before he turned up in South Shore, Kentucky, just south of the Ohio River, in 1979. Apparently, he came there as an assistant or locum to Dr. Billy Riddle, who had been the town's family doctor for many years. The two worked together for a time, and it appears that Dr. Proctor ran a regular family practice. But it seems that he and Billy Riddle did not get along, and within a couple of years, they had separated their practices and gone their own ways. Dr. Riddle had a heart attack, and that left Dr. David Proctor on his own. Because unemployment rose, families came gradually to rely on worker's compensation or welfare payments to survive. Dr. Proctor gained a name for himself as one who was sympathetic to these families and would readily sign paperwork in support of their claims. Some patients soon developed pains that were in their mind only. At the time, the opioid push was on; and soon, Dr. Proctor's prescribing habits changed.

In the late 1980s, the Kentucky Board of Medical Licensure investigated Dr. Proctor but found that he was practicing legally. He was put on probation, but his license was not withdrawn. In the subsequent decade, people's pain had increased, in parallel with Dr. Proctor's prescribing. The more he ordered, the greater the pain; and the greater the (perceived) pain, the more he ordered. His practice grew, and he found that this was an easier way to make money. A visit for pain relief (i.e., opiates) was $250 and took only a few minutes. Over time, David Proctor's behavior became more degraded. He began accepting sex from patients in return for drugs, and then he started demanding sex from them in his office.[27] In 1998, he had a car accident and claimed that he was no longer able to practice medicine. He gave up his registration in Kentucky but kept his clinic open, employing a string of other doctors to keep it going. Many of them started out in their own clinics, having learned how to do it from Proctor, earning him a reputation as the Godfather of the Pill Mill. Meantime, Proctor had developed a habit himself.

In 2002, Dr. David Proctor, a Canadian, was charged with conspiracy to distribute a controlled substance and received a twelve-year sentence in prison plus a fine of $250,000. He requested after a year that he be allowed to serve the last eleven years in Canada. His wish was not granted, as he had not paid the fine.[28,29] He was released in 2014, and his wish was then granted when he was deported to Canada.[30]

Dr. Paul Volkman

In many ways, the story of *Dr. Paul Volkman* followed but paralleled the rise of the opioid epidemic in the USA. Volkman was only one of many physicians who subsequently became caught up in the epidemic that was fueled by the opioids. If Dr. David Proctor was known as the Godfather of the Pill Mill, Dr. Paul Volkman must have earned the title King of the Pill Mill. His greed and lack of empathy surpassed all the others.

According to Philip Eil, writing in the *Cincinnati Magazine*, Paul Volkman was born in 1947 and raised in Washington, DC. He was the son of a pharmacist and a clerk in the US Treasury

Department and graduated from University of Chicago Pritzker School of Medicine in 1974 after initial training at the University of Rochester, New York. He seemed, at first, to have been a quiet person, perhaps even introverted, as his interests lay in chess, bridge, and classical music. After graduation, Volkman studied pharmacology (the effects of chemicals on the body) and then—for a time, strangely—pediatrics (specializing in children). He was licensed to practice medicine in Ohio on July 15, 1996 but was also licensed in Illinois and four other states. Dr. Paul Volkman initially started a pediatric and family practice in Chicago but, in due course, found that it was not financially sufficient to support his family or himself in any sort of lifestyle. He soon took locum employment in hospitals at nights and weekends to supplement his income. His CV shows that he flitted from hospital emergency room to hospital emergency room. He worked at numerous hospitals on a locum basis between 1975 and 2002. In places, he is described as a native of Chicago, and that is undoubtedly where he lived at the time, which interests us.[31,32]

Life was not going to get easier anytime soon, though. Before long, Volkman had accumulated four malpractice suits. According to Philip Eil, two of these cases against Volkman were lost and two were settled out of court. In either case, the insurance company lost money.[33] Whether or not Dr. Paul Volkman was at fault in those cases is of no importance now, but what was important then was that the insurance companies refused malpractice cover for him in the future. Finding employment suddenly became even more difficult. Casual work in hospital emergency rooms was impossible without medical indemnity. Dr. Volkman took employment briefly in a restaurant kitchen after six months on unemployment welfare payments.[34]

The Opportunity

Then in 2003, Dr. Volkman saw an advertisement for a physician in a pain management clinic in Portsmouth, Ohio. No insurance was required, and the starting salary was $5,500 per week. Although Portsmouth, Ohio, was 420 miles from Chicago, he applied for and got the job.[35] The work was at a clinic called the Tri-State Healthcare run by Denise Huffman and her daughter Alice. There were three addresses in Portsmouth and one in Chillicothe in Ross County. Still, it was work. Volkman still lived in Chicago, so he flew down to Columbus on Monday mornings and drove the remaining two hours from Columbus to the office in Portsmouth and did the reverse on Friday evenings after work. All seemed to be going well in the clinic.

All Might Not Be Well

The earliest suggestion that all might not be well with Tri-State Healthcare occurred in mid-2003 when the pharmacies in the area stopped filling Volkman's prescriptions. A pharmacist in West Virginia complained about Volkman's prescribing habits to the DEA, and he and others in the area stopped dispensing his prescriptions. This was a major problem, but Volkman had a solution. He suggested opening a dispensary on the Tri-State Healthcare site and distributing the prescriptions from there. Denise Huffman objected, but Dr. Volkman reassured her that "I am a doctor." Volkman's PhD in pharmacology presumably assisted in the issuance of a license. Volkman submitted an application to the Ohio Board of Pharmacy for a permit to distribute controlled substances. Board representatives conducted an inspection of the clinic grounds, during the course of which they found a Glock pistol in the safe where the drugs were stored. Despite this discovery, the board issued a license.

In spite of these setbacks, Volkman continued in business until almost the end of 2003.

Volkman's Ordering History

Some of the figures reported by Philip Eil in the *Cincinnati Magazine* are worth repeating.

In August 2003, a medical supply company notified the DEA that it had received an order for hydrocodone from Volkman that exceeded the company's ordering limits. Another reported an order that was the biggest it had ever seen. In 2004, Volkman ordered 457,000 dosage units of oxycodone, 106,100 units more than the next doctor in the USA. He ordered 96 percent of all the oxycodone sold directly to Ohio practitioners that year, ninety-seven times greater than the national average.[34] The board inspected the facility again in December 2003. They found numerous problems with the new dispensary. The records were poorly maintained, and Volkman provided little oversight over the paperwork. No licensed physician or pharmacist oversaw the dispensing process.

By February 2004, the clinic took measures to satisfy the board's concerns. But it still had its problems. Volkman was in charge of the dispensary but did a poor job of regulating access. The drug safe's security was poor, with unauthorized personnel regularly accessing the pharmaceutical stockpile contained inside. Despite these issues, the dispensary was busy. It purchased 135,900 dosage units of oxycodone in five months to December 2003; 457,100 dosage units in 2004; and 414,200 dosage units in the nine months to September 2005.

It eventually became clear that Volkman's medical practice did not follow a standard pattern. Drug addicts, drug peddlers, and individuals otherwise not complaining of pain would come to see him as his "patients." Little was done in terms of taking medical histories or conducting physical examinations. Volkman would regularly prescribe a drug cocktail consisting of opiates (such as oxycodone and hydrocodone) as well as sedatives (diazepam, alprazolam, and carisoprodol—commonly referred to as Valium, Xanax, and Soma). He tended to resort first to narcotics, disregarding first lines of treatment for pain management such as nonsteroidal anti-inflammatory drugs (NSAIDs).

A federal investigation of Tri-State led to a search of the clinic facility on June 7, 2005. Medical personnel accompanying the investigative team saw that the clinic was in complete disarray. Urine specimen cups, filled with urine, were scattered all over the floor. The clinic had no regular medical equipment. Miscellaneous pills were strewn all through the clinic premises.[35]

Three months after the investigation, Denise terminated Volkman's employment because she "could no longer get along with him" and because there was "no control." In her words, "Dr Volkman did what Dr Volkman wanted to do."

Philip Eil reports that having fallen out with the Huffmans, Volkman used a spare room in his Center Street apartment, Portsmouth, to write prescriptions but he was closed down by the police after only three weeks. Not to be put off, he opened another office in a double-width trailer by the roadside of Route 23, forty miles north, close to Chillicothe. A large sign on the trailer blared "Paul H Volkman, M.D. pain management." Volkman decided to open his own shop in Ohio, at first in Portsmouth and later in Chillicothe. Twelve of Volkman's patients died during his tenure at Tri-State Healthcare and another two during the early months of his new practice. Kristi Ross, Steve Hieneman, Bryan Brigner, and Earnest Ratcliff were four of these patients.

All Was Not Well

On Friday, February 10, 2006, agents of the DEA and Major Crimes Task Force with search warrants raided the "pain clinic" at 5565 US 23. According to the sheriff, Ron Nichols, "The raid was the result of a lengthy investigation into suspected prescription writing abuse at the clinic." No charges or arrests were made, and the Ohio and Illinois licensing boards took no action.[36] One would have thought that it would be a warning to those at the pain clinic that they were under surveillance.

Just over a year later, on Monday (May 21, 2007), Dr. Paul Volkman and two office managers were arrested and charged with illegally distributing the drug oxycodone and others, which led to the deaths of fourteen people. Volkman was accused of writing countless prescriptions for excessive doses outside the scope of medical practice. Also indicted were Denise Huffman, fifty-four, and her daughter Alice, thirty-two, the owners and managers of the Tri-State Healthcare clinic. All three faced life in prison if found guilty and $3.1 million in fines, being the sum that they are thought to have made from the illegal trading.[37,38,39,40,41]

It took four years for the trial to begin on March 1, 2011, in Cincinnati with Volkman being charged with prescribing oxycodone, hydrocodone, and other drugs for a patient named Aaron Gillespie, who died four days later from multiple drug toxicity. The charges say that the following month, the Huffmans and Volkman opened a dispensary of their own because the local pharmacists refused to dispense their prescriptions. The charges also claimed that at least eleven others died following the abuse of those prescriptions over the next two years. The indictments also claimed that patients were charged between $125 and $200 in cash after some of them had allegedly driven for hundreds of miles to see them. Prosecutors said that Volkman rarely, if ever, counseled patients on other treatments for pain. Volkman denied all the charges, saying that he had always acted in good faith.

Lisa Roberts, a public health nurse, said that Volkman had "helped to set the stage for this epidemic in which we found ourselves." She regarded him as a link in the chain of corrupt physicians who together represent an era where Scioto County became a "dumping ground for every crazed doctor who could not make an honorable living anymore and came here and just wrote prescriptions for narcotics."[42]

Sadly for Volkman and ironically for the rest of us, the Huffmans, Denise and Alice, gave evidence against Volkman in return for a plea bargain in their own case, in which they faced a charge of operating a place whose primary purpose was the illegal distribution of prescription drugs. Volkman was found guilty of causing four deaths as well as eight other accounts of illicit distribution.[42,43,44,45] Denise Huffman was found guilty of owning and operating a drug-related premises, namely Tri-State Healthcare, and remained in federal prison until September 2020. Her daughter Alice was also found guilty and was released in 2016.[46]

Philip Eil established a relationship with Volkman and intended to write a book about him but was prevented from doing so, as he could not access information despite freedom for information regulations. Instead, he made email and telephone calls to Volkman while he was within the prison.[47] During these conversations, Eil gained Volkman's confidence, but Volkman apparently continued to claim innocence, saying that he had always acted in the best interest of his patients. It seems that the jury and the appeal judges did not believe him.

On the charges of causing death, he was given a life sentence in each case to be served consecutively. On the other charges, he was given sentences between ten and twenty years to be served concurrently with the life sentences. Dr. Volkman appealed these sentences in 2013, but the judges rejected his appeal by a verdict of 3–0. In any event, he is in his seventies now, and it is unlikely that he will see the outside of a prison again.

Epilogue

Physicians must shoulder much of the blame for allowing this health crisis to develop. It seems unlikely that the blame can be placed on the shoulders of the authors of a short letter written in a medical journal in 2000. Readers of that letter usually are critical professionals who would not have missed the insignificance of it. As a group, the governmental bodies that regulated the medical and pharmaceutical professions were frozen by apathy. They should have restricted the licenses of doctors, preventing them from prescribing opiates without higher authority. It should have been anticipated that decadent doctors would fall greedily on this cruel method of acquiring wealth at dreadful expense to their fellow human beings. It is hard to know where it will all end, especially when one of the factors is an addiction, meaning that many of the victims do not want it to end.

One light has emerged. The Sackler family, owners of the giant pharmaceutical company Purdue Pharma, had civil suits lodged against them in thirty-nine states and more than 1,500 US cities and counties, claiming that the company had helped to create the opioid crisis. According to Cameron Stewart, the Washington correspondent of the *Australian* newspaper, the suit states, "The Sacklers' full understanding of opioids' abuse and addiction risk is underscored by their willingness to research, quantify and ultimately monetize opioid abuse and addiction by pursuing the development of medications to treat the addiction their own opioids created."[48] The Sackler family, owners of Purdue Pharma, have a combined wealth of US$13 billion. They are known benefactors of the arts and have museums named after them. Their names are on a slide now though, with establishments like the Metropolitan Museum of Art in New York and the Smithsonian Institution in Washington rejecting their donations.

It is claimed that over four hundred thousand Americans have died from overdoses of prescription drugs or illegal opioids in the last twenty years. It is said that eleven million Americans are addicted to opioids. For the first time since World War II, the overall life expectancy in the United States has fallen because of opioid deaths, which now kill more people in the country than guns, motor vehicle accidents, or HIV have ever done in one year. The Centers for Disease Control and Prevention reported in 2015 that 236 million prescriptions were written for opioids in the United States; that is approximately one bottle for every adult.[48]

The opioid epidemic is one of the most severe health crises in the United States for generations. There is little sign of it retreating. The large pharmaceutical companies that manufacture the opioids and the health-care providers who distribute them must carry a large proportion of the blame. As recently as early 2019, sixty people have been indicted for prescribing opioids illegally. These include thirty-one doctors, seven pharmacists, and eight nurses. The offenses include 350,000 opioid prescriptions and more than thirty-two million pills in the states of Ohio, Kentucky, Tennessee, Alabama, and West Virginia, roughly one prescription for every person in those states.[49]

The United States has 17.4 days of opioids use per person per annum compared with 6.1 days per annum in Australia, according to the International Narcotics Control Board. Prescribing of opioids in Australia is increasing, and annual deaths involving opioids almost doubled to 1,119 in the ten years to 2016. This is worrying, as it suggests that Australia and the rest of the world are not far behind the United States, and unless something is done soon, Australia and the world will become victims of the same epidemic.

Notes

1. Welsh-Huggins, A. "Scioto County Hit by Painkiller 'Tsunami.'" *The Cincinnati Enquirer*. 2010: 18.
2. World Health Organization. Management of substance abuse (internet). World Health Organization; 2018. Available from https://www.who.int/substance_abuse/information-sheet/en/.
3. Ibid.
4. Northpoint Recovery. "The Ugly Truth about Pill Mills in the United States." Northpoint Recovery (internet). 2017 (cited March 8, 2019). Available from https://www.northpointrecovery.com/blog/ugly-truth-pill-mills-united-states/.
5. Esposito, L. "Opioid Epidemic: What Brought Us Here?" (internet). US News; Health; 2018. Available from https://health.usnews.com/health-care/patient-advice/articles/2018-01- 24/opioid-epidemic-what-brought-us-here?.
6. Quinones, S. *Dreamland—the True Tale of America's Opiate Epidemic*. 1st ed. New York: Bloomsbury Publishers; 2015.
7. Eil, P. "The Pill Mill that Ravaged Portsmouth." *Cincinnati Magazine* (internet). 2017 (cited March 5, 2019): 1–10. Available from https://www.cincinnatimagazine.com/features/pill-mill-portsmouth/.
8. Welsh-Huggins, op. cit.
9. Parson, J., H. Jick. "Addiction Rare in Patients Treated with Narcotics." *New England Journal of Medicine*. 1980; 302(2): 123

10. Ibid.
11. Bergman, J. Owner's guide for humans (blog). *A pharmaceutical atomic bomb*. (cited March 26, 2019). Available from http://www.drjohnbergman.com/the-destruction-of-societys-social-fabric-and-opioid-drugs-part-22-opiates-and-the-pill-mill/.
12. Drug Enforcement Agency. "Waging the War against the Devil in Scioto County: A Grassroots Response to Prescription Drug Abuse in a Rural community." Presentation given by Lisa Roberts R.N., Portsmouth City Health Department; 2012. https://www.deadiversion.usdoj.gov/mtgs/drug_chemical/2012/roberts.pdf.
13. Welsh-Huggins, A. |Scioto County Hit by Painkiller 'Tsunami.'" *The Cincinnati Enquirer*. 2010: 18.
14. Eil, P. "The Pill Mill." p. 1.
15. LaMendola, B., W. Lucey, B. Hijek. "Doctor Saw Nine Who Died of Overdose." *South Florida Sun-Sentinel*. 2006.
16. Johnson, P. "Florida's Opioid Crisis Fueled by Pill Mills". DrugRehab.com (internet). 2017 (cited March 9, 2019). Available from https://www.drugrehab.com/2017/03/01/florida-pill-mill-crisis/.
17. Musgrave, J. "West Palm Beach Pill Mill Doctor Gets 4-Year Term." *The Palm Beach Post*. 2017: B1.
18. Freeman, M. "Defense Says Evidence Was Obtained Illegally." *South Florida Sun Sentinel*. 2016: B1.
19. Freeman, M. "Former Pain Doctor Gets Probation." *South Florida Sun Sentinel*. 2016: S13, A5.
20. Kaplan, T. "Deadly Overdose. Los Gatos Doctor Prosecuted in Rare Pill Mill Case." *The Mercury News* (internet). 2015 (cited March 27, 2019). Available from https://www.mercurynews.com/2015/06/22/deadly-overdose-los-gatos-doctor-prosecuted-in-rare-pill-mill-case/.

21. LaForgia, M. "One Twin Ordered Jailed on Gun Charge." *The Palm Beach Post*. 2010: A013.

22. Musgrave, J. "Ex-Pill Mill King Jeff George Testifies in Doctor's Murder Trial." *The Palm Beach Post* (internet). 2015 (cited March 11, 2019). Available from https://www.palmbeachpost.com/news/crime--law/pill-mill-king-jeff-george-testifies-doctor-murder-trial/Gjell6PpLZDJvM8uh4gaHI/.

23. Duret, D. "Prosecutor: Doc Pushed 'Pharmaceutical Heroin.'" *The Palm Beach Post*. 2015: B001.

24. Duret, D. "Judges Vacation Postpones Murder Trial." *The Palm Beach Post*. 2015: B002.

25. Duret, D. "Manager of Pain Clinic Admits He Falsified Doctor's Inventory." *The Palm Beach Post*. 2015: B002.

26. US Department of Justice. "Huntsville Pill Mill Doctor Sentenced to 15 Years in Prison for Illegal Prescribing and Health Care Fraud" (internet). 2017. Available from https://www.justice.gov/usao-ndal/pr/huntsville-pill-mill-doctor-sentenced-15-years-prison-illegal-prescribing-and-health.

27. Quinones, S. *Dreamland—the True Tale of America's Opiate Epidemic*. 1st ed. New York: Bloomsbury Publishers; 2015.

28. Wire dispatches. "Physician Indicted on Drug Charges." *The Courier-Journal* (Louisville, Kentucky). 2002: 12.

29. Fields, B. "Pill Mill Doctor Wants to Go Home." *The Daily Independent* (internet). 2007 (cited March 14, 2019). Available from https://www.dailyindependent.com/news/local_news/pill-mill_doctor-wants-to-go-home/article_db1a61eb-ab99-5c4d-a2bb-b663c2c7c874.html.

30. Quinones, S. *Dreamland* (internet). "Dr Proctor's House." 2016 (cited March 7, 2019). Available from http://samquinones.com/reporters-blog/2016/10/03/dr-procters-house/.

31. Eil, P. "The Pill Mill."

32. Robertson, L. "DEA Agents Search Pain Clinic." *Chillicothe Gazette*. 2006: 1.

33. Eil, P. "The Pill Mill that Ravaged Portsmouth." *Cincinnati Magazine* (internet). 2017 (cited March 5, 2019): pp. 3–4. Available from https://www.cincinnatimagazine.com/features/pill-mill-portsmouth/.

34. Eil, P. "The Pill Mill." pp. 5–6.

35. *United States v. Volkman*. August 14, 2015. No. 12 3212. http://Caselaw.findlaw.com/us-6th-circuit/1710544.html

36. Robertson, L. "DEA Agents."

37. Ibid.

38. Bush, R. "Doctor Faces Charges in 14 Deaths." *Chicago Tribune*. 2007: 2,3.

39. AP. "Government Seeks to Recover $10 Million from 'Pill Mill.'" *Chillicothe Gazette*. 2007: 1.

40. Associated Press. "Doctor Goes on Trial in Ohio Painkiller OD Deaths." *The Tribune* (Coshocton, Ohio). 2011: 4.

41. Eil, P. "The Pill Mill." p. 8.

42. Welsh-Huggins, A. "Scioto County Hit by Painkiller 'Tsunami.'" *The Cincinnati Enquirer*. 2010: 18.

43. Welsh-Huggins, A. "'Pill Mill' Doctor Is Convicted of Causing 4 Deaths." *Fort Collins Coloradoan*. 2011: 7.

44. Welsh-Huggins, A. "Doctor Gets Four Life Terms in Pill Mill Case." *The Marion Star* (Marion, Ohio). 2012: 3.

45. Musgrave, J. "West Palm Beach Pill Mill Doctor Gets 4-Year Term." *The Palm Beach Post*. 2017: B1.

46. Eil, P. "The Pill Mill." p. 8.

47. Thompson, F. "Dr Paul Volkman and the Philip Eil Saga." All Things Wildly Considered (internet). 2015 (cited March 7, 2019). Available from http://allthingswildlyconsidered.blogspot.com/2015/03/dr-paul-volkman-and-philip-eil-saga.html.

48. Stewart, C. "Opioids Epidemic: The Prophets of Pain."
The Australian (internet). 2019 (cited April 8, 2019).
Available from http://file:///F:/Dr%20Paul%20Volkmann/
Purdue%20v%20Pharma%20-%20Ausralian.htm.
49. Robertson, C. "Thirty-One Doctors, 32 Million
Pills: Sweeping Opioid Case Revealed."
The Australian. April 18, 2019.

Suggested Further Reading

Quinones, S. *Dreamland—the True Tale of America's Opiate
Epidemic*. 1st ed. New York: Bloomsbury Publishers; 2015.

Eil, P. "The Pill Mill that Ravaged Portsmouth." *Cincinnati
Magazine* (internet). 2017 (cited March 5, 2019): 1–10.
Available from https://www.cincinnatimagazine.com/features/
pill-mill-portsmouth/.

CHAPTER TWELVE

DR. HARRY BAILEY—DEEP SLEEP

Prologue

Dr. Harry Bailey's consulting rooms were in Macquarie Street, Sydney, the equivalent of Harley Street, London, where elite specialists have their headquarters. On occasions, he entertained colleagues in his office. On one of those visits, several of us were invited to take a seat and make ourselves comfortable. The room was quite dark with no window allowing daylight. Only subdued light was provided from wall and desk lamps. Dr. Bailey seated himself in a large squeaky leather chair behind a massive dark-mahogany desk decorated with several military artifacts and a bottle containing a human brain floating in formalin.

He pressed a button on his desk, and a buzzer sounded in the reception room next door. His secretary came in. She had blonde hair and was aged around twenty-five years. "Bonnie," (not her real name) said Dr. Bailey, "I want to show these gentlemen something." From his jacket pocket, he took out a monocle on a gold chain.

As soon as Bonnie saw it, her face palcd. "Oh no, Dr. Bailey," she said. "Oh no!"

Bailey began to swing the monocle on the chain.

Again, Bonnie begged, "No, Dr. Bailey, please, no."

Still swinging the monocle on the chain, Harry Bailey commanded, "Yes, Bonnie, yes, you are going to be a chicken. Crouch down. You are a chicken now."

Gradually, Bonnie bent her knees in front of herself and crouched down with her elbows bent behind her torso, flapping them like a chicken's wings, and then she started hopping around the floor on the toes of two feet in his consulting room, clucking like a chicken.

Dr. Harry Bailey was clearly gratified that his demonstration of hypnotism had gone so well in front of his amazed guests. When he was satisfied, he said to her as he put his monocle away, "Bonnie, it is over now. You can get up."

With that, Bonnie stood up and carried on as though nothing had happened. Whether she was acting or hypnotized, it was not clear to the rest of us.

Later that evening, Dr. Bailey produced a variety of drugs, among them LSD, placing them on his desk and offering them around, inviting everyone to try whatever took their fancy. It seemed this was the usual way Harry Bailey entertained guests or visitors to his consulting rooms rather than offering cheese and biscuits, and perhaps a wine or sherry, as others might do.

Dr. Harry Richard Bailey does not fit into the classic model of fraud and deceit that is usual in this book; however, he was indeed fraudulent and deceitful. And devastatingly, he was much more than that. He was wicked. The most accurate description of him is a serial killer.[1] One of the most surprising things about Bailey's story is that it took so long to be exposed. His first deaths from deep sleep therapy (DST) occurred in 1963. About twenty-four further deaths happened between then and 1979 when DST was made illegal. Over the next four years, public pressure, malpractice suits, and a manslaughter charge resulted in increasing pressure on him until he committed suicide in 1985. A Royal Commission into Mental Health Services in NSW included Chelmsford Private Hospital and deep sleep therapy. It commenced hearings in 1988 and lasted almost two years. Numerous relatives of patients who had died in Chelmsford Private Hospital realized that the deaths might have been as a result of DST. When these deaths were investigated, the true magnitude of the catastrophe was recognized by the inquiry. In the end, it was estimated that sixty-six deaths had occurred in Chelmsford and another ninety-six had committed suicide within a week of discharge and twenty-one within a year, making a total of 183 deaths. Additionally, 997 patients were considered to be brain-damaged as a result of DST.

In the Beginning

Harry Bailey was born on October 29, 1922, in Picton, New South Wales, Australia. Picton was a sleepy country village at the time, one and a half hours' or two hours' drive from Sydney's central business district (CBD). Harry's father, Jack, was a railway worker, and his mother was Ruth Smith. Harry was their eldest child. As Picton is a little out of town, it is said that Harry boarded at Christian Brothers' College in Waverley, close to Sydney's CBD, to complete his schooling. There is, however, no evidence that he was ever enrolled there. At one time, there was another Christian Brothers school in the area, and he may have attended there. At any rate, when finished at whatever Christian Brothers school he attended, he enrolled in science at Sydney University but soon ran out of money and took employment as a pharmacist's assistant. Harry Bailey married Marjorie Noonan, a cashier, in January 1945 before commencing medicine at Sydney University that year, graduating in 1951. During his studies, he won the Major Ian Vickery Prize for Paediatrics and the Norton Manning Prize for Psychiatry (for which there were only three candidates).[2,3]

After graduation, Dr. Bailey spent one year at Royal Prince Alfred Hospital in Sydney to complete his internship and then took a position at Broughton Hall Psychiatric Clinic in Lilyfield, close to the inner city. Broughton Hall had previously served as a hospital for soldiers suffering from shell shock after returning from World War I. It was located adjacent to Callan Park Hospital for the Insane, and together they were amalgamated into Rozelle Hospital in 1976. Dr. Harry Bailey was appointed assistant director of psychiatric clinical services in the Department of Public Health at the age of thirty-three years.[4]

Dr. Bailey went overseas on a World Health Organization–funded tour of the United States and Europe for fifteen months. He was already much interested in electroconvulsive therapy (ECT) as a therapeutic tool, having been introduced to it by *Dr. Cedric Swanton*, the prominent Sydney psychiatrist who was one of the first advocates of ECT in Australia. In Europe, Dr. Bailey was impressed by the neurosurgical techniques of Lars Leksell in Sweden, and he studied the other psychosurgical techniques of interventional psychiatrists and neurosurgeons of the USA, Canada, and the UK.[4] Some twenty years later, Bailey boasted to nurses in a lecture that he and another psychiatrist had used Negroes to experiment on as it was cheaper than cats because they were everywhere and cheap experimental animals.[5]

Haberfield

Dr. Harry Bailey lived in Haberfield, a suburb conveniently close to the central business district of Sydney. His house was in a rambling federation style, built of dark brick. The interior was also dark like his office in the city. The lighting was subdued, and the rooms were separated by arches with solid uncut glass blocks and quarried stone rocks of random shapes with concealed lights behind. There were many leadlight windows, in many cases with low-level concealed lighting behind them. On the walls, there were numerous artifacts of a medieval military style. Behind the house, there was a swimming pool of about two meters wide, thirty meters long, and three meters deep. Harry explained, "It works on the Bailey Principle: you can't swim longitudinally at the same time as you are swimming transversely."

He dressed in a Hawaiian shirt, short trousers, and sandals. He was quite relaxed. Harry was a charming and generous host with a great sense of humor. He only offered the best whiskey and wine. His affability concealed the monster within.

Psychosurgery

Psychosurgery is the treatment of mental health conditions by operating on the brain. Small parts of the brain are removed, destroyed, or stimulated by radiation, diathermy, freezing, or cutting the connections between them. All of the brain has a function, and in many cases, that function is not clear. Dr. Bailey believed that psychosurgery could be the treatment of choice for manic depression (now known as bipolar disorder) and obsessive-compulsive disorder as well as for psychosexual exhibitionism and compulsive antisocial behavior. He suggested that it might allow offenders to be treated in a hospital and therefore avoid prison. It has been suggested that in some cases, convicted criminals were treated with psychosurgery without giving their consent. In the case of schizophrenia, for instance, it was not known which part of the brain or which connections in the brain might be the cause. This made it difficult to know which parts of the brain should be diathermied, cauterized, or dissected. The operation would be dependent on a tiny part of the brain being the correct target. There are very few of these operations performed around the world, and in some countries, psychosurgery is illegal. Nonetheless, Dr. Bailey's brain was focused on the concept that mental disorders could be cured by surgery, just as appendicitis can be cured by removing the appendix. He believed that psychosurgery could still be very useful for other mental disorders. In Dr. Bailey's case, all his candidates for psychosurgery were referred to a psychologist, *Dr. Evan Davies*, who had been a close colleague and friend of Dr. Bailey for years. Dr. Davies would conduct a psychological assessment before and after the psychosurgery, as he attempted to measure the patients' motivation, affection, aggression, anxiety, depression, family relationships, etc. At the Chelmsford Royal Commission some years later, the commissioner commented that in his view, "The tests were of limited use." The third member of this little group was *Dr. John Dowling*, a neurosurgeon who had also been known to Harry Bailey for many years. Around 1973, psychosurgery was creating considerable interest in the medical field around the world. Dr. Dowling was keen to operate on patients referred from Bailey through Davies, and it was not long before forty neurosurgical cases were being performed every year at the Prince Henry Hospital in eastern Sydney. The results of these operations were published in the *Medical Journal of Australia*,[6,7,8,9] but they soon became the object of severe criticism by several noted psychiatrists and medical professionals because of the flawed methods of recording the findings of the study. Bailey soon found himself defending his practices.[10] In many cases, the results of the psychosurgery were simply untrue. As a consequence, the number of psychosurgical procedures dropped at Prince Henry Hospital to almost zero, to the great disappointment of Dr. Dowling.

Deep Sleep Therapy

Dr. Harry Bailey was not dependent on psychosurgery for a living.

Deep sleep therapy was introduced as a treatment regime to Australia from Europe and the USA by Dr. Bailey, who then used it with gay abandon. The risks and complications include pneumonia, deep venous thrombosis (DVT), stroke, cardiac arrest, pressure ulcers, inhaling vomit, and death. Deep sleep therapy (DST) was used in few other places in the world. The theory of combining DST and electroconvulsive therapy (ECT) seemed to be that the brain would be switched off, like a TV in those days (but like a modem being rebooted nowadays), and clear itself out, forgetting its bad habits.

When he left the salaried employment as superintendent of Callan Park, he went into private practice in Macquarie Street, where his income was derived from consulting referred patients in his private rooms. If he wanted to use DST or ECT, he would need a hospital for his patients. Deep sleep therapy and electroconvulsive therapy (ECT) were part of his plans, and he used them in combination for numerous psychiatric disorders. Anything he could think of, really. Some were not mental disorders at all, such as premenstrual tension. As well as that, the "sleep" was not a natural sleep; instead it was a drug-induced coma. Patients were heavily sedated with psychotropic or sedative drugs to keep them in a comatose or soporific state for days and sometimes weeks. Sedation or a coma was usually achieved by giving a drug called Tuinal, a combination of a very rapid but short-acting barbiturate to induce the coma quickly and a longer-acting barbiturate to keep the patient sedated.

As Dr. Harry Bailey would say, "The effectiveness of the treatment is a function of the depth of the sedation. If you keep them down deep and hold them down deep, they will do better, very much better … The real art is, of course, to watch them turn around and as they come out then you bop them again."[10] This indicated an extraordinarily cavalier, even cruel attitude, to therapy.

Once sedated, a patient might also undergo ECT by electric shock or treatment with psychotropic drugs. Patients were invariably billed for DST, ECT, and an anesthetic. Dr. Bailey seldom arranged an anesthetic, as he considered the deep sedation as adequate. This did not stop him from fraudulently billing the patient directly or indirectly through an insurance fund for an anesthetic that the patient did not have. Nowadays, DST is not approved in Australia by the Royal Australasian College of Psychiatrists, and it is illegal for any reason.

The Royal Australian and New Zealand College of Psychiatrists (RANZCP) in their November 2012 position statement on deep sleep therapy stated it "has no place in the treatment of psychiatric illness. It has not been demonstrated to be an effective treatment for any psychiatric condition and has unacceptably high morbidity and mortality rates."[11]

Electroconvulsive Therapy

Electroconvulsive therapy (ECT) is a treatment used for a variety of psychiatric illnesses, such as major suicidal depression, mania, catatonia, and personality disorders. The therapy induces seizures, and it is therefore given under general anesthetic with a muscle relaxant to avoid the patient being injured during the procedure. Once anesthetized, a low current of electricity is passed through either half of or the whole brain, depending on the condition, after having electrodes placed on the skull. ECT should be given only when the patient is anesthetized, as the body will thrash around and be injured by biting the tongue or breaking teeth, for instance. Beneficial effects may or may not follow, and the treatment might have to be repeated in days, weeks, or months, depending on the response. Some patients require regular repeat therapy. The use of ECT varies widely from country to country and from one psychiatrist to another. In some countries, ECT is illegal; in other countries, it is only used in private psychiatric facilities. In Dr. Harry Bailey's case, it was used extensively, combined with DST. He induced the electric current with a machine that he invented himself. It was called a pulsator, which he named a Minecta Mark II, and was manufactured with the help of AWA. It is said that it had no dial on it, so it was not possible to say how much electricity was being delivered. The machine could not be found after Dr. Bailey's death.

Callan Park Mental Hospital

When Dr. Harry Bailey returned to Australia from his travels to the northern hemisphere, the Department of Health was so impressed by his report that it agreed to his recommendation to establish a Cerebral Surgery and Research Unit (CSRU) at Callan Park Mental Hospital, and he was appointed director in 1957 where he had previously been assistant director. The Department of Health was so proud of its new unit that the premier himself opened the unit at Callan Park Mental Hospital. The *Sydney Morning Herald* blared, "New Sydney unit puts Australia in Front Rank of Brain Surgery. Dr Harry Bailey, the outstanding Australian psychiatrist, who is in charge of the unit, said that a new type of brain surgery would be performed at the unit for the first time outside of Sweden." It went on, "It is an operation performed by an electronic needle which can destroy damaged tissue to within half of a millimeter. Using this technique, the skull would only have to be opened by the width of the needle."[12] The unit cost over $2 million although the future of psychosurgery was doubtful.

No expense was spared. Bailey's office was huge, and he had concealed switches under his desk so that he could eavesdrop on the rooms next door through the intercom.[1] His appointment at the hospital gave him time and freedom to experiment with various techniques of ECT and psychosurgery. He was soon promoted to superintendent. Dr. Bailey was a man in a hurry, and he instituted change quickly. When he took over, Callan Park Mental Hospital was neglected and dilapidated. It had a continuous solid brick wall around it about twelve feet high to restrict the movement of the inmates. The wall was only broken by gates operated by security guards. It was a widespread view in those days that mentally ill patients should be locked up, but now they had a new superintendent, Dr. Harry Bailey, who had a different, modern view of psychiatric illness and who thought that the wall did not need to be there to contain the inmates as they were not dangerous. Dr. Bailey is credited with having the wall pulled down because of his new enlightened view of mental illness. It was not an illness that must be shut off from the public. It should be treated like any other illness. Dr. Bailey saw mental illness in a new light, and he was just the man to change things.

Not long after having the wall removed, Bailey complained to the Public Service Board that things were not all well at Callan Park, which was then the largest psychiatric hospital in Australia. He complained that there was insufficient stock, food was being stolen, staff were being cruel to patients, and patients were being neglected. The claims were investigated by police and the public service, but the outcomes were inconclusive. Bailey persisted, however, through the printed and electronic media until he embarrassed the premier, Mr. Rob Heffron, and his minister for health, Mr. William Sheehan. A Royal Commission was appointed under Mr. Justice McClemens. Dr. Bailey's claims were mostly supported by the commission, but the relationship between him and the minister for health was irreparably broken, and Bailey had to resign from Callan Park Mental Hospital.

Dr. Bailey also became a consultant psychiatrist at the Women's Hospital, Crown Street in Sydney, Australia, where I met him during the years 1968 to 1977. The Women's Hospital, as the name implies, was for obstetric and gynecologic patients. However, women are prone to postnatal depression and other mental illnesses as are men, so it was appropriate that the hospital had a Department of Gynaecological Psychiatry.

The Crown Street College of Carnal Knowledge

Dr. Harry Bailey's clinic was held on a Tuesday afternoon, starting at 1:00 p.m. It was held in a consulting room on the ground floor of the main hospital. A gynecology registrar was rostered to attend the clinic, ostensibly to learn something about gynecologic psychiatry. A large number of women would turn up by appointment and wait in a room across the corridor. Mostly, Dr. Bailey would turn up around 5:00 p.m. and go into the dining room for his dinner. The women would wait patiently under the kindly eye of the devoted, faithful, matronly nursing sister who was regularly rostered on for the clinic. She was a motherly, Italian-mamma type of woman of about sixty-five years named Sister Maria (not her real name). Most of the patients had been referred because they had been told that they were frigid. Sister Maria would gather them together like sheep and keep them calm until the great man had finished his dinner. Many of the patients had been waiting all afternoon, but there were few complaints as the solution was so close. Other patients had been to the clinic before and were back for a progress visit. Sister Maria would usher a patient into the room and invite her to lie down on a clinic trolley to wait for Dr. Bailey. It was not unknown for Dr. Bailey, when he arrived at the hospital in his white Jaguar saloon, to turn around and drive away if he found someone had parked in his parking spot. Poor Sister Maria had to rebook his entire clinic to return for another appointment.

Most treatments for frigidity (in Dr. Bailey's clinic) involved testosterone, and the patient had to return regularly to assess the effect. Dr. Bailey said that frigidity in women could be treated by increasing their testosterone levels. It was his aim that a woman's testosterone should be increased until she was "chasing her husband around the room." In the meantime, she had to return every week or two to check that she was not growing a beard and that her voice was not deepening. Dr. Bailey also assessed the effect of the testosterone by measuring the clitoris with an instrument given the descriptive name of Cliterometer.

In some cases, the woman was asked to masturbate while doctors or medical students were invited to watch. Unsurprisingly, not all women could or would comply. In spite of this, dozens of women would wait under the motherly, watchful, unflappable eye of Sister Maria, often until after midnight, to see the great Dr. Harry Bailey.

The clinic became colloquially known as the Crown Street College of Carnal Knowledge.

Private Practice

Dr. Bailey took consulting rooms in Macquarie Street now that he had to make a living separately from Callan Park Hospital. His reputation was broad, and he had no trouble securing honorary appointments to Wollongong Hospital, two hours' drive south of Sydney, as well as to Canterbury and Eastern Suburbs hospitals in the suburbs. As these appointments were honorary, Dr. Bailey derived no income from them directly; but when he saw a patient in a hospital clinic, that patient might choose to attend him in his private consulting rooms where he could charge for his services. Alternatively, as his reputation was so great, doctors in general practice referred patients to him directly.

When Dr. Harry Bailey first had to earn a living, he required access to a hospital for his inpatients, so he started at St. Anne's Private Hospital in Killara in Sydney's northern suburbs. Unfortunately for him, the nursing matron there, *Mrs. Clare Ray*, who owned the hospital, when giving evidence to the Chelmsford Royal Commission in 1989, related that she foresaw that his methods were dangerous and she made it difficult for him to admit patients to that hospital. Mrs. Ray spoke of how she "got rid" of Dr. Bailey from her hospital. She said, "I felt he was a bad man who happened to have a medical degree." She had returned from a holiday in October 1962 to find five of Dr. Bailey's patients had been admitted to her hospital for deep sleep therapy. She consulted other psychiatrists, some of whom said that they had never heard of this form of treatment. *Dr. Guy Lawrence*, who was then medical superintendent of Broughton Hall, cautioned Mrs. Ray against allowing deep sleep therapy; he said Dr. Harry Bailey was mad and warned her against him. Mrs. Ray related that when she called Dr. Bailey about a patient, his wife would answer the phone and tell her that Dr. Bailey was up a ladder or bricking up the bathroom or in the toilet and was unable to come to the phone. Mrs. Bailey herself gave advice to Mrs. Ray about how she should manage the patient. From then on, Mrs. Ray made sure that those patients who had already been admitted were not kept deeply asleep; and when Dr. Bailey requested further admissions, Mrs. Ray said that she had no beds. Being unable to admit his patients for deep sleep therapy whenever he wanted, Dr. Harry Bailey had to look around for another solution.[13]

Chelmsford Private Hospital

Dr. Bailey's attention fell on a small private hospital in the northern suburbs of Sydney that might do very well. It was in leafy Pennant Hills, a suburb in the northwestern region of Sydney. It was soon renamed Chelmsford Private Hospital and opened in January 1963. It depended on high bed occupancy to survive, and there was nothing better than to have patients of a psychiatrist to fill those beds for days on end.

The hospital was little more than a large suburban home given a license by the Department of Health to qualify it for hospital status. It had fifteen beds when first licensed, and its equipment was from the Middle Ages. Few visitors were allowed into Chelmsford, but once it began servicing patients, anyone walking through would see bed after bed, often so close that they were touching, some in the corridors, with snoring or snorting patients on their backs with tubes in their noses, lying in their own urine and feces. Some were shackled to their bed, and others were in straitjackets. Now and again, a patient would struggle and try to move—even sit up—but a nurse would come and give an injection so that the patient would collapse back in bed again, in a coma. There was no proper resuscitation equipment, such as laryngoscopes or oxygen outlets, or monitoring equipment such as electrocardiograms, blood pressure machines, or x-ray equipment.

The nurses were mostly nurse aides and not trained to care for high-risk patients. Even the registered nurses were not qualified for this sort of treatment. There was no treatment program. The medication given to patients was decided by the nurses. Bailey left blank presigned treatment sheets in the hospital. Only the patient's name had to be filled in at the top by the nurse, and then the remainder was usually completed by the nurse, often in accordance with "Dr. Bailey's Book." "Dr. Bailey's Book" was left in the ward for the nurses to fill out as they thought necessary, and it took no account of the patient's medical history, weight, or present diagnosis. The book meant that Dr. Bailey did not have to come into the hospital to start a patient's treatment. It was illegal, of course, but that did not bother Dr. Bailey. His visits to the hospital were quite rare anyway, and often he would not appear for days or weeks, and when he did attend, it was frequently after midnight. He was sometimes affected by alcohol when he came to see patients whom he had never seen before and whose treatment had already begun. It placed the nurses in the invidious position of having to make treatment decisions for which they were not trained. The procedure, in any case, was almost always the same, regardless of whether the patient was depressed, overweight, or had premenstrual tension. The treatment would be deep sleep therapy and ECT—often without a physical examination or the patient's consent.

Dr. Bailey started to use Chelmsford Private Hospital in 1963. Patients would usually be admitted for DST and ECT, often without their consent—indeed, their knowledge. Years later, in 1988, a Royal Commission of Inquiry was set up. Patients would give evidence to the commission of the atrocities that had gone on under the guise of treatment for mental illness during those years. One patient described arriving at the hospital from Dr. Bailey's consulting rooms: "A nurse led me to a darkened room and told me to undress, put on a nightgown and get into bed, which I did. She gave me a tablet to take, saying it would settle me down, and I would feel better about being there. That is all that I remember." Luckily she survived, unlike many others who woke up ten, twenty, or thirty days later and were transported to nearby Hornsby Hospital in a desperate state.

Another patient, Patricia McGuire, said, "When I arrived, I saw people sitting in the hall in a drugged state, waiting to see their doctors. I was woken about 2.30 or 3.00am and told the doctor was here to see me. He was sitting in a chair in a Hawaiian shirt and shorts. He said to me, 'Mrs. McGuire, you are having some domestic troubles; what you need is a good fuck …'" Mrs. McGuire went on, "My immediate reaction was to take my report and leave, stating that nobody speaks to me in that manner, not my husband, my sons or the men who work for us. However, I went back to my room very upset but with no money or clothes and nowhere to go. I wanted to ring my husband to come and get me. I remember the sister giving me a pill to settle me down. I did not sign consent for shock treatment or any other kind of treatment."[14]

Mrs. Ray, the matron from St. Anne's Private Hospital, later backed up Patricia McGuire's account when she related to the Royal Commission how Dr. Bailey would often tell his female patients what they needed and that he was "the one to do it."[13]

Mrs. June Brackley said, "My husband and one of my daughters drove me over to Chelmsford, where I was told I would have to stay for a couple of days for 'a little rest.' I had only been there for approximately one hour when I was given an injection and the next thing, I was coming to, nine days later, going through the most horrible vivid hallucinations. I was not told that I would be completely unconscious during this period, nor was I told that I would receive any shock treatment. I do not recall having signed any paperwork, but I was in a vague state at the time, still under the effects of the overdose of tablets. My husband informs me that he did not sign any paperwork. If I did sign any consent, I was not in a fit state to do so."

Mr. Paul Hereford-Smith said, "I cannot remember at any time that I signed any consent forms for any of the treatment that I received in Chelmsford. I was told by one of the hospital nursing aides that I had been sleeping for 31 days and that I had been given ECT. Now, please bear in mind that at no time did I sign for any of this treatment and that it was done without my knowledge."

Another patient's wife who complained that consent had not been obtained was Mrs. P. J. Ashley, who said, "Neither my husband nor I signed consent for any of this. After the fourteenth day, I was allowed to bring my husband home. He had been given shock treatment."[14]

Harry Bailey treated Chelmsford as his own personal experimental laboratory where he expounded to himself his theory of DST and ECT. He seemed to be convinced that between DST and ECT, the brain would be cleansed in the same way that we reboot a computer these days. Unfortunately, he kept no notes or accurate record of the outcome of his experiments. Often the only record of an event in a patient's treatment would be found on the back of his or her notes and then just with an enigmatic remark. No intelligible information came from Bailey's Chelmsford laboratory to explain whether it was DST that refreshed the mind or whether it was ECT that cleaned it out. Even when patients died, Dr. Bailey did not seem to let it interfere with his goal of proving that DST and ECT together could cure almost any mental derangement. The affairs at Chelmsford went on to be known as Australia's greatest psychiatric disaster.[15]

The Zombie Room

Mr. Jim Lawler, a patient, reported that he had been kept in what was known as the Zombie Room. "I was given six lots of ECT and kept against my will by means of leather gauntlets on my ankles and wrists. I cleared out of the place twice, only to be returned and strapped to my bed and, I presume, given more shock treatment."[10]

In 1973, a patient, Mr. Barry Hart, who later became the leader of the Chelmsford Victims Action Group, sued a doctor and the hospital for brain damage that he claimed was due to temporary deprivation of oxygen while under treatment with DST and ECT. He said that he had become depressed after unsuccessful and unrelated plastic surgery. The court found in his favor and awarded him damages of $60,000 although it cost him several times more than that in legal fees and court costs to prosecute the case. Pre-Chelmsford, Barry Hart was "blessed with a muscular physique and trained as an actor, he donned the iconic leotard for a Lifesavers television commercial in 1971."[16] Barry made numerous TV appearances; perhaps his most notable role was, ironically, in a local production of the 1975 *One Flew over the Cuckoo's Nest*. Barry was offered the part by director Stanley Walsh, and although initially reluctant, he later agreed and was praised for his role. Barry wanted to be involved because of the subject matter; his role was to read the words of the Indian chief Bromden. He must have felt a sense of empathy with the chief, a "once-powerful man silenced by forces beyond his control," and it's no wonder Barry became emotional during the reading.[17]

Post-Chelmsford, Barry was left with pneumonia, pleurisy, and a pulmonary embolus after his treatment, for which he never consented; instead, he was "drugged after refusing to sign a consent form." The awarded $60,000 was compensation for false imprisonment, assault and battery, and damages for several physical ailments.[16]

Stevie Wright, English-born musician and songwriter, joined the Easybeats at age sixteen in 1964 as their lead singer. Wright has been called Australia's first international pop star. The Easybeats were popular, with several hits in the Top 10 in Australia, and their international hit "Friday on My Mind" peaked at No. 1 in Australia in 1966 and made the Top 10 in the UK, France, Germany, Italy, and the Netherlands. Affectionately known as Little Stevie during these years, he was the lead vocalist with the band until 1969.[18] Stevie was admitted to Chelmsford by Harry Bailey in the late 1970s for DST and ECT for treatment of drug addiction. He was alarmed when he could hear people shrieking, so he jumped out the window in the middle of the night to escape and took off down Pennant Hills Road hoping for a lift. It's no wonder nobody picked him up, as he was naked, except for a jumper. He was horrified to see the night nurse drive past; she stopped and ordered Stevie to jump in, and with one click of the automatic switch, she locked all the doors and returned him to the hospital. Stevie recalls, "Three blokes held me down, and they chained me to the bed. In the end they broke my will."[19] Wright had fourteen shock treatments over two weeks at Chelmsford. After his release from the hospital, it took him ten years to write another song.

Dr. Harry Bailey was not known for his empathetic character. It was clear he felt he could help some of his female patients by giving them a dose of the amazing Bailey sexual prowess; however, his drug-addicted patients would cop verbal abuse. He would ask them why he should bother to treat them and told one patient that he hated junkies.[20]

And so it went on. Numerous patients had not signed consent for DST or ECT. In essence, many of them had been hijacked or kidnapped. It seemed standard practice to treat patients with whatever suited Dr. Harry Bailey. Additionally, he never bothered to explain the treatment or its effects. He signed blank treatment sheets, which could be completed by nurses later. In all, 1,127 patients would be treated with DST and ECT by Dr. Harry Bailey and his offsider between 1963 and 1977, when the treatment was terminated. At least twenty-four would die as a direct result of treatment, and nineteen others would commit suicide within a year of being discharged. Many of those who survived went home with illnesses, such as pneumonia, that they did not have before treatment began. In the meantime, Dr. Harry Bailey also referred many patients (said to be over three hundred) for psychosurgery (lobectomies) for such conditions as homosexuality, pedophilia, and postnatal depression.[21] It appeared Harry Bailey considered himself to be very special. Former nurse Mrs. Lesley Hosi said he would instruct staff,

"Don't call me Harry, call me God." He also told them he could walk on water.[22] Bailey believed the world was divided into two types of people—Martians and earthlings.[20]

The Deaths

But back in Chelmsford, Julie Myers was the first to die. She died on October 31, 1963, only days after her eighteenth birthday. She committed suicide four days after being taken home from Chelmsford by her parents who had visited her in the hospital and found her to be in "an infantile state of mind" after shock therapy. Six patients died in 1964 and then another fourteen until at least a total of twenty-four had died by 1978. Muriel Kell was the second. She died in July 1964, and five others followed her that year. Disquiet about drug policy in the hospital started to spread in 1967 following the inquest into the death of a young plumber, Ronald Carter, aged twenty-three. On the advice of the professor of psychiatry at Sydney University, Professor D. Maddison, the coroner said that "in his opinion nurses should not be left to decide how much drug should be administered to patients in deep sleep or the time between doses." Still, nothing was done by the Health Department, Medical Board, police, or media.

The Whistleblower

On March 22, 1970, a nurse at Chelmsford wrote anonymously to the Health Department and separately to the NSW Public Service Board, suggesting "that procedures at Chelmsford Hospital should be investigated." She was quickly identified as Mrs. M. Pett, a nurse at the hospital only recently employed. Nurse Pett went on, "The treatment of all patients takes place at all hours of the night and in the early hours of the morning, with machines imported from America. I believe doctors are experimenting with patients. I have known patients to be under deep sleep sedation for 21 days and being fed intravenously during that time." Nurse Pett gave much other information that resulted in an inquiry by the Health Department. The investigation was conducted by Dr. G. Procopis, the director of establishments. However, the inquiry was far from thorough and resulted in little being done. The study reported, "Dr Bailey's practice of deep sedation is well known, and although it is not generally accepted as a desirable form of therapy, the Under-Secretary of the Health Department does not consider the method should be stopped." As the manager of the Health Care Complaints Unit, Merrilyn Walton said later in relation to Nurse Pett's allegations, "No investigation took place into the clinical appropriateness of this treatment and, had it done so, many of the deaths since 1970 may have been prevented."

Again, a whistleblower was ignored, and a government department was derelict in its duty.

Michael Perry, writing for the *Jakarta Post* in 1990, believed "the horrors of Chelmsford would never have been exposed had it not been for the courage of one person, nurse *Rosa Nicholson*." It was not until 1977 when Nicholson replied to an advertisement in a Sydney newspaper that she landed herself a job at Chelmsford. Following the death of a friend after deep sleep treatment, she spent eighteen months trying to get a job there. Over the next two years, Nicholson smuggled hospital and patient records out of the hospital and copied them before returning them. For ten years, she remained undercover, leaking damning evidence against Bailey to anybody who would listen. Nicholson would later tell the Royal Commission about deep sleep patients frequently suffering from internal bleeding and severe infections, having ECT every day except Sunday. The staff remembered how Bailey would have sex with female patients, often having them sent by taxi late at night to his office or home.[23]

The Deaths Went On

On March 14, 1976, Audrey Francis died. She was the nineteenth death and a patient of one of the other doctors who wrote her death certificate, and at the inquest, her cause of death was recorded as cardiac and respiratory failure *due to natural causes*. That inquest was in 1976. There was much disquiet over the years as rumors of the events at Chelmsford became known. Another inquest into the death of Ms. Francis was held twelve years later, in 1988. The coroner, Mr. Greg Glass, on this occasion, found that she had died of cardiac and respiratory failure due to *barbiturate intoxication*. The coroner went on, "The administration of drugs at Chelmsford was based on a form of therapy not acceptable to reputable scientific opinion in 1976." Although no criminal charges and no particular action was recommended, this finding and these comments gave heart to a group of Chelmsford victims who had been agitating for an inquiry. Sadly, only those victims who had survived could agitate for an inquiry. Those who had died were silent.

Another Death

John Adams, aged twenty-three, booked into Chelmsford in September 1977 for his seventh attempt to overcome drug addiction to narcotics. This time he did not leave alive. The cause of death, which the coroner reported after a second inquest two years later, was "Respiratory failure while under deep sleep therapy." Again, this revelation caused increasing alarm among the medical fraternity and the Health Department, including the minister for health. Still, the attitude of the bureaucracy was that it was the fault of the person "who introduced him to the drugs at the age of 15."[24]

Then on August 12, 1977, Miriam Podio died. The coroner's inquest in 1982 found that her death was from treatment and suggested that Dr. Harry Bailey was negligent and should be charged with manslaughter and referred his findings to the attorney General. Many of the deaths at Chelmsford attracted two inquests because the first one was subsequently thought to be unreliable, as seen in the case of Audrey Francis, and public pressure demanded that the deaths be reviewed. Dr. Bailey, therefore, faced a serious charge, which, if proven, could land him in prison.[25]

The deaths went on until Sharon Hamilton died on February 15, 1978. Sharon was a singer and dancer who had worked briefly for Harry Bailey. She had been a patient in Chelmsford herself, first in 1974 when she sought treatment after being assaulted while performing in prison. Bailey developed a relationship with Sharon that saw her hopelessly dependent on him. She attempted suicide more than once. Bailey also dominated Sharon Hamilton sexually, and she became pregnant. He claimed to be infertile because of infantile mumps and that he could not be the father. He arranged for an abortion. He also dominated her physically and threatened to have her committed to a psychiatric institution. She was hopelessly in love with him and could not resist his advances. Sharon became pregnant again, and Bailey made her have another termination. Sharon Hamilton committed suicide three weeks later.[26]

At the same time, a complaint was lodged against Dr. Bailey by Ms. Jan Eastgate, president of the Citizens Commission on Human Rights, a social reform group sponsored by the Church of Scientology. The Scientologists had been opposed to all types of psychiatric treatment for years, especially DST, ECT, and psychotherapy. This complaint related to having a sexual relationship with a patient and the signing of blank prescriptions so that patients' names and details could be filled in later by unqualified people. Ms. Eastgate had been trying to have this complaint heard under the Medical Practitioners' Act since 1980. The pressure was building on Dr. Harry Bailey.[27]

Suicide

Although the charge of manslaughter of Miriam Podio was dismissed, the allegations of medical malpractice remained. Then another case of medical malpractice raised by Mrs. Patricia Vaughan against Bailey was to be heard on Monday, September 9, 1985, when he was to face the charges. Harry Bailey committed suicide that day. Three weeks previously, he had held a meeting with his estranged wife, his two adopted daughters, and his lover, Ms. McArthur. He planned to break up his assets and distribute them, ensuring that his lover, Ms. McArthur, would have occupancy of one of the houses. At the same time, he would ensure that he had no assets that could be attacked by the impending action because he would be bankrupt. The courts later reversed that plan and ruled that his assets were distributed in favor of the daughters.[28] He clearly knew at that time that he was going to commit suicide, and he was organizing his estate before his death. Three weeks later, on the ninth of September 1985, he drove his car about two hours north of Sydney and parked in a remote area about fifty meters from the roadway. He then took a massive overdose of the drug Tuinal, a combination of two barbiturates that he had commonly used on his deep sleep patients.[29] He left a message saying, "I would rather be having a scotch, but this bottle of German beer will have to do," and in another note, he said, "Let it be known that the Scientologists and the forces of madness have finally won."[30,31]

The Royal Commission

Bailey was still described by some as "a brilliant psychiatrist,"[32] and he had many admirers, such as Ms. Helen McArthur, who was living with him when he died. She defended him to the last at the Royal Commission, saying, "Personally, I think that everyone is pleased to slander him because he is not around and he is the ideal scapegoat." [33] His own wife, from whom he had been separated for years, defended him to the last. In spite of the small number of supporters, rumors and public exposures in the press persisted; and in August 1988, the minister for health, Mr. Collins, announced there would be a public inquiry. This, he said, would not be a Royal Commission, just a "public enquiry into mental health but it would include Chelmsford Hospital." Further pressure came from the pen of John O'Neill and Robert Haupt, writing for the *Sydney Morning Herald* in Sydney and the *Age* in Melbourne.[10,14,34] Public opinion, however, soon mandated that it would be a Royal Commission, which has many more powers than a public inquiry. A Royal Commission has the power to subpoena witnesses. In this case, it was to be one of the biggest and longest in Australian history, finally lasting 288 days. It commenced on October 4, 1988, employed twenty-eight staff, and cost about $50,000 a day. Halfway through, in April 1989, it had taken evidence from 178 witnesses and two million documents, but this evidence already revealed the magnitude of the disaster. By October 1988, another nine deaths were linked to DST and ECT at Chelmsford, bringing the total to thirty-three. It was also revealed that Dr. Bailey himself had been admitted to Chelmsford and had undergone DST and ECT in 1974 under the care of an associate using similar treatment techniques, who kept a close eye on him, contrary to the care that Dr. Bailey had shown regarding his own patients. Dr. Bailey had been depressed after a previous complaint against him had been made and was yet to be heard in court. His suicide in 1985 may have been the result of his own treatment methods.[29]

One mother who visited her son in the hospital described the scene: "Men and women lying undressed in beds side by side, most of them restrained and with tubes in their noses. They were making moaning noises. No one bothered to put a dressing gown on the patients as they were dragged between two nurses to the toilets." The next time she visited her son, he was in the same state as the others had been, being restrained and with a tube in his nose. The boy died after four months from bronchopneumonia, according to the death certificate written by Dr. Bailey. There was another death (by suicide) of Dianne Britton in 1987 while waiting for the outcome of a civil case for compensation.

Another patient, visiting the hospital, said that she saw some patients naked, some with sheets over them—strapped to their beds—and some in straitjackets, groaning. She thought that she had walked into a set from the film *One Flew over the Cuckoo's Nest*. As the commission went on, more people realized that a relative who had died in Chelmsford might have died from DST and ECT; and by November 1988, the death toll had risen to forty-one.[35] By the time the Royal Commission was finished, the death toll was up to 183 deaths during or shortly after DST in Chelmsford. Sixty-six patients died in Chelmsford Hospital, another ninety-six committed suicide within a month of discharge, and twenty-one others committed suicide within a year, a total of 183. This was 5.2 percent of all patients who underwent deep sleep therapy in Chelmsford Private Hospital.[36] Another 997 patients were said to be brain-damaged.[37]

Epilogue

Dr. Harry Bailey was nefarious. On the one hand, he could be charming and hospitable, generous and amusing; but on the other, he was totally devoid of empathy for his patients. He was gregarious, and he was a callous, devious bully. At the same time, his prescribing of drugs was fraudulent, and his billing of patients and insurance companies was dishonest. He covered his tracks by writing false death certificates showing that patients had died from natural causes when, in fact, they died from the effects of his treatment. There is strong presumptive evidence that he was responsible for the destruction or removal of the medical records of patients who had died. Bailey did not seek the counsel of his colleagues or of ethics committees. Bailey sought no guidance from his peers but preferred to project an image of himself as being above reproach. He was a sadistic psychopath who had no boundaries and no conscience. He knew that his treatments were causing death, but he went on causing deaths by experimenting on them. Bailey did not kill for pleasure, like Harold Shipton or Michael Swango. He killed because he did not care. He should never have been a doctor. It would have been better if he had never been born. The commission, under Justice John Slattery, described Bailey as "two-faced, devious, dissembling and unprincipled. It accused him of a disgraceful breach of all standards of principled medicine in relations with female patients. Bailey had brought the profession of psychiatry into disrepute." He has been described as a serial killer, a description that seems entirely appropriate.[1]

Notes

1. Kaplan, R. *Medical Murder: Disturbing Cases of Doctors Who Kill*. Sydney, NSW: Summersdale Publishers; 2011.

2. Garton, S. *Bailey, Harry Richard (1922–1985)*. 17th ed. *Sydney: Australian Dictionary of Biography* vol. 17 (MUP); 2007. National Centre of Biography, Australian National University.

3. Bromberger, B., J. Fife-Yeomans. *Deep Sleep: Harry Bailey and the Scandal of Chelmsford.* 1st ed. East Roseville, NSW: Simon and Schuster; 1991. p. 2.

4. Garton, S: *Harry Bailey*. 2007.

5. Cheeves, H., and D. Cheeves. *Legacy*. Trafford Publishing (UK); 2004. p. 234.

6. Bailey, H. R., J. L. Dowling, C. H. Swanton. "Studies in Depression: Cingulo-Tractotomy I the Treatment of Severe Depressive Illness." *Med. J. of Aust.* Jan. 2, 1971; 1(1): 8–12.

7. Bailey, H. "Studies in Depression. II. Treatment of the Depressed, Frigid Woman." *Med. J. of Aust*. April 28, 1973; 1(17): 834–837.

8. Bailey, H., J. Dowling, E. Davies. "Studies in Depression. 3. The Control of Affective Illness by Cingulotractotomy: A Review of 150 Cases." *Med. J. of Aust.* August 25, 1973; 2(8): 366–371.

9. Dowling, J. L., H. R. Bailey. "Cingulotractotomy and Leucotomy." *Med. J. Aust.* Dec. 15, 1973; 2(24): 1,101.

10. O'Neill, J., and R. Haupt. "The Chelmsford Nightmare." *The Age* (Melbourne). July 30, 1988: 163, 170.

11. "Royal Australian & New Zealand College of Psychiatrists (RANZCP) Position Statement No. 34—Deep Sleep Therapy." Nov. 2012. Committee for Therapeutic Interventions and Evidence-Based Practice. Available from https://www.wpanet.org/uploads/News-Zonal-Representatives/wpa-policy-papers-from-zone-18/ZONE%2018-RANZCP.34_PS-2012-Deep-Sleep-Therapy-web.pdf.

12. Staff. "New Sydney Unit Puts Australia in Front Rank of Brain Surgery." *Sydney Morning Herald*. December 6, 1958: 3.

13. Fife-Yeomans, J. "Dr Bailey Scared Me, Says Matron." *SMH*. January 25, 1989: 2.

14. O'Neill, J., R. Haupt. "We Accuse." *SMH*. July 30, 1988: pp. 1, 74, 170.

15. Citizens Committee on Human Rights (Sydney, NSW), 1986. *The Chelmsford Report: Australia's Greatest Psychiatric Disaster*.

16. Walters, C. "Chelmsford Victim Gets a Legal Ray of Hope, but It's 36 Years Overdue." *SMH*. September 7, 2009.

17. The New Theatre History. Person of interest— Barry Hart. Available from http://newtheatrehistory. org.au/wiki/index.php/Person_-_Barry_Hart.

18. McFarlane, I. Encyclopedia entry for "Stevie Wright." *Encyclopedia of Australian Rock and Pop*. St. Leonards, NSW: Allen & Unwin; 1999.

19. Browne, R. "The Addiction that Took Everything from Stevie Wright." *SMH*. December 28, 2015.

20. Coulton, M. "Dr Harry Bailey's Bizarre Life and Death." *SMH*. September 1985: 1

21. Birnbauer, B., J. Davies. "The Doctors Who Play God." *The Age* (Melbourne, Victoria, Australia. February 14, 1999: 9.

22. Fife-Yeomans, J. "Ex-Nurse: I Thought Dr Bailey Was Mad." *SMH*. September 26, 1989: 4.

23. Perry, M. "Horror Tales Emerge from Australian Hospital." *The Jakarta Post* (Indonesia). December 28, 1990.

24. Franklin, R. "The Deep Sleep Therapy from Which John Did Not Wake." *SMH*. February 17 1980: 15.

25. "Doctor Charged over Death." *SMH*. March 10, 1983: 47.

26. Dean, A. "Bailey Used Dancer's Love for Own Gain." *SMH*. December 21, 1990: 6.

27. Staff. "Doctor Seeks Inquiry Delay." *SMH*. December 4, 1984: 5.

28. Lagan, B. "Deep Sleep Doctor's Death Wish Annulled." *SMH*. November 21, 1987: 9.

29. Staff. "Psychiatry's Stormy Petrel Dies a Lonely Death in His Car." *SMH*. September 11, 1985: 3.

30. Coultan, M. "The Bizarre Life and Death of Dr Harry Bailey." *SMH*. September 14, 1985: 11.

31. Bromberger. *Deep Sleep*. p. 1.

32. Soper, H. "Obituary: Psychiatry Suffers Great Loss." *SMH*. September 22, 1985: 144.

33. Fife-Yeomans, J. "Dr Bailey, an 'Ideal Scapegoat.'" *SMH*. August 8, 1989: 8.

34. O'Neill, J., R. Haupt. "Collins Announces Public Inquiry in Response to Herald Disclosure." *SMH*. August 1, 1988:4.

35. Fife-Yeomans, J. "Deep-Sleep Toll Now Put at 41." *SMH*. November 1, 1988: 3.

36. Fife-Yeomans, J. "First Statistics on Therapy in Report to Commission." *SMH*. December 20, 1989: 14.

37. Reuters. "Mental Hospital Horrors Shock Australia." *The Vancouver Sun*. BC, Canada; December 20, 1990: 8.

Suggested Further Reading

Kaplan, Robert M. *Medical Murder: Disturbing Cases of Doctors Who Kill*. Allan and Unwin. June 30, 2009.

Bromberger, Brian, and Janet Fife-Yeomans. *Deep Sleep: Harry Bailey and the Scandal of Chelmsford*. Simon and Schuster. 1991.

CHAPTER THIRTEEN

DR. GRAEME REEVES—THE BUTCHER OF BEGA

Prologue

"Until now, I thought the law was to protect the public and the people. I have now learnt otherwise." *Carolyn DeWaegeneire* was livid! On the morning of July 1, 2011, outside Sydney's Downing Centre District Court, the fifty-eight-year-old widow had heard that *Dr. Graeme Reeves* could be released from jail as early as 2013.[1] We can only imagine how Ms. DeWaegeneire felt when she discovered he was released on parole from Sydney's Long Bay Jail just before Christmas only two years later, having served only eighteen months of his original three-and-a-half-year sentence despite a non-parole period of two years.[2,3]

Initially from the United Kingdom, now a resident of Wolumla—near Bega in New South Wales, Australia—in 2002, Carolyn sought treatment for a small patch of discolored skin on her labia from Dr. Reeves, an obstetrician and gynecologist in Bega. She could not have known upon entering his rooms that restrictions had been placed on his registration, that a raft of serious complaints hounded him, and that this consultation would result in the removal of her clitoris and labia without a medical reason or consent.

The conversations alleged to have occurred around the time of this surgery might have come straight out of a B-grade horror movie. Carolyn DeWaegeneire says she had consented to a "simple vulvectomy" to treat a precancerous lesion on her labia and at no time was there any discussion of the need to remove her clitoris. In the seconds before she succumbed to the anesthetic, she recalls Dr. Reeves leaning over her and whispering in her ear, "I am going to take your clitoris, too."[4] This story is simultaneously incredible and cringeworthy.

Dr. Graeme Reeves

Born on July 28, 1950, Graeme Stephen Reeves graduated in medicine from the University of New South Wales in 1975.[3] He was elected to the Royal Australasian College of Obstetricians and Gynaecologists in 1981.[4] He married Sharon McGrath, whose parents had announced their engagement in the *Sydney Morning Herald* on November 24, 1973.[5] His father had died in Reeves's arms of a heart attack at age fifty-five the previous year, before he was able to see him graduate from medical school.[6] Reeves was the only male among six siblings.[7]

Northern Sydney Area Health Service—Hornsby Hospital, 1985–2000

Reeves worked at several hospitals in and around Sydney between 1977 and 1998, including Hornsby Hospital, Sydney Adventist Hospital, and the Hills Private Hospital to the north of Sydney as well as the Royal Hospital for Women–Paddington near the central business district (CBD).[8] He also worked at Richmond, about forty kilometers from Sydney's CBD, as a family practitioner from 2001 to 2003 and illegally at the Bega

Hospital and his private office in Bega on the far south coast of NSW between 2002 and 2003.

Dr. Reeves worked at several of these centers simultaneously. It seems that after he burned his bridges at one, he moved on to the next until such time as he was well known around Sydney, from where he moved on to the south coast, perhaps hoping that word would not have spread that far.

Banned from Obstetrics—1997

By 1986, complaints were gathering at an alarming rate. In 1997, The NSW Medical Board banned Reeves from practicing obstetrics after he was found guilty of professional misconduct.

In December 2000, he was suspended from practicing gynecology at Hornsby Hospital after working relations reached the point where midwives refused to work with him.[9]

In 2004, he was deregistered entirely as a doctor by the Medical Council for continuing to practice obstetrics despite having been banned for seven years. In 2008, the press exposed Reeves when they dubbed him the *Butcher of Bega* after he mutilated Ms. DeWaegeneire. Subsequently, his medical career ended in jail time amid a host of complaints from former patients, medical colleagues, and nursing and midwifery staff.[10]

It is alleged that former doctor Graeme Reeves has mutilated or sexually abused as many as five hundred female patients during his time working as an obstetrician and gynecologist at various hospitals across Sydney and the NSW south coast.[8]

The Northern Sydney Area Health Service covers Hornsby Hospital, the Sydney Adventist Hospital, the Royal North Shore Hospital, and others. Graeme Reeves was appointed to the position of visiting medical officer in obstetrics and gynecology at Hornsby Hospital on December 20, 1985. NSW

Health policy required the hospital to check his qualifications and registration, but there is no evidence that they did.[11]

Although Reeves may have been quite pleased with himself, landing this new appointment five days before Christmas, the women of Hornsby would have been unsettled if they had known how Reeves might turn out. Only six months after his first appointment at Hornsby, the picture began to unravel.

Complaints related to his behavior and clinical practice included bullying and aggression toward staff and patients, his condescending attitude toward junior medical and nursing staff, sometimes in the presence of patients, his failure to communicate clinical information to other staff, and his failure to offer pain relief. By July 1986, only six months after his commencement at Hornsby, an internal memorandum referred to a proposed meeting at which Reeves would be told that he might not be recommended for the full term of three years if his behavior did not improve. He was reminded that he was serving a probationary period during the first twelve months of his appointment.[10]

Spreading the Misery over the Next Fifteen Years

Reeves secured this position at Hornsby because authorities failed to conduct the required preemployment checks. The NSW Health Department review that would take place some twenty-two years later provides an unsettling insight into Reeves's practice during his time in the hospitals of North Sydney.

In 2008, the New South Wales Health Department engaged a retired federal court judge, the Honorable *Deirdre O'Connor*, to conduct a review of the behavior of the deregistered Reeves. Her report, released in May 2008, covers twenty-three years. Her findings are disturbing.[11]

In November 1986, less than twelve months after his commencement, Hornsby Hospital sent Reeves a letter drawing his attention to previous complaints and incidents and invited him to respond, "as they may reflect on your ongoing appointment and service." He did not reply.

Between 1986 and early 1989, the number of complaints had risen to eleven, relating to seven different incidents.[12] The hospital management met with Reeves on three occasions to address these issues; however, amazingly, he was reappointed to the hospital in 1988.

Three more incidents occurred between February and April 1990. The review by Justice O'Connor could find no evidence that the hospital had taken any action.[13] Again, Reeves was reappointed in 1991!

Over the following years, complaints accumulated. Further meetings were held between management and Reeves to discuss these incidents. At one meeting, in July 1995, he was advised to seek professional counseling and was offered referral to the Impaired Registrants Program at the NSW Medical Board, which he declined.[13] (NSW Medical Board is the organization with authority to license a medical practitioner. It is illegal to practice in NSW without being registered with the board. Other committees mentioned in this chapter are committees convened by hospitals or government—Ed.)

Twelve months later, for the first time since 1986, a formal written warning letter was sent to Dr. Reeves. His aggressive and unacceptable behavior had raised serious concerns. One of the consequences would be a "formal review," the letter warned, if the behavior continued, another being the termination of his appointment as a visiting medical officer.[14]

In late 1995, a pediatric registrar and two midwives complained about Dr. Reeves's attitude and manner toward a couple after the woman had given birth to a nonviable fetus. They complained that Dr. Reeves attempted to remove the placenta without adequate pain relief and that he refused offers by the pediatric registrar and nursing staff as they attempted to resuscitate the patient after she had a massive postpartum hemorrhage.[13]

The hospital convened a Medical Advisory Committee (MAC) to investigate this and several other recent incidents. In March 1996, they found Reeves had demonstrated a "lack of professional conduct and unacceptable behaviour." They noted that personal and health issues might have contributed; however, as the pattern could not continue, action had to be taken.[14]

As the committee had not been informed of any other major incidents involving Dr. Reeves, they simply issued him with a formal warning. The hospital had not been informed that three further patient complaints about Reeves had been referred to the Health Care Complaints Commission (HCCC), two of which had originated from the Hornsby Hospital.

After studying all documentation related to the incidents, the Medical Board advised the committee that Reeves had reduced his work commitments and was managing his health-related issues.[14] It seems that Reeves was off the hook again!

Warnings and Reappointments

Justice O'Connor discovered that Reeves had been sent a letter as long ago as January 1997 inviting him to reapply. Despite the adverse findings against him, a formal reprimand by the MAC, and several incidents investigated by the NSW Medical Board for prosecution before a Professional Standards Committee (PSC), he was again invited to reapply.[12] The incompetence beggars belief!

The Medical Advisory Committee recommended in August 1997 that Dr. Reeves should be reappointed "for a temporary period of twelve months, subject to review, with privileges limited to gynaecology, provided that Dr Reeves complied with the conditions imposed by the Committee." Accordingly, this reappointment process did not consider his performance of any importance in relation to Dr. Reeves.[13] After three more complaints between September 1999 and June 2000 relating to the gynecology clinic, the hospital wrote to the Medical Board, saying, "The hospital foreshadows that, subject to due process, it was likely to discontinue Dr Reeves' clinical privileges" as he had still failed to provide the information required to support his compliance with the conditions of the Professional Standards Committee.[9,14]

Termination from Hornsby Hospital in 2000—Unsafe Environment

Medical administration at the hospital could not guarantee a safe working environment for midwifery staff or a safe place for patients while Reeves was around, so they had no choice but to suspend him from attending the gynecology clinic or caring for patients in the hospital, pending an investigation. His temporary reappointment at the hospital with restricted privileges soon expired, leaving him devoid of any privileges at Hornsby Hospital. Reeves did not work at Hornsby Hospital after December 2000. As he had failed to supply the hospital with the requested information relating to his appointment, they refused to renew his credentials, and the hospital did not hear from him again.[9]

The Hills Private Hospital (1983–1996)

The Hills Private Hospital was "a landmark on Windsor Road, a major arterial route through the Hills District of North

Western Sydney for over 40 years."[15] Reeves worked there between 1983 and 1996, at which time the NSW Medical Board received notice of a "marked deterioration" in his performance. Reeves became very aggressive and made "unprovoked verbal attacks" on nurses, without a care about who else could hear his tirades. These outbursts often occurred within earshot of patients, relatives, and visitors.[16]

His time at the Hills ended that year after the death of *Kerry Ann McAllister* in May 1996.[16,17] Ms. McAllister had given birth to her third son when she developed septicemia, and despite nurses begging Reeves in vain to give her antibiotics, she died after he refused. Ms. McAllister had mentioned multiple times that her son and husband had both been sick with the flu, and although she complained of a sore throat and congested lungs, the court heard that Reeves refused to enter her room to examine her as he did not want to "catch it." Worried nurses reported that her temperature had climbed to 40.3 degrees; it is alleged that Reeves retorted, "I am well aware of her temperature, she has got a virus."[1]

When the case came before the NSW District Court, it heard that Reeves continued to dismiss the nurses' concerns about her rising temperature and pain. According to his barrister, Ragni Mathur, Reeves believed that Ms. McAllister had a viral infection. Ms. Mathur suspected the trial would hear evidence that viral and bacterial infections produced symptoms that were "indistinguishable" from one another.[18] Mathur also claimed that other doctors who had seen Ms. McAllister had also neglected to prescribe antibiotics.

Prosecutor David Price had a different view. He said a "reasonably competent" obstetrician could have diagnosed Ms. McAllister as having a bacterial infection. Price continued, "His failure to take steps to investigate Kerry's condition appropriately and his failure to assume and treat for bacterial infection was a gross deviation from the standard of care expected of a reasonably competent obstetrician."[18] He continued, "It seems evident that Kerry had a bacterial infection from the outset. If Dr Reeves had acted differently, it is highly likely that Kerry would have received appropriate treatment much earlier."

Reeves eventually organized for Ms. McAllister to be transferred to Westmead Hospital, only after he saw results of blood tests ordered by another doctor. In need of intensive care, suffering from organ failure, sadly it was too late. Kerry died at Westmead Hospital the next day, leaving behind her husband and three sons.[17,18,19] In 1999, Ms. McAllister's family sued the hospital and reached an out-of-court settlement.

Reeves was found not guilty of manslaughter, but he did admit that his failings had led to her death.[17] Countless victims suffered at his hands—women, men, boys, babies, nurses, and midwives, to name a few. A midwife who had worked for several years with Reeves at the Hills told the *Sydney Morning Herald* that often nurses were too afraid to confront him about his "rough" treatment of patients. She indicated the bizarre behavior had gone on over several years "in the late 1980s and early 1990s." She said, "He was super aggressive when nursing staff informed him of their concerns."[16]

On July 31, 1996, a few months after Ms. McAllister died, Dr. Alfred Lewis (chairman of the Medical Advisory Board at the Hills Hospital) had written a letter to the Medical Board explaining that the hospital had seen Reeves "decline" over the previous twelve months. Dr. Lewis was most concerned about the increasing verbal attacks, a "marked deterioration in his performance," repeated transgressions at the Hills, and the knowledge that both Hornsby and Sydney Adventist hospitals had observed similar behavior.[16] Dr. Lewis noted that Reeves was on antidepressants after having been discharged from the Medical Board's Impaired Doctors' Program. Review by the Department of Obstetrics and Gynaecology concluded that Ms. McAllister had not received adequate care. Lewis advised that the hospital had decided to suspend Reeves's privileges as a visiting medical officer at the Hills Private Hospital indefinitely.

It was another year before Reeves was found guilty of professional misconduct and banned from obstetrics but allowed to continue practicing gynecology if he agreed to get psychiatric help.[16,20] This privilege came to an end on December 14, 2000, when the hospital suspended him from the gynecology clinic after midwives refused to work with him. By 2001, complaints were rolling in, spanning the previous fifteen years. Among them were bullying, rudeness, angry verbal outbursts, and failure to provide adequate pain relief. Reeves had gained an appalling reputation around Northern Sydney.

It was time to move on, and so he did, down to the far south coast of NSW. Perhaps Reeves thought nobody would know him down there? Perhaps he thought he'd just keep quiet and hope they did not check. It had worked for Dr. Death—Jayant Patel, also featured in this book. Patel had blatantly lied on his CV, scoring himself a position with Queensland Health. And check? Southern Area Health Service and Bega Hospital did not check either.

Southern Area Health Service (SAHS)

The 1990s had taken their toll on Reeves. Aside from the obvious professional problems he was having, he was also "impaired by personality and relationship problems and depression, which impinged on his capacity to practice medicine."[21] In 2002, Reeves moved to the NSW south coast as he wanted a "lifestyle change,"[8] so he worked in the town of Bega and at the Bega District Hospitals from April 2002 until July 2003.

Bega is the urban center of the Sapphire Coast. Famous for cheese making since 1900, it is surrounded by lush dairy country, rivers, creeks, lagoons, and national parks. The farmers market brings the town's center to life, featuring locally produced fruit, vegetables, meat, egg, honey, and wine.[22]

Reeves's appointment to the Bega Hospital with the Southern Area Health Service (SAHS) was possible due to his "intentional and calculated dishonesty."[23] The health service was unaware that the Professional Standards Committee had ordered in June 1997 that Reeves was not to practice obstetrics.[24] Background checks were inadequate. SAHS did not check with the NSW Medical Board whether Reeves was qualified to practice in the areas for which he was employed.[25]

A hospital executive had a phone conversation with an unnamed referee of Reeves in April 2002. Handwritten diary notes state that the referee told the executive that they had "last heard Reeves was not meant to do obstetrics." The notes also referred to Reeves's depression and "arguments with nursing staff and junior registrars."[25]

The Medical Tribunal recognized that Dr. Reeves had deliberately set out to deceive the health service and that he had done so successfully. The advertisement required an obstetrician and gynecologist, so in his written application, Reeves referred to himself as a gynecologist. He also provided the letter from the medical board, which did not refer to the conditions imposed by the Professional Standards Committee, nor did he make any mention on his curriculum vitae that there were any such conditions.[26]

Not only did they fail to check, but they also ignored that warning from a referee. The senior health department executive who had spoken to one of Reeves's referees on the phone and had been told he was "not meant to do obstetrics" proceeded to employ him anyway. It was with this background that Reeves was appointed and continued practicing on the south coast of NSW.[25] Reeves was "regarded as a prestigious addition to the Bega Valley hospital services" and given a red-carpet welcome.[8]

The chief executive officer of SAHS, Dr. Denise Robinson, told a local newspaper, "We are delighted that Dr Reeves has come to the area and we are delighted to see local women with access to this (gynaecological and obstetric) service in Bega Valley once again."[8]

Reeves might have felt quite pleased with himself thinking his deceitful nature had won him another chance to continue his rogue ways; however, life did not improve for Reeves after his sea change. While the CEO of SAHS thought it was a boon for the south coast, Reeves was all set to spread the misery. Perhaps a boon for the women of Northern Sydney who were rid of him, not so for the women of the south coast.

Carolyn DeWaegeneire

Carolyn DeWaegeneire was a resident of Wolumla on the south coast of NSW who consulted her family doctor, Dr. Salisbury, about a two-centimeter area of thickened skin on her vulva.[27] A biopsy was taken, revealing an area of vulval intraepithelial neoplasia 3 (VIN 3) on her left labia minora. (VIN 3 indicates a precancerous lesion that can progress to cancer if left untreated—Ed.) Dr. Salisbury referred Ms. DeWaegeneire to Dr. Reeves for a consultation. Carolyn consented to a simple vulvectomy (removal of the vulva and nothing else), and the operation went ahead on August 8, 2002, in nearby Pambula Hospital.[8] DeWaegeneire recounts the panic she felt when Reeves leaned over her in the seconds before she succumbed to the anesthetic and said, "I'm going to take your clitoris too."

Nurse Demmery was in attendance during the operation. While giving evidence, Nurse Demmery said she had questioned Dr. Reeves about the amount of tissue he was taking and that he explained he was taking that much so that the cancer couldn't spread. When she retorted with "You wouldn't be taking my clitoris, no matter what," he said it did not matter as Carolyn's husband was dead.[28]

DeWaegeneire claims Reeves never mentioned the clitoris to her at all, and she was completely unaware it would be removed. She said that she would never have walked through the hospital door had she known that was what was intended.[29,30]

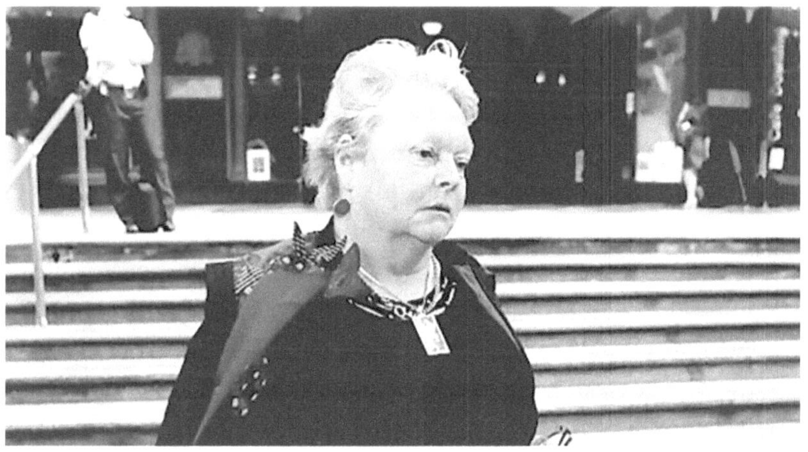

Carolyn DeWaegeneire
Photo by Simon Alekna (with permission)

While giving evidence in the High Court of Australia in July 2013, Reeves claimed he had taken a history from Carolyn DeWaegeneire during that initial consultation and used a colposcope to examine her. A colposcope is a binocular microscope. Ms. DeWaegeneire denied he used such an instrument but said he told her he would excise the lesion, drew her a diagram, and told her it would be a simple operation.[31,32]

Expert Evidence

Earlier, during the hearing in the Criminal Court of Appeal in 2012, two expert witnesses—Dr. Andrew Pesce, a specialist obstetrician and gynecologist, and Dr. Andrew Korda, a professor of obstetrics and gynecology—gave evidence. They explained that generally, every effort is made to preserve the clitoris and, if removing it is unavoidable, the implications should be discussed with the patient. They each stated they felt the surgery was excessive.[33] Dr. Korda said the operation could have been performed without removing the clitoris.[34]

Three gynecological oncologists—Drs. Davy, Dalrymple, and Professor Hacker—said that "the extent of the surgery was not appropriate for the presentation of a single lesion."[33]

Two pathologists called by the Crown, Dr. Edwards and Dr. Jain, each examined specimens taken from Ms. DeWaegeneire. Apart from VIN 3, they said none of it, not even the clitoris, had evidence of lichen sclerosus, which would have been a more notable finding. Dr. Jain said it was not an invasive malignancy.[35]

Carolyn DeWaegeneire's GP concurred she only saw VIN 3, not dystrophy or lichen sclerosus, and the letter Reeves wrote her made no reference to lichens sclerosus or dysplasia.[36] During the hearing, Reeves, in an attempt to explain why he took so much tissue, claimed he had seen evidence of dystrophy; he explained this is thinning and reddening in the vulval area. Reeves added that there was "quite a degree" of dystrophy and it meant abnormal growth and appearance. He continued, stating it was also known as "lichen sclerosus et atrophicus," and it is sinister when localized on the vulva. And in combination with VIN 3, it is more likely that invasive cancer would follow in the future.[37]

The presence of dystrophy would be an essential finding, but Dr. Reeves failed to note the presence of dystrophy in the letter he wrote to the referring doctor, Dr. Salisbury, and he also failed to note it on the consent form that Carolyn DeWaegeneire signed and on the operation record.[38] The prosecutor alleged that Reeves had forged the clinical notes by adding, after the fact, a notation of "DYS" and the words "lesion on vulva noticed in the past two years."[39]

Ms. DeWaegeneire woke up with a clitoridectomy for which she had not consented. Her whole genitalia—including her labia majora, her labia minora, her clitoris, and her perineum—had been removed, all without her knowledge or consent, a form of female circumcision or genital mutilation. Female genital mutilation (FGM), unless medically necessary, is a crime under section 45 of the Crimes Act.[40,41,42]

During the high court hearing of July 2013, the prosecution pitched their case to the jury on two bases. Firstly, they asked, was the operation necessary, and did Reeves believe it was necessary? Did he obtain DeWaegeneire's informed consent, and did he believe he had? And secondly, did Graeme Reeves perform an unnecessary operation without gaining consent, and was he aware he was committing one or both of those offenses? At some points, the prosecution suggested that Reeves's actions might have been motivated by spite, as he thought Carolyn DeWaegeneire could do with being "put in her place" as he "thought she was a bit uppity."[43]

In any case, while the truth behind this evil act may never be discovered, one must wonder if Dr. Graeme Reeves knew—indeed, still knows—why he did what he did that day. The question of intent was raised by Associate Professor Paul Macneill from Sydney University's Centre for Values, Ethics and the Law in Medicine. Macneill speculates that due to the volume of complaints and pattern of behavior, the "prosecution may be able to build a case based on circumstantial evidence, to suggest that he set out to intentionally harm these women." Macneill also noted that newspapers had suggested Reeves was a misogynist.[41]

There is, however, no question about the physical and emotional scars Ms. DeWaegeneire and many of Reeves's patients live with. Carolyn woke up in agony and said it was months before she could sit on a chair and a year before she could use toilet paper. She told the *Herald* that "every nerve ending was screaming."[41] When she woke up in the ward after having lost one-and-a-half liters of blood, Reeves told her, "The fun bits always bleed a lot."[44]

Like many women who have had the misfortune of suffering at the hands of Graeme Reeves, life for Carolyn DeWaegeneire had changed forever. Indeed, Reeves's life was not getting any less complicated. His mother died in November 2002, and he was said to be so distraught he was unable to deliver the eulogy.[7] In the same month, the Medical Board discovered he had been practicing obstetrics, and they wrote to him to remind him of the Professional Standards Committee order. His reply was, according to the Medical Tribunal, "a litany of lies and deceptive statements." Reeves assured them he would not practice obstetrics again; however, he continued to do so illegally and recklessly, a butcher, aggressively and sexually assaulting patients until his contract was terminated in July 2003. When the Area Health Service discovered he had been practicing illegally, "it failed to take appropriate steps to enforce this ban."[45]

Termination from Southern Area Health Service—2003

An inquiry held by the Medical Board in February 2003 reaffirmed that Reeves was not permitted to practice obstetrics. The health service gave him three months' notice that his contract would not be renewed. Reeves commenced an appeal against the decision to terminate him, but he did not pursue it.[46]

A Law unto Himself

Despite having been ordered by the Professional Standards Committee of the NSW Medical Board in 1997 to "cease the clinical practice of obstetrics," Reeves continued to practice obstetrics at Bega Hospital and in his private offices in Bega between 2002 and 2003.[47]

Reeves carried on until he was deregistered in 2004 for continuing to practice obstetrics despite the ban. Reeves claimed he continued to work as women needed him. The Health Care Complaints Commission (HCCC) set up an inquiry into the delivery of patient and hospital care in NSW chaired by Peter Garling, SC. It was convened in January 2008. Reeves told the Garling Commission of Inquiry in May 2008 that he "felt, in all conscience that I could not stand back and watch disaster after disaster after disaster happen." He added that the "standard of care had improved in my presence, not become worse." It seemed that Graeme Reeves was seriously deluded.[19]

Deregistered—July 23, 2004

By 2004, the NSW Medical Board had noticed his "bare-faced lies" and "deceptive conduct" and subsequently struck him off for "gross professional misconduct of the most serious kind."[8] The period between 2004 and 2007 saw complaints continue to roll in with no action taken, as Reeves had been deregistered.[41] Over these years, Carolyn DeWaegeneire did some research and mustered the courage to speak up. She was initially told there was no benefit in pursuing the matter, but she commenced civil proceedings and eventually complained to the police. DeWaegeneire became frustrated that so many women had been ignored for years; she said, "Marriages have been broken up, women have been so traumatized they won't let their partners touch them."[41] Carolyn was allegedly told by staff at the Complaints Commission in NSW to go and have her hair done so she might "feel better."[48]

Christine Griffin, another of Reeves's victims, was told in 2004 there was no use pursuing a charge at the time even though she would later testify: "I knew what he had done to me was rape." Marilyn Hawkins, who believes Reeves sexually assaulted her and ruined her surgery, received a similar response.[49]

Strike Force Tarella—February 2008

A police investigation called Strike Force Tarella involving fifteen full-time detectives from the Child Protection and Sex Crimes Squad was established on February 27, 2008, to investigate 113 allegations of abuse and misconduct. The investigation took seven months and is unique in the history of the sex crimes squad.[20]

Mrs. Jillian Skinner (North Shore, deputy leader of the opposition) reported to the Legislative Assembly that she was in the Bega electorate for a conference when *Andrew Constance*, member for Bega, asked her to meet with Carolyn DeWaegeneire, which they did in July 2007. Ms. DeWaegeneire had proceedings before the court; she asked them to keep her story in confidence, which they did until after the media exposure that was to come.[49]

Exposed—the Media Frenzy of 2008

Lorraine Long, the founder of private watchdog Medical Error Action Group (MEAG), had received many complaints about Reeves and had been ignored for years by the NSW Health Department. In 2007, out of sheer desperation, she approached respected investigative journalist *Ross Coulthard*, who worked for Channel 9's *Sunday* program. They eventually exposed the government's failings and cover-ups when they aired "Who Watches the Doctors?" on February 17, 2008.

Harmed patients came forward in droves, prompting Nine television Network to follow up with "The Butcher of Bega: Australia's Worst Medical Disaster?" which aired on March 2, 2008. Prompted by further information, Nine Network aired a third cover story on May 4, 2008, called "Questions Surround the Butcher of Bega over Deaths." In conjunction with the timings of Nine Network's TV programs, the *Sunday Telegraph* ran front-page stories: "Hundreds Betrayed by Doctor—NSW Specialist Who Butchered Women," "The Butcher of Bega—the Government Finally Acts," and "Butcher Linked to Fifteen Deaths."[48] Reports said Reeves had "committed such monstrous acts that hundreds of terrified victims remained silent for over five years."[8]

Media attention focused on the case of Carolyn DeWaegeneire as they dubbed Reeves *the Butcher of Bega*. Ms. DeWaegeneire had finally broken her five-year silence, along with two other women on Channel Nine's *Sunday* program, and this started an avalanche of further complaints.[8] Media attention related to more than five hundred complaints by former patients who alleged he had mistreated them, sexually assaulted them, and/or performed unnecessary and mutilating gynecological surgery on them.

The *Daily Telegraph* in Sydney reported that Dr. Reeves was still not under investigation by police, the NSW Medical Board, or the Health Care Complaints Commission (HCCC). They continued, "Women who had placed their trust in the new doctor were soon allegedly being betrayed in the most intimate of ways. The litany of complaints included losing a kidney, having genitals sewn up or cut up, inappropriate examinations, fondling and lewd comments."[8]

After the media exposure, Jillian Skinner, with whom Carolyn DeWaegeneire had spoken in July the previous year, wrote to Commissioner Garling and the HCCC, asking them how it could be that Graeme Reeves was employed by SAHS and why none of the patient complaints had been investigated by the commission. The HCCC said they would work with the police, and Garling agreed to investigate, which he did, taking six months to compile a report, handed down at the end of July 2008.[49]

Lorraine Long, of MEAG, became very busy following that media frenzy. MEAG received five hundred emails from women expressing their "humiliation and pain after parts of their genitals were removed or sewn up without their consent."[8]

Surgical Horrors—Disaster after Disaster

Other alleged surgical errors include a woman who underwent an operation on an ovarian lesion but who awoke to find she had lost both ovaries and both fallopian tubes, and after complications arose, she lost a kidney. Another woman who had an abnormal Pap smear (a routine screening test for early-onset cancer of the cervix) says she was in pain while Reeves took more than an hour attempting to insert an IUD, saying, "I haven't got this right." No cervical biopsy was done, and her pelvis was subsequently found to be full of cancer.[50] It would seem that the reason he could not "get this right" was probably that the pelvis was full of cancer.

Gail Small, fifty-five, alleged he failed to diagnose ovarian cancer in 2003, resulting in her admission to Liverpool Hospital a year later for an emergency hysterectomy.[25] Gail was given twelve months to live. She said that she was very traumatized.[51] In another patient, Reeves removed the wrong breast in a mastectomy operation.[52] Several other women say that they discovered their uterus had been removed without their knowledge or consent.[48]

Another woman went to her doctor several months after seeing Dr. Reeves, having had no period since. She told her doctor she would like to have another baby and attended a fertility clinic where an ultrasound was performed. The woman was told, "You do not have a womb."[48]

A fifty-eight-year-old Ms. Hawkins "was having a great life" before she was betrayed by her gynecologist, Dr. Reeves. Ms. Hawkins trusted him, as she should. Speaking from her home on the south coast, she struggled to control her emotions as she related her story to the *Australian* newspaper. Ms. Hawkins had visited Mr. Reeves in 2002 with complaints of a "slight leakage." She recalls as she lay on the operating table, Reeves rested his penis, still inside his trousers, on her arm as he stroked her fingers.

Ms. Hawkins's recovery from the surgery found her condition "a hundred times worse," her bladder more difficult to control, leading to depression, thoughts of suicide, and a mental breakdown in 2004. Writing to the HCCC at the time, their response was a similar one to that which many other women had received. There is no benefit in pursuing this, as Reeves has already been deregistered.

"He stitched me up like an old blanket," she said. "I was in such agony after the operation that I could hardly sit down for about a month. He also stitched up my vagina so tight that I couldn't have sex."

Ms. Hawkins later required a major gynecological operation to fix Reeves's work; she received a disability pension and required medication for the psychological trauma he caused.[53]

As the horror stories pile up—leaving women in pain, rough handling, rudeness, using frightened and vulnerable women for his sexual gratification, more-than-required stitching to the vagina—it becomes increasingly easy to form a picture of a man who has a severe dislike for women and perhaps a deep hatred for himself.

Babies

In addition to the allegations of the deaths of at least seven women, new allegations of the deaths of ten babies came to light, along with those of "barbaric" handling of babies at birth. In one example, Lorraine Long was told that Reeves "ripped" a baby out with such force that he fell back on the floor with the baby, leaving the mother to believe her baby had been strangled.[52,54]

Ms. Jillian Skinner, MP, told Parliament of the story one woman told of the forceps delivery Reeves had performed on her when she was only eight centimeters dilated. Using all his strength, he applied such tremendous force that he had his foot on the end of the bed as he "dragged her baby out of her body." Skinner heard a similar story from another woman who has never spoken of the experience to anyone except her husband but who lives in constant pain and has trouble wearing clothes.[55]

Iwona Taborek's twins died at Hornsby Hospital, and she came close to death due to uncontrolled bleeding under the "care" of Reeves in 1995. Mrs. Taborek, a former registered nurse, related how frightened she felt as Reeves attempted to remove her placenta, causing severe lacerations to her vagina and cervix, and refused to provide pain relief medication. She said, "His voice was so rough, and he was so rude." After two blood transfusions, a cardiac arrest, and acute renal failure, Reeves "also performed an unnecessary hysterectomy without her permission."

It was alleged that Reeves was again negligent in that he failed to treat an infection before Iwona's twins were born. According to the *Sydney Morning Herald*, her waters (membranes) broke in the hospital, and the first twin was stillborn a week later. Almost a month later, while Mrs. Taborek was in labor, Reeves examined her and left. Eleven minutes later, the second twin was born and died at five minutes of age.

Court documents said Reeves had "exhibited a conscious and contumelious disregard" for her rights. The state government was forced to compensate Iwona and Arthur Taborek with hundreds of thousands of dollars after they sued the Northern Sydney Area Health Service and Mr. Reeves in 1999 for $750,000. Mrs. Taborek never returned to work as a nurse.[56]

Nothing could have prepared Ray Williams, member for Hawkesbury, for the day that Margaret Russell and her husband, Geoff, visited his office. They told him of their dream of having a big family, a dream that ended abruptly with the birth of their third son. Mrs. Russell said that during labor, Reeves had pushed on her abdomen to force the baby out; he "grabbed the baby's head and 'twisted it at several angles' in an attempt to dislodge the baby's shoulders after he became stuck for 40 minutes."[56]

Mrs. Russell told Williams she could "'feel her baby's heartbeat between her legs during the entire time of the birth." Dr. Reeves told her that the baby would weigh between eight and nine pounds, but their baby was over fourteen pounds at birth.[57] She was in excruciating pain and continued screaming in agony, and at one point, Dr. Reeves shouted at her, "Shut up and stop f——king screaming. Your baby's dead—just push." Dr. Reeves had hold of the baby's head, with his leg on the bed, and was pulling the baby from Mrs. Russell. The Registry of Births, Deaths and Marriages shows the birth on September 1, 1996, of Langdon Francis Russell—weighing fourteen pounds four ounces, length 61.5 centimeters, head circumference thirty-eight centimeters; his birth was documented as a stillbirth. Mrs. Russell said she was never offered a cesarean section.[57]

After being told her claim was not enough to warrant further action, Mrs. Russell was eventually awarded approximately $185,000 for damages and $130,000 for legal costs; however, it is reported she never received a cent.[58]

Lisa McCann reports she was at high risk of having a uterovaginal prolapse due to a congenital pelvic abnormality, but despite this, she alleges Reeves advised her to continue a pregnancy and proceed to vaginal birth. After her baby's birth in April 1995 at Hornsby Hospital, she did suffer a uterovaginal prolapse as predicted. Reeves "unsuccessfully tried to fix her uterus surgically to her abdominal wall and she suffered a serious postoperative infection." Lisa abandoned her claim against Reeves after he was declared bankrupt.[56]

The *NZ Herald* reported in May 2008 that "Reeves reported deaths as stillborn, escaping formal inquiries because neither death certificates nor coronial and other investigations are required in such cases."[52] Some mothers told police they heard their baby cry after the birth but were told by Reeves they had "imagined" it.[54]

Allegations of Sexual Assault

It was reported that Reeves had performed a gynecological examination on a woman without wearing gloves; she said he used an "intimate, sexual" touch and touched her breasts unexpectedly.[50] Further allegations followed, one from a complainant known as CA who said that during an internal examination, Reeves "just kept rubbing my clitoris, and he did not stop. I thought I was being masturbated.[59] I have been stimulated before, and I know how it feels. I was not there to be pleasured in any way. I was there for a Pap smear and a Pap smear only."[60]

Another woman known as RF recounted her story of having Reeves perform an internal ultrasound. He told her to "just rip your knickers off." She remembered Reeves helped her remove her underwear and her feeling of embarrassment that there was no sheet on the examination table and lack of a modesty cover or any attempt by him to cover her body or protect her privacy.[61]

These stories have been corroborated by many other women over the years.

RF went on to explain the touching she experienced on her clitoris as Reeves examined her, which made her feel very uncomfortable. This complainant went on to see Reeves for surgery later. When she was having the spinal anesthetic inserted, wearing only a hospital gown, Reeves placed himself between her legs and suggested she wrap her arms and legs around him so he could support her to keep still during the insertion. RF recalls, "I actually felt his penis flex against like the inside of my leg and the side of my fanny ... right up near my—where your knickers go in your groin there, in that area."[62]

Reeves continued to practice on the south coast even after the NSW Medical Board had warned the Area Health Service in November 2002 that Reeves was working illegally. Maree Germech and Christine Griffin both allege that he sexually assaulted them in 2002 in his office.[25] Griffin said she knew what Reeves had done to her was rape and molestation; it affected her sex life and made her afraid of doctors.[49] Evidence was given by experts, Drs. Korda and Pesce, who both stated that Reeves's touching in these cases "could not have been incidental to the gynaecological procedure."[63]

NSW health minister Reba Meagher would later be questioned about how Graeme Reeves came to be employed by SAHS and would be criticized for not doing enough to legislate against people like Reeves. Meagher did apologize to the women for "the awful experiences you suffered at the hands of someone who acted so despicably" and announced a helpline for former patients to call.[51] Workers at the helpline were to assess the needs of the caller and arrange for follow-up counseling services as appropriate.

Meagher also instructed the director general of health to direct all New South Wales Health CEOs to conduct an urgent audit aimed at identifying all doctors registered and practicing in NSW public health facilities who have restrictions on their practice as a result of disciplinary proceedings.[64]

For many, including member for Bega, Mr. Andrew Constance, Meagher's actions were too little too late as he called for her sacking, exclaiming her to be not only incompetent but also insensitive. Called to order by the parliamentary speaker, Constance dropped that line of thought and proceeded to verbalize his displeasure about the way *Jon Mortimer*, as deputy director of clinical standards at SAHS, failed to act upon warnings about Reeves's practice.[65]

The Health Care Complaints Commission has the power to refer doctors to the NSW director of public prosecutions but decided in Reeves's case to simply refer a complaint to the Medical Board for possible deregistration. Lorraine Long of MEAG recommended complainants bypass the Medical Board and go instead to MEAG or the police.[66]

Failing Health

Confidential records obtained by the *Sunday Telegraph* reported that warning signs detected by Reeves's psychiatrist had revealed the full extent of his disturbed mental state. These included paranoia, fear of criticism, insomnia, uncontrolled anger, aggression, and an eating disorder that resulted in his weight dropping from a hefty 106 kg to a mere fifty-nine kilograms after he commenced a total fat-exclusion diet and exercised at a gym. Reeves slept two to three hours per night and paced the floor, read, or lay awake thinking. He battled to "tolerate" midwives and claimed that pregnant patients tried to blackmail him emotionally.[6,7]

The report revealed that authorities within NSW Health were aware of these issues but employed him regardless. Psychiatrist Dr. John Woodforde explained that Reeves had an unresolved problem with his late father. Reeves's father had been an army officer; and Graeme, a medical student at the time, was a conscientious objector to conscription in the Vietnam War. His father had subsequently died in his arms as a result of a heart attack in 1972 at age fifty-five.[7] Another psychiatrist, Dr. Anthony Samuels, said Reeves had formed an attachment to a man he viewed as a type of "surrogate" father figure and felt "hurt and rejected" when this man refused to accompany him to a disciplinary hearing with the Medical Board.[6]

Drs. Woodforde and Samuels both diagnosed Reeves with a personality disorder. Dr. Samuels said he was at times severely depressed and had prominent narcissistic features.[7]

It was said that Reeves refused to take a holiday for two years and often worked weekends and became anxious in situations where he was not directly in charge. He also had severe visual problems exacerbated by unstable diabetes. Dr. Samuels reports Reeves felt actively suicidal and was prescribed Zoloft to treat depression, initially at a dose of fifty milligrams, later increased to one hundred milligrams.[6]

NSW Health Department Review—May 2008

When retired judge Deirdre O'Connor was asked to conduct a review, her report for the NSW Health Department spanned about twenty-three years. In the report, she acknowledged that as the period in question was the 1980s, her findings that some files and records did not appear to be complete could be explained, in part, by their age.[11]

O'Connor noted that historically, it seemed that during the 1980s and the early 1990s, health services managed complaints locally as much as possible. In February 1998, the *Better Practice Guidelines for Frontline Complaints Handling* were issued by NSW Health and set out specific requirements relating to the investigation of complaints. While O'Connor found evidence that the hospital administration acted to address complaints with Dr. Reeves, she felt "matters should have been better managed at the time."[12,13]

The hospital management met with Reeves to discuss specific issues on three occasions between July 1986 and December 1989. Three more incidents occurred between February and April 1990; however, it is unclear what action, if any, was taken.

The catalogue of complaints continued ad nauseam and included incidents relating to

- his behavior toward an obstetric patient during her labor,
- aggressive and inappropriate conduct toward staff in the presence of patients,
- rude behavior toward a patient.

In the fifteen years between 1986 and 2001, thirty-five complaints were lodged, relating to twenty separate incidents. Complaints were made by nursing staff, medical staff, and patients.[10]

Identified Gaps and Suggested Improvements[67]

On October 13, 1995, NSW Health issued a policy saying that health system managers would be required to "make a referral to the Health Care Complaints Commission when a matter

a. raises an important issue of public health or safety,
b. raises an important question as to the appropriate care or treatment of a client by a health system provider,
c. provides grounds for disciplinary action against a health practitioner, or
d. involves gross negligence on the part of a health practitioner."[14]

Legislative Changes—Medical Practice Amendment Bill (2008)[68,69]

In June 2008, the NSW Parliament passed the Medical Practice (Amendment) Act. The then minister for health said that NSW "now has the strongest legislation in the country to protect patients against misconduct by doctors."[70]

Review of the legislation included increasing the powers of the Medical Board and the HCCC.[46]

The legislation made the following notable changes:

- "expanding the circumstances in which the Medical Board can suspend medical practitioners
- formally requiring the Commission and the health registration authorities (Registration Boards) to consider previous complaints and adverse findings when dealing with a current complaint about a health practitioner
- increasing the transparency of disciplinary proceedings against medical practitioners before Professional Standards Committees of the Medical Board
- introducing mandatory reporting requirements for the medical profession—medical practitioners must report other practitioners whom they believe have engaged in sexual abuse, drug or alcohol abuse, or a gross departure from accepted standards of professional practice or competence."[69]

Mandatory Reporting

October 2008 saw the introduction of mandatory reporting of misconduct by medical professionals.[69] This applies to three critical areas of serious misconduct: sexual abuse in the practice of medicine, being intoxicated by drugs or alcohol while practicing medicine, engaging in conduct while practicing medicine that is a departure from accepted standards of professional practice and competence and risks harm to another person.[71]

Service Check Register for NSW Health

NSW Service Check Register was released on January 30, 2009, to set out rules related to the creation, maintenance, and deletion of records when dealing with certain misconduct matters and the recruitment process.[72] The policy applies to applicants, employees, and contractors and contains information about suspension from duty, dismissal from a public health facility, resignation pending serious action, and any conditions imposed following disciplinary processes.[70]

The NSW Health Care Complaints Commission (HCCC) uses the title *Mr.* when referring to Reeves rather than *Dr.* since his deregistration. Mr. Reeves features heavily in their 2007–2008 annual report, which cites him as the main reason for the 11.4 percent increase in inquiries they handled over that period. The HCCC's Inquiry Service dealt with 8,831 inquiries in 2007–2008, up from 7,927 inquiries handled in 2006–07. This represented a considerable rise in the number of calls to the commission, especially during the second six months of that year. The commission acknowledged that factors affecting this rise in complaints included the extensive media coverage concerning Reeves and the concerns voiced at the hearings of the Garling Inquiry.[73]

Garling Commission of Inquiry—July 31, 2008

In January 2008, the minister for health announced there would be a Special Commission of Inquiry into the delivery of patient care in NSW.[73] The inquiry, headed by Mr. Peter Garling, SC, known as the Garling Inquiry, was to investigate the adequacy of NSW hospital services. Garling handed down his findings on the Reeves case on July 31, 2008 and concluded that Reeves's "intentional and calculated dishonesty" led to his employment by SAHS and recommended the case be referred to the public prosecutor.

Garling also concluded that *Jon Mortimer* and *Robert Arthurson* of SAHS should have carried out better background checks on Reeves. Dr. Mortimer was publicly reprimanded and suspended from duty pending the outcome of further inquiries.

Garling made ten recommendations aimed at tightening recruitment procedures. Health executives had failed to conduct background checks and failed to check his registration status. Garling explained that while he found dangerous system failures related to Reeves's hire, it was his dishonesty that was the key reason he was recruited.[74]

Finally, the Arrest and Criminal Charges—September 2008

Reeves was arrested at his Baulkham Hills home in Sydney early on the morning of September 11, 2008. He was taken into custody and charged with seventeen offenses: nine counts of aggravated sexual assault, six counts of indecent assault, and one count each of female genital mutilation and of maliciously inflicting grievous bodily harm. The offenses were allegedly committed between June 2001 and December 2003 in his office in Bega, at the Bega Hospital, and in Richmond, New South Wales.[20]

Police launched an investigation into the rogue doctor. He ignored a committal hearing and was ordered to stand trial in August 2009. By October that year, Reeves appeared to be in hiding, last known to be living in Castle Hill, north of Sydney.

He was eventually arrested on additional charges in December 2009.

In early 2011, Reeves pleaded guilty to obtaining financial benefit by deception. As a result of his dishonesty, he gained employment as a specialist obstetrician and gynecologist and was on an on-call roster. "He received a total remuneration of $229,249.39, of which $23,104 related to obstetric services and $44,720 to his participation in the on-call roster."[75]

Reeves was found guilty by a district court jury in 2011 for maliciously inflicting grievous bodily harm with intent on Carolyn DeWaegeneire. NSW district court judge *Greg Woods*, after hearing evidence from Reeves's longtime psychiatrist, Dr. Stella Dalton, was in "no doubt that at some point in the early 1990s Dr Reeves suffered a breakdown involving a major depressive illness."[76]

Woods believed Reeves was so deluded that he had convinced himself he was "doing the right thing" and acting in the interests of his patient. Justice Woods went on to say that it was "very likely" that Reeves's actions had "undermined the confidence of thousands of women in obstetricians, gynecologists and other doctors."[1]

In 2011, Woods sentenced Reeves to the maximum three-and-a-half years in Sydney's Long Bay Jail, with a non-parole period of two years, labeling his crimes "reprehensible."[77] Reeves successfully appealed to the high court and was released on parole in December 2013, only eighteen months later.[27]

Release from Prison (2013)

After previous rulings that the original sentence was "manifestly inadequate," Crown prosecutors were calling for the sixty-four-year-old to be back behind bars for another year.[78] Premier Barry O'Farrell said that his early release would be a "kick in the guts" for his victims.[2] As news of Reeves's release from jail spread, it was also revealed that the public prosecutor had dropped sixty charges against him, including allegations of sexual assault. "These women are not angry—they are furious," said patient advocate Lorraine Long. "What has gone on is horrific."[2]

Carolyn DeWaegeneire described Reeves's original sentence as "the biggest joke of all time." Outside the court after the hearing, she was tearful. "My life has been devastated—totally. I should be enjoying life as an older person—I'm not, I have got my medical records. I know damn well what I had before I went in (to the hospital). I know damn well what he did."[27]

Gabrielle Bashir, Reeves's lawyer, argued that he was in poor health and, among other conditions, he suffered vascular disease, chronic kidney disease (requiring dialysis), and chronic depression and should not go back to jail. A doctor's report tendered by the prosecutor stated his health conditions could be adequately treated in prison.[27,79]

When hearing of his suffering, Carolyn DeWaegeneire said simply, "Great;" she explained that she was living a life sentence of her own and she would be angry for the rest of her life. Carolyn DeWaegeneire felt the justice system had failed her too. "It's not bloody good enough," she said. "If a man had his penis chopped off, the doctor would probably get several life sentences."[80] Carolyn was awarded $154,000 in damages; however, Reeves said he was bankrupt and could not pay. In 2014, she was planning to sell her house and leave her adopted country Australia as she believed there is no justice here. She was planning to move back home to England to write a book about Reeves.[44] It is estimated Reeves has received about $1.6 million in legal aid.[81]

The Murky Waters of the Land of Informed Consent

It was paramount to establish whether informed consent was obtained in this case. Here are questions to be answered: Did Ms. DeWaegeneire understand what would occur? Did Reeves believe she understood? Did Reeves believe the operation he performed was necessary and in her best interests?

Reeves's sentence imposed in 2011 by Judge Woods in the district court was said to be "lenient," as the judge had placed undue emphasis on Reeves's depression.[78,82] Judge Woods was "not satisfied beyond a reasonable doubt that the offender deliberately intended to perform an unnecessary and unjustified operation."[83]

Two years later after Reeves had appealed to the high court in July 2013, the trial judge held that Reeves had "failed in his important duty to explain to the patient the full extent of what he intended to do."[84] No case could be found in which a doctor had been criminally liable due to a failure to disclose the extent of a surgical procedure as opposed to the nature of the procedure. "No case has been found where a doctor acting in what he believed were the best interests of the patient was found to be guilty of a crime involving malice or specific intent."[85] As there was no precedent, the case was dismissed.

Lessons Learned?

Gross negligence, incompetence, and brutality were recurring themes throughout the career of Graeme Reeves, leading to his infamy as the "Butcher of Bega" or as "Chopper Reeves" as he became known to some of the general practitioners around Bega.[41,56]

Apart from the women harmed and whom he failed in his duty of care and in spite of the women he had mutilated and the babies who had died under his care, Reeves was able to escape detection for almost twenty years due to a series of bureaucratic failures.[6] Many led to Reeves being able to carry on as he did for so long. There was much debate about whether his credentials checks were carried out. Records of phone conversations warning about Reeves were ignored.

In any case, just as Dr. Jayant Patel (also known as Dr. Death) did in the Queensland debacle, Reeves lied on his CV. Anne-Maree Farrell, an academic who used to work as a lawyer specializing in mass torts and medical negligence, noted in her 2017 book *Health Law: Frameworks and Contexts*, "Administrative failures of public hospitals and the Medical Boards of New South Wales and Queensland enabled Doctors Graeme Reeves, Jayant Patel and Abdalla Khalafalla [another unregistered 'doctor' who worked for years in Queensland] to continue practicing medicine."[86] Tony Morris, QC, who ran the commission of inquiry into Bundaberg Hospital in the wake of the Jayant Patel scandal, said of the Khalafalla case, "It is absolutely terrifying, it is like reliving a bad nightmare."[87] Reading the story of Dr. Khalafalla draws an uncanny resemblance to the Patel case, and indeed, Morris continues, "It is almost a complete replica of what happened in Bundaberg." One year before he was deregistered, a "damning report" raised issues about his competence, but nothing was done for a further twelve months when whistleblowers went to a member of the federal parliament.

Khalafalla, an Egyptian-trained surgeon, worked at Mackay Hospital from 2004 to 2006, when he was deregistered. It was believed he was living in Victoria in 2008 and able to seek registration in another state.[87] Khalafalla lacked insight into the detrimental effects of his behavior, and like Graeme Reeves and Jayant Patel, he was often rude and aggressive to female staff and patients.[88]

The NSW Medical Board was criticized at the time for being "more worried about their reputation than the patient," according to Lorraine Long of MEAG.[66] Ms. Long received 832 complaints about Reeves over twenty years.[2,44] She remarked that Reeves's case is the most notorious they have ever exposed.[89]

Judge Woods pondered over Reeves's arrogant disregard for any opinion regarding Carolyn DeWaegeneire and found himself at a loss to explain why Reeves acted in this way year after year.

Regarding the operation on Ms. DeWaegeneire, the district court heard that Reeves was suffering from a personality disorder, major clinical depression, and impotence at the time and was bankrupt in 1999.

Regarding the indecent assaults, Judge Woods could not explain why Reeves had offended in this fashion, but he suggested that the impotence might have had some "causal role in his rash behaviour" in that he "took the opportunity to touch the clitoris unnecessarily" of two patients. Woods said, "The story is a disaster." He described the case as a "Shakespearean tragedy" in which "intellectual pride and the fanatical pursuit of professional perfection led to mental illness and grave injury to patients."[78]

Patient advocate Lorraine Long was disappointed with Reeves's original sentence, and Ms. Long thought Reeves had "played the depression card" and succeeded.[78]

Supposing he did believe that he was doing Carolyn DeWaegeneire a service by removing her whole external genitalia "in case the cancer spread," supposing he believed Mrs. McAllister had a viral infection, supposing he really did believe that the community needed his help, this man was clearly unwell and should have been stopped earlier. Understandably, the general public may lack confidence and feel anxious about the prospect of themselves or their family being at the mercy of the health system, as it appears that one department does not always inform the other departments of their position. How can we be confident that critical information is passed on, references are checked, restrictions are enforced, and unacceptable practice is reported and stopped?

Thankfully, times have changed—or have they?

Graeme Reeves's behavior led directly to the foundation of at least three bodies designed to address complaints arising from unprofessional behavior:

- Medical Appointments and Credentials Advisory Committee (MAC)
- NSW Health's *Better Practice Guidelines for Frontline Complaints Handling*
- Medical Practice Amendment Bill (2008)

In addition to these changes, there was also the enforcement of mandated notification in 2008 and the Service Check Register in 2009.

As recently as June 2018, the *Guardian* reported that Marie Bismark, a doctor and health lawyer, warned that a decade after Reeves's exposure, red flags are still being missed. Bismark cited the case of Emil Shawky Gayed, an obstetrician and gynecologist who performed unnecessary surgeries on the reproductive organs of women for almost two decades. It was reported that Gayed often worked in small regional and rural Australian towns where it can be challenging to attract specialist doctors, which make them a haven for doctors who have failed to secure positions in larger centers.

Four NSW public hospitals were under the scrutiny of a major investigation in this case. Bismark has spent many years researching clinical governance and patient complaints. She acknowledged that there are barriers to patients and practitioners raising concerns for patients, especially if they are elderly, from a low socioeconomic group or of minority ethnicity. Barriers for practitioners include concerns about repercussions for whistleblowers, concern for future career prospects, and "organisations turning a blind eye if the problem doctor is a high earner or in a hard-to-fill role." Bismark says that "under-reporting of adverse events is rife."[90] The NSW mandatory reporting legislation was not adopted in Queensland, a state that could have benefited most, so was not included in the national law.[91]

It is unsettling to consider how one man can create so much suffering. Like others in this book, it leads one to ponder the incongruence of the picture. How is it that somebody can be altruistic, curious, creative, and caring—graced with the gifts and blessed with the talents required to graduate in medicine— yet, sooner or later, can morph into a toxic individual capable of such greed, selfishness, cruelty, and complete lack of empathy?

Doctors nowadays may not be bound by the Hippocratic oath; however, the Australian Medical Association has adopted a modern version called the Declaration of Geneva, now formally known as the Physician's Pledge.[92,93] Even a cursory glance at the pledge triggers a cerebral tick-off list and reminds the reader of other chapters in this book. The case of Reeves conservatively ticks off ten out of thirteen items in the pledge that he failed to achieve. It is reproduced here from the World Medical Association website for reference.

The Physician's Pledge

AS A MEMBER OF THE MEDICAL PROFESSION:

I SOLEMNLY PLEDGE to dedicate my life to the service of humanity;

THE HEALTH AND WELL-BEING OF MY PATIENT will be my first consideration;

I WILL RESPECT the autonomy and dignity of my patient;

I WILL MAINTAIN the utmost respect for human life;

I WILL NOT PERMIT considerations of age, disease or disability, creed, ethnic origin, gender, nationality, political affiliation, race, sexual orientation, social standing or any other factor to intervene between my duty and my patient;

I WILL RESPECT the secrets that are confided in me, even after the patient has died;

I WILL PRACTISE my profession with conscience and dignity and in accordance with good medical practice;

I WILL FOSTER the honour and noble traditions of the medical profession;

I WILL GIVE to my teachers, colleagues, and students the respect and gratitude that is their due;

I WILL SHARE my medical knowledge for the benefit of the patient and the advancement of healthcare;

I WILL ATTEND TO my own health, well-being, and abilities in order to provide care of the highest standard;

I WILL NOT USE my medical knowledge to violate human rights and civil liberties, even under threat;

I MAKE THESE PROMISES solemnly, freely, and upon my honour.[93]

While working on this book, I have marveled at how many of these doctors continue to receive support from spouses, partners, or colleagues even in the face of such damning evidence. It appears Reeves's wife, Sharon, is another loyal supporter.

The Life and Times of Graeme Reeves

1986—thirty-five complaints related to twenty different incidents.

1990 to 1996—fourteen complaints heard by HCCC. Nine serious matters go to a hearing, including the death of Kerry Ann McAllister at Hills Private Hospital and death of a baby after a traumatic delivery.[41]

1996—Hills Private Hospital no longer allows him to work there.[41]

1996 to 2004—psychiatric reports reveal a personality disorder and speak of prominent narcissistic features and severe depression at times.[27]

1997—three more complaints to the commission, including a baby born with cerebral palsy. No further action was taken.[41]

1997—banned from practicing obstetrics but continued to do so, as he believed "his help was desperately needed."[19]

2000—suspended from the gynecology clinic, as midwives refused to work with him. Sacked from Hornsby Hospital.

2001—took a full-time GP position at Marketplace Medical Centre in Richmond.

2002—employed by Greater Southern Area Health Service after they failed to verify his registration status.

2002—complaint of sexual harassment at his Bega office.[41]

2002—complaints made by staff about Reeves; Pambula Hospital ceased providing obstetric services.[27]

2002 to 2003—continued to practice obstetrics and gynecology in hospitals around NSW's south coast until the termination of his contract.

2003—Complaint to the commission about a 1999 post-surgery death is dismissed.

2003—Bega Hospital received similar complaints, and Bega Hospital (SAHS) terminated his contract.

2004—deregistered by the NSW Medical Tribunal for breaching orders not to practice obstetrics.

2004 to 2007—no action on complaints due to deregistration.[41]

2008—MEAG has received 1,200 emails and over five hundred complaints.[41]

2008—exposed by the media. Alleged to have routinely mutilated or sexually abused as many as five hundred female patients.[8]

2008—Strike Force Tarella investigated the deaths of ten babies and seven women under his care.

2008—arrested and charged.

2011—found guilty of inflicting grievous bodily harm with intent on Carolyn DeWaegeneire. Sentenced and jailed.[27]

2013—Medical Error Action Group (MEAG) received 832 complaints about Reeves spanning the previous twenty years.

2013—released from jail.

2014—deteriorating health. Lives in quasi custody since his release on parole, now living in a community offender support program center.[27,94]

Epilogue

It is clear from the preceding chapter that Graeme Reeves was mentally ill. He could not avoid that, but the numerous regulatory organizations that should have assessed him failed to filter him out as a result of sheer incompetence and the lack of courage to act. They are at fault for allowing this failure of a man to practice as a doctor. They are to blame.

Notes

1. Bibby, P. "Victim Livid at Bega Doctor's Sentence." *The Sydney Morning Herald*. July 1, 2011. Available from https://www.smh.com.au/national/nsw/victim-livid-at-bega-doctors-sentence-20110701-1gttl.html.

2. Carroll, L. "'Butcher of Bega' Graeme Reeves Released from Jail." *The Sydney Morning Herald*. December 28, 2013. Available from https://www.smh.com.au/national/nsw/butcher-of-bega-graeme-reeves-released-from-jail-20131228-300fo.html.

3. High Court of Australia. July 12, 2013. p. 1, part V, para. 5. Available from http://www.hcourt.gov.au/assets/cases/s44-2013/Reeves_App.pdf.

4. Ibid. p. 5, lines 11–12.

5. "Engagement announcements. Reeves–McGrath." *The Sydney Morning Herald*. November 24, 1974. p. 174.

6. Weaver, C. "Bega Butcher Warnings Ignored." *The Sunday Telegraph*. May 31, 2008. Available from https://www.dailytelegraph.com.au/news/nsw/bega-butcher-warnings-ignored/news-story/87641bfe6121c3b551b1b0392d49f3ee.

7. Wallace, N. "The Bega Butcher: A Depressed, Distrustful, Volatile Man." *SMH*. June 1, 2008. Available from https://www.smh.com.au/national/the-bega-butcher-a-depressed-distrustful-volatile-man-20080601-gdsg3p.html.

8. Weaver, C., C. Melouney. "Revealed: The Butcher of Bega." *The Sunday Telegraph* (Sydney). February 23, 2008. Available from https://www.couriermail.com.au/news/national/revealed-the-butcher-of-bega/news-story/c43ee56259713df4bb6f6a0826c8e8bf.

9. O'Connor, D. "Review of Appointment, Management and Termination of Dr Graeme Reeves as a Visiting Medical Officer in the NSW Public Health System." NSW

Department of Health. May 2, 2008. p. 7. Available from https://web.archive.org/web/20080822053023/http://www.health.nsw.gov.au/resources/news/pdf/oconnor_2.pdf.

10. Ibid. p. 3.

11. Ibid. p. 2.

12. Ibid. p. 4.

13. Ibid. pp. 4–5.

14. Ibid. p. 6.

15. Healthscope *The Pulse*. Private Health Magazine. Edition no. 3, 2015, p. 32. Available from http://www.healthscope.com.au/index.php/download_file/view_inline/188.

16. Wallace, N. "Hospital Warned Board against Butcher." *SMH*. March 10, 2008. Available from https://www.smh.com.au/national/hospital-warned-board-of-butcher-20080310-gds4ih.html.

17. Brown, M. "Former Obstetrician Graeme Reeves Found Not Guilty of Manslaughter of Patient." ABC News. June 16, 2017. Available from https://www.abc.net.au/news/2017-06-16/former-obstetrician-found-not-guilty-of-manslaughter/8624054.

18. Kembrey, M. "Notorious Ex-Gynaecologist Graeme Reeves on Trial for Manslaughter of Patient." *SMH*. February 24, 2017. Available from https://www.smh.com.au/national/nsw/notorious-exgynaecologist-graeme-reeves-on-trial-for-manslaughter-of-patient-20170224-gukqzg.html.

19. Wallace, N. "My Help Desperately Needed: Reeves." *SMH*. August 2, 2008. Available from https://www.smh.com.au/national/my-help-desperately-needed-reeves-20080802-gdsorm.html.

20. Welch, D., A. Ramachandran. "Bega Butcher Denied Bail on Sex Charges." *SMH*. September 11, 2008. Available from https://www.smh.com.au/national/bega-butcher-denied-bail-on-sex-charges-20080911-gdsuhc.html.

21. Supreme Court of New South Wales (NSW) Court of Criminal Appeal. *Reeves v R; R v Reeves [2013] NSWCCA 34*. Hearing before Bathurst CJ, Hall J, Hulme J. August 13, 2012, para. 6. Available from https://www.caselaw.nsw.gov.au/decision/54a6396f3004de94513da619.

22. Sapphire Coast Destination Marketing Pty Ltd. Destination NSW. *The Region–Bega*. Available from https://www.sapphirecoast.com.au/the-region/towns/bega/.

23. NSW Government. "Health Care Complaints Commission (HCCC) Report 2007–2008." p. 12. Available from https://www.hccc.nsw.gov.au/Publications/Annual-Reports.

24. O'Connor, D. op. cit. p. 11.

25. Tadros, E., N. Wallace, and B. Robins. "Butcher of Bega's File Was Marked 'No Obstetrics.'" *SMH*. May 15, 2008.

26. O'Connor, D. op. cit. p. 12.

27. Lee, S. "Victim of Butcher of Bega Breaks Down in Court after Coming Face to Face with Doctor Who Mutilated Her as Prosecutors Try to Get Him Thrown Back in Jail." *Daily Mail Australia*. May 23, 2014. Available from https://www.dailymail.co.uk/news/article-2637062/Mutilation-doctor-jail.html.

28. High Court Australia. op. cit. p. 5, line 23.

29. High Court Australia. op. cit. p. 4, line 10.

30. Supreme Court of NSW Court of Criminal Appeal. op. cit. para. 23.

31. Supreme Court of NSW Court of Criminal Appeal. op. cit. paras. 31–32.

32. High Court Australia. op. cit. p. 3, lines 4–9.

33. Supreme Court of NSW Court of Criminal Appeal. op. cit. para. 28.

34. High Court Australia. op. cit. p. 3, notation 5.

35. Supreme Court of NSW Court of
Criminal Appeal. op. cit. para. 27.

36. Supreme Court of NSW Court of
Criminal Appeal. op. cit. para. 26.

37. Supreme Court of NSW Court of
Criminal Appeal. op. cit. para. 31.

38. Supreme Court of NSW Court of
Criminal Appeal. op. cit. para. 40.

39. High Court Australia. op. cit. p. 15, para. 59.

40. Supreme Court of NSW Court of
Criminal Appeal. op. cit. para. 14.

41. Wallace, N. "Patient Battle to Prove
Malice." *SMH*. March 10, 2008.

42. Shiel, W. C., Jr. MedicineNet Inc, WebMD.
Available from https://www.medicinenet.com/
script/main/art.asp?articlekey=33610/

43. High Court Australia. op. cit. p. 6, para. 22.

44. Sutton, C. "'I Woke Up Mutilated': Butcher of Bega's
Sinister Act." News.com.au. June 26, 2017. Available
from https://www.news.com.au/national/courts-law/i-
woke-up-mutilated-butcher-of-begas-sinister-act/
news-story/2b4331e2f358029d26447f781c2b9de8.

45. NSW Gov't. "HCCC Report 2007–2008." p. 13.

46. O'Connor, D. op. cit. p. 16.

47. Supreme Court of NSW Court of
Criminal Appeal. op. cit. para. 6.

48. Medical Error Action Group—June Long Foundation.
"The Butcher of Bega Scandal." Available
from http://www.medicalerroraustralia.com/
medical-disasters/the-butcher-of-bega-scandal/.

49. Parliament of New South Wales. Legislative Assembly
Report. Hansard. May 15, 2008. p. 7,708.

50. Lauredhel. "Graeme Reeves: Medical Rape Culture and
Collegiality." Hoyden About Town. February 18, 2008.

Available from https://hoydenabouttown.com/2008/02/18/graeme-reeves-medical-rape-culture-and-collegiality/.

51. Wallace, N. "'Butcher' Doctor's Victims Relive Horror." *The Age*. February 29, 2008. Available from https://www.theage.com.au/national/butcher-doctors-victims-relive-horror-20080229-ge6saa.html.

52. Ansley, G. "'Butcher' Accused of Deaths at Birth." *NZ Herald*. May 4, 2008. Available from https://www.nzherald.co.nz/world/news/article.cfm?c_id=2&objectid=10507956.

53. Wilson, A. "'Butcher of Bega' Betrayed Me: Victim." *The Weekend Australian*. March 5, 2008. Available from https://www.theaustralian.com.au/archive/news/butcher-of-bega-betrayed-me-victim/news-story/f0263e7f5420b36964f403ea7f5ec3d3.

54. "Police Yet to Interview 'Butcher of Bega.'" *Herald and Weekly Times*. May 11, 2008. Available from https://web.archive.org/web/20080913191009/http://www.news.com.au/heraldsun/story/0%2C21985%2C23679389-662%2C00.html.

55. Parliament of New South Wales. op. cit. pp. 7,708, 7,710.

56. Wallace, N. "Revealed: Payouts for Surgical Horrors." *SMH*. March 15, 2008.

57. Parliament of New South Wales. op. cit. p. 7,766.

58. Parliament of New South Wales. op. cit. p. 7,767.

59. Supreme Court of New South Wales (NSW) Court of Criminal. op. cit. para. 367.

60. Supreme Court of New South Wales (NSW) Court of Criminal. op. cit. para. 370.

61. Supreme Court of New South Wales (NSW) Court of Criminal. op. cit. para. 306.

62. Supreme Court of New South Wales (NSW) Court of Criminal. op. cit. para. 319.

63. Supreme Court of New South Wales (NSW) Court of Criminal. op. cit. para. 393.

64. NSW Government Department of Health. Media Release. February 28, 2008. Available from http://www5.health.nsw.gov.au/news/2008/20080228_01.html.

65. Parliament of New South Wales. op. cit. pp. 7,762–7,763.

66. Fife-Yeomans, J., K. Sikora. "The 'Butcher of Bega' Graeme Reeves Is in Hiding." News.com.au. October 23, 2009. Available from https://www.news.com.au/national/butcher-of-bega-in-hiding/news-story/85b44c335a8098548bd85f003fbed876?sv=fc12c75fbf19bbbc59b8b0e5f2b080d5.

67. O'Connor, D. op. cit. pp. 15–16.

68. O'Connor, D. op. cit. pp. 9–10.

69. NSW Gov't. "HCCC Report 2007–2008." p. 15.

70. NSW Gov't. "HCCC Report 2007–2008." p. 18.

71. Durack, L. "Mandatory Misconduct Reporting Now Law." June 11, 2008. 6minutes.com.au. Available from https://web.archive.org/web/20080612181203/http://www.6minutes.com.au/articles/z1/view.asp?id=174103.

72. NSW Government Health. "Policy Directive– Service Check Register for NSW Health." Document no. PD2013_036. October 31, 2013. Available from https://www1.health.nsw.gov.au/pds/ActivePDSDocuments/PD2013_036.pdf.

73. NSW Gov't. "HCCC Report 2007–2008." p. 7.

74. Wallace, N. "I'm Sorry: Butcher of Bega." *SMH*. August 1, 2008. Available from https://www.smh.com.au/national/im-sorry-butcher-of-bega-20080801-gdsokm.html.

75. High Court Australia. op. cit. p. 7, para. 25.

76. High Court Australia. op. cit. p. 7, para. 26.

77. Madden, J., A. Priestley, M. Nadin. "Victim Carolyn Dewaegeneire Outraged at Lenient Sentence for Rogue Surgeon Graeme Reeves." *The Weekend Australian*. July 2, 2011. Available from https://www.theaustralian.com.

au/news/nation/victim-carolyn-dewaegeneire-outraged-at-lenient-sentence-for-rogue-surgeon-graeme-reeves/news-story/03b19bb76a746fd17d024c8b15420d48.

78. Hall, L. "Genital Mutilation Sentence 'Manifestly Inadequate,' Court Told." *SMH*. August 13, 2012. Available from https://www.smh.com.au/national/nsw/genital-mutilation-sentence-manifestly-inadequate-court-told-20120813-24439.html,

79. High Court Australia. op. cit. p. 8, para. 29.

80. Weaver, C. "Surviving the Butcher of Bega." *The Australian Women's Weekly*. May 23, 2014. Available from https://www.nowtolove.com.au/celebrity/celeb-news/its-not-good-enough-victim-9865.

81. Wells, J. "Jail Time Extended for Genital Mutilation Doctor." ABC News online. February 21, 2013. Available from https://www.abc.net.au/news/2013-02-21/jail-time-extended-for-genital-removal-doctor/4532374.

82. High Court Australia. op. cit. p. 7, para. 28.

83. High Court Australia. op. cit. p. 9, para. 36.

84. High Court Australia. op. cit. p. 8, para. 33.

85. High Court Australia. op. cit. pp. 10–11, para. 43.

86. Farrell, A., J. Devereux, I. Karpin, P. Weller. 2017. *Health Law: Frameworks and Context*. Cambridge University Press. p. 75. Accessed on May 25, 2019.

87. "Qld Health Rocked by Another Doctor Scandal." ABC News online. August 5, 2008. Available from https://www.abc.net.au/news/2008-08-05/qld-health-rocked-by-another-doctor-scandal/464474.

88. Queensland Government. Health Quality and Complaints Commission. "An Investigation into Concerns Raised by MRS De-Anne Kelly MP about the Quality of Health Services at Mackay Base Hospital." 2008. p. 133, para. 9.4.3. Available from https://cabinet.qld.gov.au/documents/2008/Aug/HQCC%20Report%20

into%20Mackay%20Hospital/Attachments/HQCC%20
report%20on%20Mackay%20Hospital.pdf.

89. Medical Error Action Group–June Long Foundation.
"How MEAG Began." Available from https://www.
medicalerroraustralia.com/about-us/how-meag-began/.

90. Davey, M. "Emil Shawky Gayed. A Decade after the
Butcher of Bega, Red Flags Are Still Being Missed." *The
Guardian.* June 28, 2018. Available from https://www.the-
guardian.com/australia-news/2018/jun/28/a-decade-after-
the-butcher-of-bega-red-flags-continue-to-be-missed.

91. Australian Medical Association (NSW) Ltd.
"Mandatory Reporting—Looking to the Future."
2017. Available from https://www.amansw.com.au/
from-the-ceo-mandatory-reporting-looking-to-the-future/.

92. Moy, Chris. Australian Medicine. "AMA Fully
Supports Physician's Pledge Update." Feb. 13,
2018. Available from https://ama.com.au/ausmed/
ama-fully-supports-physicians-pledge-update.

93. World Medical Association. "WMA Declaration of
Geneva." 2019. Available from https://www.wma.
net/policies-post/wma-declaration-of-geneva/.

94. Gardiner, S. "'Butcher of Bega' Graeme Reeves
Won't Go Back to Jail." *SMH*. August 18, 2014.
Available from https://www.smh.com.au/national/
nsw/butcher-of-bega-graeme-reeves-wont-
go-back-to-jail-20140818-1059xn.html.

CHAPTER FOURTEEN

THE TROUBLE WITH DOCTORS—GREED AND DECEIT

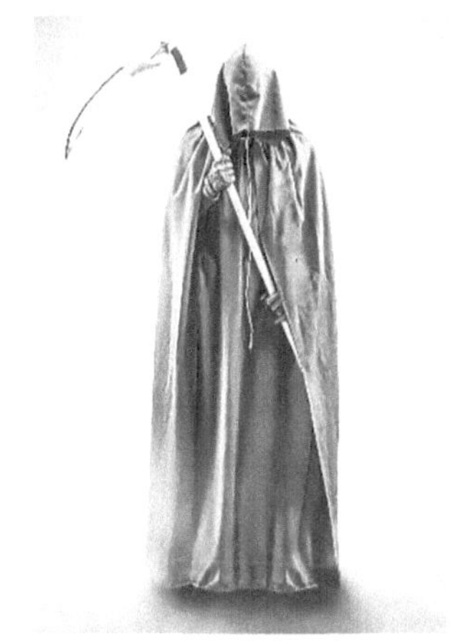

Shutterstock (with permission)

So How Did We Get Here?

With the exception of Dr. Yoshiki Sasai, the doctors in this book were not scientists. They were dishonest miscreants who, with the exception of Dr. William McBride, contributed nothing to medical knowledge. Even in McBride's case, the discovery of the effects of thalidomide was a clinical observation rather than the result of some rigorous scientific study. Scanning the pages of this and the many other books covering deceit, one finds that greed is a defining factor. Whether this greed is simply for monetary gain or for academic recognition, it is still greed. Deceit is the nefarious vehicle most often used to satisfy this egregious greed. Deceit may range from forgery of tertiary qualifications to fraudulent alteration of a curriculum vitae, to dishonestly altering the results of scientific experiments. In all cases, it is harmful because it challenges the honesty of the perpetrator. Examples of all can be found in this book.

Hippocrates was a Greek physician who lived on the island of Cos about 2,500 years ago. He is best remembered for his writings on ethics, the most important of which is the *Hippocratic oath,* which has been modified over the centuries since it was first credited to him although others may have been involved. The oath forms the basis of proper behavior for a doctor to this day although it has been updated from time to time depending on social and medical practices as they existed at the time (see last chapter for a modern version). It has been the practice for generations for most medical schools to have the graduands recite the oath at graduation ceremonies. The original version of the Hippocratic oath is reproduced here:

1. I swear by Apollo, the physician, and Asclepius, and Hygieia and Panacea and all the gods and goddesses as my witnesses, that, according to my ability and judgement, I will keep this Oath and this contract.
2. To hold him who taught me this art equally dear to me as my parents, to be a partner in life with him, and to fulfil his needs when required; to look upon his offspring as equals to my own siblings, and to teach him this art if they shall wish to learn it, without the order that by this set rules, lectures, and every other method of instruction, I will impart knowledge of the art to my own sons and those of my

teachers and to students bound by this contract and having sworn this all to the law of medicine but to no others.

3. I will use those dietary record regimens, which will benefit my patients according to my greatest ability and judgement, and I will do no harm or injustice to them.

4. I will not give a lethal drug to anyone if I am asked nor will I advise such a plan; and similarly, I will not give a woman a pessary to cause an abortion.

5. In purity and according to divine law, I will carry out my life and my art.

6. I will not use the knife even upon those suffering from stones, but I will leave this to those who are trained in this craft.

7. Into whatever homes I go, I will enter them for the benefit of the sick, avoiding any voluntary act of impropriety or corruption, including the seduction of women or men whether they be freemen or slaves.

8. Whatever I see or hear of the lives of my patients whether in connection with my professional practice or not which ought not to be spoken of outside I will keep secret as considering all such things to be private.

So long as I maintain this Oath faithfully and without corruption may it be granted to me to partake of life fully and the practice of my art, gaining the respect of all men for all time.

However, should I transgress this Oath and violate it, may the opposite be my fate. (Translated by Michael North, National Library of Medicine, 2002)

Note that the phrase "First, do no harm" does not appear in the oath, to which it is often incorrectly attributed, but the words "do no harm" do appear in this translation in the third paragraph.

The oath prohibits physicians from assisting in euthanasia and abortion. These activities occur in various parts of the world nowadays. Rather than lay down rules by which physicians can determine whether a particular procedure may or may not be performed, the oath is directed at defining a preferred style of life to guide the physician. By following these guidelines, the physician can expect to live his life after having gained "the respect of all men for all time."

Regrettably, some of the doctors in this book have lost the "the respect of all men for all time." The reason for that is greed. Greed can be monetary or academic, and it is satisfied by deceit or fraud. The physicians and surgeons in this book fit into one of these categories with the possible exception of Graeme Reeves, who may have been mentally deranged.

What Is Happening Now?

Nobody knows how much dishonesty and fraud is still going on. It is probably more than we all would like. As Merrilyn Walton says, "The system is still largely dependent on the attitude of the institution and the personality of the players. If a case similar to that of William McBride surfaced today, the same difficulties would arise in relation to investigative responsibility."[1] Although these words were written twenty years ago, the same is likely to apply today. If we cannot rely on the personality of the players, what can we do?

Medical Students

Firstly, medical students should be interviewed before admission to medical school. Only those who seem suitable should be admitted.

Licensed Doctors

Then surely we can confirm that they are doctors. The human resources department of any hospital or health organization should insist on visualizing the original certificate (or a certified copy) from the graduating medical college of the candidate. Additionally, any certificate for postgraduate degrees or training should be viewed and certified. These should be confirmed with the records of the relevant training institutes. Even so, doctors who lack moral character can reach the position of a trusted physician.

Consider the position of *Dr. Donald Cline*, a fertility specialist in Indianapolis. He was aged eighty years at the time of writing and retired in 2009, aged seventy-one, but it has been revealed that in the 1970s and 1980s he used his own sperm to impregnate over fifty women without their knowledge. This only came to light when one of his unsuspecting offspring was given a gift of Ancestry.com by her husband. She took a sample from her cheek and sent it off, only to find that she had eight siblings! Subsequent investigations revealed that Dr. Cline fathered at least forty-eight children through his clinic. At that time, there was no law against fertility clinics donating sperm from staff who worked in the clinic, so Dr. Cline had committed no offense, but it was an offense to donate sperm anonymously. As he had repeated egregious lies about the source of his sperm, he was convicted on two counts of obstruction of justice and sentenced to one year in prison, the sentence being wholly suspended. He spent no time in prison.

Anonymous use of sperm was immoral and unethical, but it was not illegal in the '70s and '80s. It leads to the chance of two half-siblings meeting each other and parenting a child who would be at substantial risk of genetically inherited disorders. Fortunately, in many cases, the affected offspring have identified their half-siblings on social media.[2,3,4] An even more extreme example is that of *Dr. Cecil B. Jacobson* of Vienna, Virginia, USA, who is alleged to have fathered as many as seventy-five children using his own sperm without consent in the 1970s and 1980s. He was given five years in jail for fraud and perjury.[5] There are many other examples known of sperm donations without authority. *Dr. Jan Karbaat* in the Netherlands has recently been shown to have fathered at least forty-nine children to women without their knowledge or consent. Dr. Karbaat died in 2017.[6] It is likely that there are many more instances of children who have been born to unscrupulous doctors without their knowledge and who have never, and will never, be exposed. It is unlikely that any checks or balances could be put in place that would detect these examples of unethical behavior if the miscreant is determined to keep their offense secret.

To say whether these examples of unethical behavior are due to pure monetary greed is challenging. Some have argued that sympathy for the infertile couple was the motivation for their inappropriate donation. In the 1970s, DNA analysis was unknown or in its infancy, and the donor doctor was probably totally unaware that he might be exposed in thirty- or forty-years' time. In regulated, legal sperm banks, donations from one individual are limited because of the risk of siblings meeting and parenting a child. Unregulated donations are therefore unwise. Monetary greed or altruism will be challenging to separate, but there is little doubt that altruism will be used to conceal financial greed.

Unfortunately, the doctors described would not have been detected regardless of how much official investigation had been carried out, as their qualifications and certifications would have been perfect. Even a whistleblower would not have recognized this behavior. The fault lies in a flaw in the character of the doctor. A test needs to be devised for that. Professor Merrilyn Walton, in her book *The Trouble with Medicine*, suggests that the medical boards should be responsible for maintaining medicine as a vocation and that better legislation is required. She indicates that accreditation should be mandatory and that information about doctors who have been disciplined should be freely available to anyone who asks.[1] This might go some way to prevent doctors from straying from ethical guidelines, but it is unlikely to uncover those who are intent on concealing their behavior. That relates to almost every doctor in this book.

Unlicensed "Doctors"

Secondly, surely we can confirm that doctors are accredited for the position for which they apply. *Mr. Sudip Sarker*, aged forty-one, was keen to be appointed as a consultant general surgeon at the Worcester Crown Hospitals NHS Trust when it was advertised. The position carried an annual salary of almost £100,000. Worcester is not far from Birmingham in the West Country, England. As is their cute little habit in England, highly qualified surgeons are referred to as "Mr." instead of "Dr.," a hangover from the barber-surgeon days. It seems, however, that Mr. Sarker was not as highly qualified as he might have liked, and he was concerned that his application might be unsuccessful. Mr. Sarker, therefore, did not hesitate to falsify his logbooks, exaggerating the number of surgical procedures he had carried out—including eighty laparoscopic (keyhole) operations in total, of which fifty-one had been solo—and he falsified the amount of broad experience that he had when interviewed for the position. Mr. Sarker's appointment to the Alexandra Hospital in Redditch, Worcestershire, was successful. He commenced work in August 2011, but it did not last long, as he was suspended on full pay in October 2012 when a number of colleagues stopped him from operating due to the high rate of complications. In the meantime, the police were investigating a number of patient deaths after Sarker had operated on them, and the NHS trust was investigating ways to recover funds fraudulently obtained. The hospital set up a dedicated helpline when concerns became known, and it is said that there were over fifty calls from relatives of concerned patients of Mr. Sarker.[7,8,9]

In the meantime, Mr. Sarker complained that the trust had dismissed him for gross misconduct after he alleged that there had been "senior management failings" in the hospital. He claimed that urinary catheters and nasogastric catheters had been left in patients longer than recommended and one of his patients had to drink from a flower bowl. It seems that he thought that the best form of defense was attack. This all resulted in the trust taking a closer look at his clinical behavior and character. Contemporaneously, the Royal College of Surgeons (RCS) carried out a clinical review. Mr. Sarker was dismissed by the trust in January 2015. He lost his case for unfair dismissal.[10]

Things were about to get worse for Mr. Sarker, though. In early 2017, he was charged with fraud by misrepresentation, an offense that carries a maximum penalty of ten years in prison.[7] Sarker had fraudulently exaggerated his experience and training during his interview for the position. He had claimed to have won a prestigious surgical prize in Glasgow and that he had previously worked with the World Health Organization, but no evidence could be found to support either of these claims. During the trial, it was revealed that the NHS trust had paid damages of over £1.9 million to twenty of his former patients.

The prosecution showed that one in five of those patients underwent operations that had not been discussed with them and a quarter of his patients developed chronic complications, showing a tenfold increase in surgical complications compared with other surgeons. Over half of his cancer patients who were considered suitable for reconstructive surgery to avoid a permanent colostomy awoke to find that they did have a permanent colostomy despite them having specifically indicated before the operation that they did not want a permanent colostomy. The RCS review commented that "the review team has never in their collective experience seen anything similar to this."[7,8,9,10] Of course, the RCS team had never been to Bundaberg in North Queensland where they would have seen a similar performance from the authorities (see chapter 2: "Dr. Jayant Patel—Doctor Death").

Regardless, the court was not sympathetic to Mr. Sarker's submissions, and he was sentenced to six years in prison.[11,12] Mr. Sarker was not reaching for academic recognition; he was simply after a position in which he would be rewarded with money. He was greedy. It was a flaw in his character. To detect Mr. Sarker's fraud, a more rigorous form of checking his qualifications should have been in place.

Dr. Richard G. Paolino of Philadelphia, Pennsylvania, was not so lucky when he was found guilty of *forgery*, *delivery of a controlled substance*, and *practicing medicine without a license*. Paolino lost his medical license in 2000 due to bankruptcy, but he continued to practice medicine using blank prescription pads that he bought from two other doctors and then often wrote them for OxyContin. He could have received life in prison. Instead, he got 120 years with a minimum of thirty years, upheld on appeal! He was aged fifty-nine when sentenced.[13] The two other doctors who supplied the blank prescriptions were *Dr. Wesley Collier*, who was sentenced to twenty-seven months to twenty years in prison, and *Dr. David Harmon*, who was given a suspended sentence of twelve years to be served in community service in Ghana. It seems extraordinary to take such a risk when the penalty is so high. Generally, it appears that penalties of all sorts are higher in the USA than in other countries.[13]

In Australia, for example, up until July 2019, there was no penalty involving jail time for doctors who practice medicine without being licensed. Those who were imprisoned did so because of fraud or deception. New laws introduced will allow up to three years' jail time and fines of $60,000 for those impersonating a doctor or nurse. The Australian Health Practitioner Regulation Agency (AHPRA) has over 1,300 reported possible offenders since 2014 on its books and has successfully prosecuted fifty individuals, so the problem seems alarmingly common.[14,15]

These individuals can only be prevented from entering the professional community by carefully and strictly checking their credentials.

Academic Fraud

It is said that more than anything, scientists value the truth. They are motivated by a constant struggle to find the truth. The doctors in this book, with the possible exception of Dr. Yoshiki Sasai, were not scientists but, instead, doctors misbehaving. They all ended up deceased or deregistered. Most doctors in this book seem to be motivated by greed and do not care much about truth. Nobody knows how prevalent academic misconduct is, but it is likely to be more frequent than we want to believe.

Stephen Lock and *Frank Wells*, in their book *Fraud and Misconduct in Medical Research*,[16] describe forty-six cases of academic fraud in Australia (4), the United Kingdom (11), and the United States (31) from 1974 until 1993, when their book was published. These cases are described as "known or suspected," and cases under investigation at the time were not included. Since then, Frank Wells has reported a further twenty-six cases of fraud to the General Medical Council (GMC) in the UK alone, so the problem is widespread. Scanning the names and positions of the offenders is interesting. All of them were single operators, and many were senior in their discipline. Eleven of them carried the title of professor, eight were psychiatrists or psychologists, seventeen were of consultant or specialist status, seven were family doctors, and nine were research fellows, scientists, or of similar rank. (The groups above are not complete or mutually exclusive.) The areas of investigation involved crossed the whole divide of medicine from biology to virology.

The fraud occurred mostly in a university laboratory or research institute, but six cases occurred in family clinical practice. The offenses included plagiarism (11), forgery (6), fraud (33), and total fabrication of work (2). Some of the forgeries involved forgery of a coworker's signature as well as forgery of their own qualifications and of scientific data. Some of the published fraudulent work was so ridiculous that it should have been unbelievable. The penalties meted out by the authorities varied from being struck off the medical register through resignation, suspension, retraction of the work to nothing at all. It is surprising that once an offense was uncovered, the veracity of the offender would not be questioned forever and therefore their data never trusted again. It is apparent that the problem is so complex that a simple solution will not suffice to protect against it.

Dr. John Darsee was an undergraduate at Notre Dame University and then became a research cardiologist at Emory and, later, Harvard University. He was one of the most infamous fraudsters of all time. In 1981, other scientists at cooperating multicenter universities began to notice discrepancies in Darsee's data. His head of department, the highly regarded cardiologist Dr. Eugene Braunwald, investigated and decided there was no serious misconduct. This was an aberration but allowed Darsee to continue to work under supervision for ten years but terminated his NIH fellowship.

The NIH demanded the return of $122,000 in grant money. Emory and Harvard universities and the NIH separately investigated and found that data had been fabricated as long ago as his undergraduate days. This was embarrassing for Harvard, as it had given reassurances that the work had been closely supervised. It was surprising that it took so long to be detected, as some of the data seemed impossible to gather. For example, Darsee claimed in one study that he drew blood from the tail veins of two hundred rats every week for ninety weeks and that he collected venous blood from forty-three members of a family on two consecutive days twice a year, as well as complete twenty-four-hour urine collections, including a two-year-old child.[17] How anyone can believe that these are possible is difficult to comprehend. Collecting a total sample of urine in a two-year-old child in one hour, never mind twenty-four hours, would be quite tricky!

Darsee's fabricated data became infamous because his were among the earliest falsified scientific works to come to the attention of the scientific world, which believed that the search for truth was without fault. Ultimately, fifty-two of Darsee's papers were retracted; but sadly, many of them are still cited positively today. This reflects how the harmful effects of fraudulent research persist for decades, although Darsee lost his license to practice medicine in New York in 1984.[18,19,20]

Other claims—such as those of *Dr. William Summerlin*, a young research dermatologist of the Memorial Sloan Kettering Cancer Center (MSK) in New York—were so outrageous that they were thought by some to be a joke. Attempts to transplant skin from one individual of one species to another of the same species had been going on for decades without success even though kidney, liver, and other organ transplants were becoming possible. Dr. Summerlin claimed that after having grown the graft cells in a culture medium, which he never properly described, he had grafted cells from the skin of a donor black mouse onto a recipient white mouse. Summerlin had been working on this for more than a year and was keen to show his new director, Dr. Robert Good, how successful it was.

At a regular meeting of the department, he was to show Dr. Good the animals themselves. He took several shiny steel bins with several of the subject mice to the office of the director one day in 1974. Before leaving the laboratory, he checked the mice so that he would take only the best to demonstrate his technique by showing that the white mouse with a black spot on its back had accepted the transplant. Unfortunately, not all the mice showed up as good examples. Most of them displayed a natural smudgy gray instead of a really dark black. He was somewhat disturbed by this, as it might not impress his boss as he wished. Impulsively he took a black permanent ink pen and blackened up the patch of gray on two of the white recipient mice. If this had been real, it would have been a triumph in the treatment of burns, as it would show that healthy skin from one individual could be transferred to another (burnt) individual. Dr. Summerlin took the bin containing the two grafted (inked) mice to show his boss, Dr. Robert Good, several floors above. Dr. Good had other things on his mind and took scant notice of the mice. Summerlin returned the mice in their bin back to the laboratory and gave them to Mr. James Martin, a laboratory assistant. Mr. Martin noticed that the black spots were not the same spots that had been there when the mice left. He applied an alcohol scrub, only to find that the black color came off. The black patch had been marked on the white mouse with an indelible black felt pen! The scientists confronted Summerlin with the evidence. They had simply washed the ink off with alcohol.[21]

Interestingly, Summerlin admitted the charges and pleaded excuses such as overwork, misjudgment, and mental illness. He was sent on leave pending a report into his findings.[22] It seems that Summerlin was not careful with the truth in other ways.

The Strange Case of the Spotted Mice

Sir Peter Medawar, in his book *The Strange Case of the Spotted Mice*, relates an earlier occasion when he visited Summerlin's laboratory as part of a scientific investigation committee. He was shown a rabbit into which Summerlin claimed he had transplanted an untreated cornea from a human cadaver into the rabbit's left eye. The left eye had a cataract. Summerlin claimed that he had transplanted a human cornea into the rabbit's right eye after keeping it for several weeks in a special solution. There was no cataract in the right eye. Medawar did not believe that the cornea had been transplanted, as gazing into the right eye of the rabbit, he could see the undisturbed vasculature of the rabbit's own circulation. One senses that Peter Medawar wished that the rabbit could speak while gazing out through the allegedly transplanted cornea with a "candid and unwavering gaze of which only a rabbit with an absolutely clear conscience is capable." Sir Peter later admitted that he thought that it was a hoax and that he did not have the "moral courage" to speak up at the time "for fear of trampling on his juniors in public." A brave admission.[23]

The importance of transplanting a fresh human cornea into a rabbit will be obvious. If a cornea can be transplanted to a rabbit, it is possible that a cornea could be transplanted to another human. The trouble was that nobody had been able to transplant human corneas to rabbits anywhere outside of Summerlin's laboratory. He explained that after removing the cornea from the human cadaver, it had to be cultured for several weeks before transplantation or it would be rejected. His theory was that if a fresh cornea was transplanted into a rabbit, the recipient rabbit's immune system, after a while, would detect the foreign material and send out tiny blood vessels carrying the leukocytes (white cells) into the cornea to destroy the foreign material there. In the process, these tiny blood vessels would cross the limbus (the junction between the cornea, which is clear, and the sclera, which is white, entering the cornea where they would be easily seen). In due course, the cornea would turn white as it forms a cataract. The theory was that if the cornea had been cultured, it would have lost some of its antigen-antibody status and would not develop into a cataract.[24]

Among Summerlin's other busy duties, he had set up an animal study in which he, or ophthalmic research assistants, had grafted fresh human cadaver corneas into the left eye of several laboratory rabbits. Into the right eye of the same rabbits, (he said) he grafted human cadaver corneas, but only after they had been cultured for several weeks. That way, the difference would be visible. He presented his results at numerous clinical review and scientific meetings, showing that if the cornea were cultured, it would not be rejected. Nobody else could repeat his results, so they came from all over to see how it was done.

Among those who came to Sloan Kettering was *Dr. John Ninnemann*, a PhD from Colorado State University. He was most interested in the mechanism that might allow the transplant of human corneas to rabbits. Plans were afoot to complete the experiment by forming another group of rabbits in which the left eye was a fresh human cornea and the right eye was a cultured human cornea even at the risk of blinding the animal because both eyes would be transplants. When Dr. Ninnemann attended a clinical meeting, he heard Dr. Summerlin describe the experiment and claim that both eyes had been transplanted. Dr. Ninnemann raised the subject with Dr. Summerlin, saying that only the left eye had been transplanted, but Summerlin contradicted him, saying he was sure that both of the rabbits' eyes had been transplanted. They agreed to go to the animal house immediately to check. When they arrived there, they examined every animal and could not find one that had both eyes transplanted. Summerlin apologized to Dr. Ninnemann and admitted that he had been wrong.

Some time went by, and still, Summerlin presented rabbits to visiting fellows and others saying that the left eyes had been operated on with a fresh transplant and the right eye with a cultured transplant and that was why it was clear. Then, by chance, Ninnemann found himself in the laboratory where the transplants were being done, and he was able to speak to the research assistant who was doing the surgery. He confirmed that only one eye, the left, in each rabbit was transplanted. But back at the meetings, Summerlin went on showing beautiful clear slides of a cornea and saying that it had come from Minnesota where he had previously worked. He did not care about the truth, and it was not long until he was exposed as a fraud (when the black ink washed off his mice).[25]

Then, of course, there was *Dr. Paolo Macchiarini*, an Italian thoracic surgeon. Paolo became famous in the mid-1980s when he began transplanting replacement bronchi (windpipes) in patients whose windpipe had been damaged, usually by cancer or tuberculosis. The donor windpipe came from a deceased person and was chemically stripped of the donor's cells before the remaining cartilaginous support was covered with the recipient's own cells (said to be stem cells) removed from the bone marrow, usually of the hip. Dr. Macchiarini claimed that this covering of the patient's cells would prevent rejection of the windpipe.[26] One of the earliest operations was carried out at Dr. Macchiarini's unit in a hospital in Barcelona, Spain. The windpipe came from Padua, Italy, and the cells were collected in Bristol, England, while an instrument (a bioreactor) was used to coat the cells on the windpipe in the University of Milan. It was quite an exercise.[27]

Further operations occurred as the popularity of the operation gained favor around the world. Surgeons took up the procedure in the US, the UK, Sweden, Italy, Iceland, Belgium, South Korea, Russia, and elsewhere. Dr. Paolo Macchiarini was soon appointed to the Karolinska Institutet (KI), the home of the Nobel Prize, and worked from the hospital there. He was famous and continued to develop the artificial windpipe. It was not long before he produced a glass and then a plastic scaffold because windpipes from deceased persons were in short supply. The whole process was called regenerative medicine.[28,29,30,31]

Macchiarini was famous. The literature records that commencing in 1989 until 2018, he had 202 scientific papers published, fifty as the first author in his earlier career and the vast majority of the remainder as the last author. These figures reflect his personal involvement in his earlier career and then his seniority in his later career as he gained gift authorship. His procedures and techniques were in use around the world, but around this time, events in his personal life took a turn. While it may not have affected his professional development, it does give us an interesting insight into the man himself.

While preparing for a television documentary on his success, he met and became romantically involved with a television producer named Benita Alexander, who later reported their ventures in the magazine *Vanity Fair*.[32] Benita Alexander's self-effacing article in *Vanity Fair* reports that early in the relationship she had come across some irregularities in Macchiarini's CVs. He apparently had more than one, and they often contradicted one another. These irregularities usually related to his professional positions and achievements.

Alexander reported that during their interlude, they traveled to Greece, Turkey, Mexico, Italy, and the Bahamas. Macchiarini proposed marriage to Alexander, and they planned to marry in 2015 in Rome. No expense was to be spared. Macchiarini's divorce had come through (he said), and (although Alexander was already divorced) they asked to be married in the Catholic Church. Macchiarini claimed to have had a four-hour meeting with Pope Francis who had agreed to allow the wedding and, indeed, had offered to officiate and to host the wedding at the Apostolic Palace of Castel Gandolfo! After all, according to Macchiarini, he was the pontiff's "official doctor." Guests at the wedding were to include Bill and Hilary Clinton, President and Mrs. Obama, as well as Emperor Akihito of Japan, all of whom he had operated on. President Putin from Russia and France's Nicolas Sarkozy would also be attending, and Andrea Bocelli would sing at the service (even though he had not operated on them).

Alexander reports that during the wedding preparations, Macchiarini told two of the dressmakers who were homosexual married men that the pope had agreed to take confession and communion from them. She says, "I nearly fell off my chair." That was it for her. She later, with the help of friends, anonymously visited Macchiarini's home in Barcelona. Macchiarini came to the door but was shortly followed by his wife and two children. Dr. Paolo Macchiarini was a confidence man of the highest degree.[33]

Professionally, things began to get on the nose in 2014 when a group of surgeons complained that he did not have either ethics committee approval or animal evidence to support his procedures or, in many cases, consent from the patients themselves. Additionally, he was falsely reporting his results. Many patients died months after their operation, and many of the rest had to have their windpipes replaced with painful surgery. Strong stuff.[34,35]

There followed several inquiries into Macchiarini's scientific claims by the KI. Some initially did not implicate Macchiarini in scientific misconduct, but some did. Some cleared him. There were claims and counterclaims. Four of Macchiarini's colleagues were critical of his work. Professor Bengt Gerdin from Uppsala University announced that he was "not guilty of scientific misconduct," but KI contradicted this judgment and said that he had only acted "without due care."[36]

Macchiarini himself had a letter published in *The Lancet* with a compelling and convincing rebuttal of the charges, a sign of his ability to convince others of his alleged skills.[37] The controversy raged back and forth from 2014 to 2018. In 2016, the Royal Swedish Academy of Sciences accused Dr. Paulo

Macchiarini of "ethically indefensible working methods." In March that year, Macchiarini was dismissed from his position at KI. Professor Anders Hamsten, vice-chancellor of KI, resigned, saying that his own judgment "should be amended to indicate that it was scientific misconduct, in other words, research fraud." The collateral damage did not end there. The dean of research at Karolinska and the secretary-general of the Nobel Committee lost their jobs, as well as Harriet Wallberg, the chancellor of all Swedish universities, who lost hers.[33,38]

The story seems to be coming to an end with an expression of concern followed by a retraction of the original 2011 *The Lancet* article and three others attributed to Macchiarini, although one never knows with a man like him. Four of his articles have now been retracted as fraudulent. Will we ever know how many of the others are false?[39]

Big Business

Doctors are not the only ones affected by greed. Big business also likes to have its snout in the trough. One of the smallest companies in the USA was among the first to get in, eventually becoming one of the largest. It started out in the early 1990s when a small company was bought by the brothers *Arthur, Mortimer, and Raymond Sackler* who turned it into *Purdue Pharma LP*, one of the wealthiest family-owned companies in the USA. All three brothers were doctors and made their fortunes when they developed a slow-release form of an opioid, oxycodone hydrochloride, which they marketed as OxyContin. OxyContin was claimed to provide relief from pain for twelve hours compared with the better-known narcotics, such as pethidine, which only lasted for three to four hours. Oxycodone hydrochloride was developed in Germany in 1916, and being an opioid, the medical profession was wary of it and reluctant to prescribe it as opioids were known to have addiction risks.

Purdue recognized that this reluctance had to be overcome and released a massive marketing push. *Patrick Keefe*, in his masterful piece "The Family that Built an Empire of Pain," says that the company "paid doctors to make the case that concerns about opioid addiction were exaggerated and that OxyContin could safely treat an ever-wider range of maladies."[40] In 1995, the Federal Drug Administration (FDA) helped things along by approving OxyContin for use in treating mild to moderate pain. They went further and approved an enclosed leaflet that asserted that the pills were safer than other drugs as the delayed-release mechanism was thought to reduce the liability for abuse.[41] There was no empirical evidence to support this claim. In 1996, Purdue followed this up by sending hundreds of trained sales representatives out into the marketplace (i.e., to the doctors) to reassure them and overcome their objections and ensure that their prescribing habits changed in favor of the opioids. Follow-up studies showed that after a visit from a sales representative, prescribing of opioids had doubled; and by the year 2000, the opioid epidemic was in full bloom.

Most doctors just wanted to relieve their patients' pain, and that is what it did for many, but some patients began to return, complaining that the pain relief only worked for eight hours, not twelve. The advice that they got was to increase the dosage frequency to eighth hourly! This advice was the first sign of addiction in those patients. Other patients read the insert with the packet of pills and found that "if the pills were crushed and taken, it could result in a potentially toxic dose." In other words, do not do it. But some users found that crushing the pills and taking them resulted in a narcotic rush, so they crushed the pills and swallowed them. Purdue Pharma LP knew all this but still promoted their business, which grew at a frightening pace; as more and more opioids came into use, more and more became addicted and more and more died.[40,41] Now more people die from opioid overdose in the USA than die from motor vehicle accidents!

The business became huge, with an estimated value of US$13 billion. The Sackler brothers became philanthropists, supporting the arts and medicine. There is a Sackler Wing in the Metropolitan Museum of Art in New York. It houses a monument of the Temple of Dendur, a gift from the government of Egypt. There is an Arthur Sackler Gallery in the Smithsonian Institution in Washington, a Sackler Museum in Harvard, a Sackler Center for Arts Education at the Guggenheim, and a Sackler Wing at the Louvre, as well as Sackler wings at Columbia, Oxford, and other universities. But there is evidence that the largesse shown by the Sackler brothers is no longer appreciated. The Guggenheim Museum announced that it would no longer accept donations from the Sackler family, and similar rejections have come from London's Tate Gallery and New York's Columbia University.[42,43]

As the company finds itself the target of lawsuits in thirty-six states and more than 1,500 cities, this may be only the first sign of trouble. Not that it might bother the company much. It has already settled recent lawsuits for US$600 million and US$270 million.[17] Company policy is to pay in preference to court action, as the latter would bring to light the company practices. All three brothers are now dead, but the remaining eight family members still own the company and will likely soon be facing the charges.

The other industrial giants involved in the opioid business are Cardinal Health, McKesson, and AmerisourceBergen, which distribute more than 90 percent of the nation's drug and medical supplies. They, along with Johnson and Johnson, may become involved in the Purdue Pharma lawsuits.[44,45,46,47] There is some evidence that federal agencies—such as the FBI, the FDA, and the DEA—are taking more of an interest in the opioid problem.

As recently as December 2018, the Appalachian Regional Prescription Opioid Strike Force—consisting of prosecutors, federal agents, and data analysts—reported that charges were laid against sixty people, including thirty-one doctors, seven pharmacists, and eight nurses who were involved in schemes that included prescribing opioids for unnecessary medical procedures or in exchange for sexual favors and, in some cases, handing out blank prescription forms. The charges were aimed mainly at health professionals in the states of West Virginia, Ohio, and Kentucky (see chapter 11: "Dr. Paul Volkman—The Pill Mill Man").[19,20]

The Media and Their Editors

The editors of the popular print and electronic media must bear some responsibility for distributing misinformation, or "fake news" as ex-president Trump would say. In their anxiety (greed?) to sell copy and attract viewers, they are prepared to headline allegedly breathless new information before it has been confirmed. How often do we read or hear a report of some new development "which might be available in five years after further tests"?

One purpose of an editor is to accept or reject whatever he/she receives. If it seems to be a genuine beneficial discovery, the editor would be derelict in his/her duty not to publicize it. On the other hand, some discretion should be shown when publishing material that has not been confirmed. Consider the breathless announcement made by Professor Zuckerman concerning the MMR vaccine (see chapter 7: "Dr. Andrew J. Wakefield—Profit from Measles"). The newspapers trumpeted, "For the first time, MMR vaccine has been linked to a bowel disorder and the onset of autism in children." This claim had already been shown to be false, yet it was published, and the news went viral. Parents around the world jumped on the bandwagon, claiming that their child had developed autism due to the MMR vaccine. Even ex-president Trump helped the misconception by stating that he had a niece who had developed autism after receiving the MMR vaccine, although now he seems to have reversed his position.

Announcements such as that by Professor Zuckerman concerning MMR can be harmful by spreading false news. Inevitably, this led to increases in the incidence of measles corresponding with the drop in vaccination. Although the misconception has been largely overcome and vaccination rates have recovered, there are still pockets of resistance of parents who believe that their rights have been infringed; and in some cases, they have formed political parties called Anti-Vaxxers.

Hopefully, then, the editors of the print and electronic media can bear this heavy responsibility and focus their attention more on purveyors of truthful and reliable information rather than unfounded gossip.

The Peer Reviewers

Peer reviewers are used extensively by editors of scientific journals to assess the value and suitability of submitted works for publication in a journal. Authors of scientific work may feel pressured to publish or perish in pursuit of academic advancement. The reviewers should check that the data is correct and that it has passed through an appropriate ethics committee. The reviewers are usually anonymous but generally familiar with the field of work to be reviewed. The authors are typically unknown to the reviewer also. Elsevier, the publishing company of *The Lancet*, has issued some valuable comments on peer-reviewing. They are produced in part below:[48]

Single-Blind Review

In this type of review, the names of the reviewers are hidden from the author. This is the traditional method of reviewing and is the most common type by far. Points to consider regarding single-blind review include:

1. Reviewer anonymity allows for impartial decisions—the reviewers should not be influenced by the authors.
2. Authors may be concerned that reviewers in their field could delay publication, giving the reviewers a chance to publish first. [Dr. Robert Slutsky recorded examples of this in a paper in 1985 in which the reviewer noted that data was identical when Slutsky was applying for a promotion. In this case, the reviewer was uncannily observant. A reviewer would not usually pick up something like that.][49,50]
3. Reviewers may use their anonymity as justification for being unnecessarily critical or harsh when commenting on the authors' work.

Double-Blind Review

Both the reviewer and the author are anonymous in this model. Some advantages of this model are listed below.

1. Author anonymity limits reviewer bias, for example, based on an author's gender, country of origin, academic status or previous publication history.
2. Articles written by prestigious or renowned authors are considered on the basis of the content of their papers, rather than their reputation.

3. But bear in mind that despite the above, reviewers can often identify the author through their writing style, subject matter or self-citation—it is exceedingly difficult to guarantee total author anonymity.

The Whistleblowers

The word *whistleblower* derives from the days when a police officer blew his whistle to attract the attention of another officer who came to help. Nowadays, the name whistleblower can be given to someone who raises a concern about wrongdoing.[51] Unfortunately, the officer who responds nowadays may not want to help but would instead let things lie in the knowledge that to speak up in many cases will only cause friction. With this knowledge, the whistleblower is less likely to blow the whistle. In some circles, a "whistleblower is still presumed to be in a powerful professional regulatory position, to be a disaffected, antisocial, incompetent pariah 'not a team player' who fails to appreciate the damage he or she is causing to the hard-earned reputations of their professional colleagues and employer."[52] Nothing could be further from the truth. This is a sad situation because it highlights a culture where institutional self-regulation has failed, and it hinders any change in health care.

Whistleblowers are probably the largest group to expose the fraud. They are usually insiders who work in the same field as the fraudster but are junior in rank (see *Ms. Toni Hoffmann* in chapter 2, *Mr. Philip Vardy* and *Ms. Jill French* in chapter 8, and *Rosa Nicholson* in chapter 12). They may be scientists or nurses. Often they are dependent on the goodwill of their superior for their position and income. For this reason, it is dangerous if they speak up. They may have a family to support.

In other cases, they may be dependent on an organization or institution for employment or advancement in their career. In the case of Mr. Vardy and Ms. French, they had an additional problem. Dr. McBride essentially controlled Foundation 41, and the risk to them of speaking out was doubly difficult as they and other scientists found out to their chagrin. Mr. Vardy's marriage dissolved, and he moved to Tasmania. More than any other, they often have more to lose by speaking out. *Ian Freckelton*, in his hugely informative book *Scholarly Misconduct*, cites several examples of whistleblowers and the difficulties they face.[53]

Not all whistleblowers are junior in rank, but regardless, the consequences can be extensive. For example, *Dr. Stephen Bolsin* was a senior anesthetist at the Bristol Royal Infirmary–England. He became worried about the length of time taken to operate by the cardiothoracic surgeon, *Mr. James Wisheart*. This resulted in the deprivation of oxygen to the heart for lengthy periods with increased risk of damage not only to the heart but also to the brain. Between thirty and thirty-five children probably would not have died at the Bristol Royal Infirmary between 1991 and 1995 if their operation had been at another institution. Numerous others were brain-damaged. Dr. Bolsin started collecting data about the mortality and morbidity of the cardiac service at the Infirmary. When complete, he considered reporting his findings to senior administrators, but they advised him that such action would be hazardous to his career and might result in them suing him for defamation.

Later, when he pursued his complaints, much friction was caused between him and some of his colleagues, especially between the anesthetists and the surgeons. After the resultant imbroglio in June 1998 and after an investigation by the General Medical Council, three doctors (*Mr. James Wisheart, Mr. Janardan Dhasmana*, and *Dr. John Roylance*) were struck off the medical register.[54,55,56,57,58,59,60]

The subsequent tension and controversy resulted in Dr. Bolsin applying for other positions in the UK, but he found himself to be unemployable. He relocated himself and his family outside of the UK and is now at the Geelong Hospital near Melbourne where he also holds the title of professor at the Deakin University.[37] Professor Bolsin may be one of the more fortunate whistleblowers, compared with Mr. Phil Vardy and Ms. Jill French (described in chapter 8 of this book).

Dr. Margot O'Toole from Tufts University and the Massachusetts Institute of Technology (MIT) blew the whistle on her supervisor, *Dr. Thereza Imanishi-Kari* and *Dr. David Baltimore* (a Nobel laureate and president of Rockefeller University) who coauthored an article in *Cell* that relied on falsified data. Senior scientists at both institutions reviewed the paper, and they told Dr. O'Toole that "it was not possible to correct the material, and any correction would damage Dr. Imanishi-Kari's reputation, and the literature was so full of errors that one more would not matter." Dr. Baltimore himself said that the paper was grossly defective and that he would never trust Dr. Imanishi-Kari's work again! It is extraordinary that such an attitude can exist among scientists aiming at the truth. Dr. O'Toole was vilified and driven from her profession.[61]

Walter F. DeNino blew the whistle on *Dr. Eric T. Poehlman*, his previous mentor, when the latter asked him to proofread a study that claimed that in certain circumstances, women's health declined after the menopause. After analysis, DeNino found that the women's health improved in those circumstances. Having been told that, Poehlman changed the data to suit his theory. DeNino blew the whistle on Poehlman. In 2005, Poehlman resigned from his position at the University of Minnesota, was prohibited from ever again applying for funding grants, and had to repay $180,000, facing jail time in default.[62]

Many in the profession regard whistleblowers among those who make an important, even essential, contribution to the improvement of patient safety and health care. In 2002, inquiries into whistleblowing at three hospitals in Australia were revealing. The hospitals were the Canberra Hospital–

Australian Capital Territory; King Edward Memorial Hospital–Perth, Western Australia; and the Campbelltown and Camden hospitals in New South Wales. (The NSW hospitals are under conjoined management.) Some features were common to the findings in all three hospitals:

1. Sentinel-event reporting failed to detect the problem.
2. Senior clinicians viewed clinical governance as adequate.
3. *Whistleblowers were discouraged and criticized by the institution.* [Italics added—JA.]
4. A direct approach to politicians was needed to bring about any action.
5. A poor institutional culture was proven.[63]

Legislation in Australia, the UK, and the USA has been introduced to protect whistleblowers but with variable success.[27] This variable success suggests that the position of whistleblower should be strengthened and supported, even formalized and protected, not weakened and obliterated. A survey of whistleblowers in the USA in 2000 found that of eighty-seven whistleblowers, only one did not experience retaliation.[63] This culture and that expressed in point 3 above need to change. The whistleblower, perhaps more than any other, has a vital part in the removal of fraud. The whistleblower may be the key to the whole fraudulent situation. Whistleblowers are not greedy, and greed is where the problem lies.

Although that study was written twenty years ago, the same is likely to apply today. If change is to come about, it will need to come from the beginning.

Regardless of how many rules and regulations there are, it is likely that there will always be those among us who cannot control their greed and who will have to be controlled by our poor suffering patients unless we can find a way to control them ourselves. Otherwise, there will always be bad apples among us in the crop.

So What Are the Problems?

Fraud and deceit fall into two categories in this book. There is fraud in academia—searching for status, such as was seen with Dr. Hwang Woo-Suk, for example—and fraud in commerce, searching for money, as with Dr. Jayant Patel, who dishonestly found employment for himself. In either case, greed was the motivation that fueled the fraud. Most of the doctors in this book are in one category or the other.

When it comes to dealing with honest people, one would have thought that it would not be necessary to guide them along the straight and narrow. All the groups described below have a part to play in eliminating greed, causing deceit and fraud. But will they?

How, for instance, can one be expected to detect the fraud perpetrated by *Dr. Jon Sudbø* of Norway's Comprehensive Cancer Centre who claimed that common pain-relieving drugs, like ibuprofen, lowered the risk of oral cancer but increased the risk of serious cardiovascular events? He claimed that his study covered 454 people with oral cancer. The findings were published in *The Lancet* because it was thought to hold important information.[64]

He later admitted that the findings of all 454 so-called participants were a total figment of his imagination, yet in the article in *The Lancet,* he had ten coauthors! The editor of *The Lancet* later said that he thought that Sudbø was a "very clever fabricator. He fooled his colleagues, he fooled his hospital, he fooled his funding agency and he fooled the journal."

When it comes to deliberate, planned deceit and fraud, detection is not so easy.

The Doctors

Most doctors are honest folk who want to help others. Honesty is traditionally taught at home, making it unnecessary to teach in medical school, but medical schools should include ethics as a subject. The Hippocratic oath or the Physician's Pledge (see chapter 13) should be the basis of ethics as a subject. It may make little difference but should be taught anyway. An interview before admission to medical school may give a glimpse into a character. Once registered, every practitioner should be accredited in their field of expertise. It is no longer practical for a physician to be an expert in all areas of surgery. We have reached a stage where specialists need to be subspecialists. In orthopedics, for example, surgeons now specialize in knees or elbows or hands, and there are fewer generalists than there were years ago. More and more physicians are extending their areas of expertise into interventional medicine, and surgeons are moving into laparoscopic (keyhole) surgery. All practitioners should be accredited in more specialized areas of expertise. Also,

1. (forgery) scientific work should include the certified signatures of all authors,
2. gift authorship should not be permitted,
3. institutional ethics committee approval should be visualized,
4. plagiarism should be easily excluded nowadays with software programs.

The Supervising Institutions

The sponsoring institutions bear much of the blame for allowing fraud and deceit in scientific research. They are often protective of the fraudsters for several reasons. They worry that exposure will affect funding. The University of California failed to act when it suspected that Ricardo Asch was stealing human eggs. They feared that exposure would jeopardize their reputation and their budget. Dr. Eugene Braunwald of Harvard University downplayed the seriousness of John Darsee's fraud. He worried that senior people would lose their jobs. The dean and vice-chancellors of the famous Karolinska Institutet did lose their jobs. The Department of Health in Queensland worried that Jayant Patel would be lost to a system short of doctors, so they kept him on. The Sloan Kettering allowed William Summerlin to continue to work after his fraud was exposed. They may be merely careless as was Dr. Robert Good in his supervision of William Summerlin. They may be overworked and unable to cope. These famous institutions' reputations have suffered as a result of attempting to conceal the fraud. Hopefully, lessons have been learned from the fraud, and there is some evidence that things are changing. *Anesthesia and Analgesia*, for example, require that all authors sign to confirm that they have seen the raw data and that the work has been approved by the Institutional Ethics Committee.

The Governments and their Departments of Health

The departments of health, starting with the politicians, should be responsible for the appointment of appropriate senior personnel who will oversee the medical registration and licensing boards.

The Medical Registration/Licensing Boards

Original secondary and tertiary qualifications should be visualized by law before employment. These boards should check the applications of each candidate forensically. References and CVs are of secondary importance and should only be considered subsequently after the tertiary qualifications are certified.

The Investigative Journalists

Investigative journalists have played an essential role in exposing scientific fraud. They are similar to whistleblowers but do not work within the establishment and move in a freelance environment, enabling them to expose the fraud. If their findings are important and worthy of publication, they are paid for their work. Consider the efforts of Mr. Brian Deer, who exposed the fraudulent work of Andrew Wakefield. If Mr. Deer had not persisted in his investigative work, Wakefield's dishonesty might never have come to light. Also, the work of Mr. Hedley Thomas chronicling the sad situation in Queensland Health (see chapter 2) and Dr. Norman Swan in the case of William McBride. These journalists and others have been instrumental in improving the standard of health care, but they have no regulatory body to which they are responsible or one that oversees them. And neither should they because they are part of the solution.

The Editors of the Scientific Journals

The editors of the scientific journals perhaps have the most difficult task of all. They are pressured to publish as soon as possible, but at the same time, they have to satisfy themselves that the work is worthy of publication. In most cases, they do not see the raw material; and therefore, the detection of fraud is not likely from the material they receive. And if they did detect fraud, they would not publish it.

The Peer Reviewers

It is the task of the peer reviewer, using his or her specialized knowledge in the field, to recommend whether the work is worthy of a place in the journal. The peer reviewer, therefore, has an opportunity to observe whether there is fraud. However, a determined fraudster can usually conceal his work, as the peer reviewer has not had the opportunity to observe the raw data firsthand in the laboratory or workplace.

The Popular Press and Their Editors

The popular press and their editors are also in a difficult position. They are at the mercy of their readers and shareholders to maintain copy and profit and, at the same time, publish the truth, some of which they may not know. How can they know?

The Pharmaceutical Companies

The pharmaceutical companies perhaps care less than anyone (see chapter 11: "Dr. Paul Volkman—the Pill Mill Man"). They have, in many cases, spent many millions of dollars developing drugs that are now valuable, and they want their money back. They have shareholders too. But what if the drug is harmful? As patients and shareholders learned, we need to be wary of pharmaceutical companies that have doctors or researchers in their pay or on their boards. They may publish material that influences the marketing of medications, such as rofecoxib, sold as Vioxx, a drug used in the treatment of arthritis that was found, after many years, to have an increased risk of causing cardiovascular events. As Harlan Krumholz said in the *BMJ*, "In considering articles for publications, journals should understand that studies with immense financial implications require a higher level of scrutiny than others."[65] The raw data of these studies should perhaps be freely available. In 2011, Dr. Annette Katelaris, the editor of the *Medical Journal of Australia*, said that she was considering requiring authors to submit their raw data in cases of randomized controlled trials of drugs that could be practice changing. Others suggested that more public funds should be directed to drug research to reduce the reliance on support from the pharmaceutical industry, where researchers were often rewarded financially, either directly or in the form of stock options.[66]

Is there any way we can make them take notice?

The Whistleblowers

A constant thistle keeps sticking a thorn in every story in this book. It is the whistleblower. These are the people who see the default and eventually report it. Sadly, they usually end up suffering from their actions. They should be protected by law (and are in some countries), but they often still end up suffering, yet they are doing the best of all when it comes to defending the truth.[67] In an ideal world, all scientific work should be audited, as is our tax return. Regrettably, that is not possible, as the scientists want us to trust their work. If we are to trust them, then they must audit themselves and convince the rest of us that we can trust them.

What Can We Do about It?

The problem is multifactorial, so the solution must be multifactorial. A large part of the solution might be found by starting at the beginning of the problem.

Prospective medical students should be interviewed by an appropriate committee appointed by the school to establish their aptitude for the profession.

Medical schools should include ethics in their curriculum.

Universities and research institutes should tighten their standards for admission to research projects and should submit them for independent review before starting and again before publication.

Government regulators and employers need to be careful in checking qualifications. Penalties should apply for failure to do so.

Pharmaceutical companies are more difficult to control. They are driven by their shareholders. In many cases, they have made discoveries at great cost to them but at great benefit to the community at large.

Peer reviewers should be alert to dishonest data.

Whistleblowers should be protected by law. As Mr. Hedley Thomas said, talking about Ms. Toni Hoffman, "Don't scare whistleblowers into silence."[68] Ms. Hoffman achieved much as a whistleblower, including the right of nurses to report directly to the coroner or to a member of parliament.[69] Yes, strong stuff indeed.

It may be time to appoint a whistleblower officially. This individual could be appointed by the funding body—such as the NIH in the US, the NHT in the UK, or the NHMRC in Australia—and would be empowered to act at the most senior level, having excluded vexatious whistleblowing. He or she could be a confidante, a comfort, and maybe a guide with the powers of an auditor where necessary and the ability to block funding when deceit or fraud is detected but the researchers will not cooperate. I hear a deep inhalation of breath through pursed lips. "Cannot be done," you say. I say that it can. Accountants do it all the time. For our patients' sake, I say, let us do it. Otherwise, the system will rely on us hoping that the researchers are telling the truth.

Notes

1. 1. Walton, M. *The Trouble with Medicine*. Allen & Unwin: St. Leonards, NSW. 1998. pp. 173–175.
2. Andrist, E. "Fertility Doctor Uses His Sperm for Impregnations." The Patient Safety League (internet). 2016 (cited May 3, 2019). Available from http://4patientsafety.org/2016/09/13/dr-donald-cline/.
3. Maheshwari, P. "Donald Cline, Doctor Who Fathered Dozens of Children, Avoids Jail." The International Business Times (internet). 2017 (cited May 3, 2019). Available from https://www.ibtimes.com/donald-cline-doctor-who-fathered-dozens-children-avoids-jail-2628807.
4. Jolly, B. "Fertility Doctor Used Own Sperm to Father 48 Children without Parent's Knowledge." *The Daily Mail* (internet). 2019 (cited May 3, 2019). Available from https://www.mirror.co.uk/news/us-news/fertility-doctor-used-sperm-father-14156179.
5. Archives. "Doctor Found Guilty in Fertility Case." *The New York Times* (internet). 1992 (cited May 4, 2019); A00014. Available from https://www.nytimes.com/1992/03/05/us/doctor-is-found-guilty-in-fertility-case.html.
6. Associated Press. "Dutch Fertility Doctor Used His Sperm to Father Dozens of Children." *The Australian*. 2019.

7. Dyer, C. "Surgeon Faces Trial for Lying about His Experience in Keyhole Technique." *British Medical Journal*. 2017; 356: 513.

8. Dyer, C. "Surgeon Who Faked Keyhole Experience Is Jailed for Six Years." *BMJ*. 2018; 360(February 5): k574.

9. Oldham, J. "Rogue Surgeon Sudip Sarker Jailed for Six Years–Hospital-Trust Pays Out £2M Damages to Patients." *Birmingham Mail*. 2018.

10. Staff. "Former Cancer Surgeon Investigated over Patient Deaths Loses Unfair Dismissal Case." *Bromsgrove Advertiser* (internet). 2016 (cited April 30, 2019). Available from https://www.bromsgroveadvertiser.co.uk/news/14836601.former-alex-cancer-surgeon-investi-gated-over-patient-deaths-loses-unfair-dismissal-case/.

11. Dyer, C. "Police Investigate Work of UK Colorectal Surgeon after Patients Die." *BMJ*. 2014; 348(Feb. 25): g1,751

12. Mitchison, O. "The Trial of Rogue Doctor." The Hippocratic Post (internet). 2018 (cited May 2, 2019). Available from https://www.hippocraticpost.com/junior-doctors/the-trial-of-a-rogue-doctor/.

13. Marcovitz Hal. "Doctor Gets Virtual Life Term in Drug Case. He Sold OxyContin Prescriptions; Can't Be Paroled until Age 89." *The Morning Call*. June 21, 2002.

14. Cunningham, Melissa. "Fake Doctors to Face Jail Time under Tough New Penalties." *SMH*. July 1, 2019.

15. Parnell, Sean. "Harsher Laws for Impersonating Doctors, Nurses." *The Australian*. Oct. 8, 2021.

16. Lock, S., F. Wells. "Fraud and Misconduct in Medical Research." 1993. p. 6 et seq.

17. Ibid. pp. 10–11.

18. Dingell, J. D. "Special Article: Shattuck Lecture—Misconduct in Medical Research." *NEJM*. June 3, 1993.

19. "Fraudulent Harvard Researcher Loses Medical Practice License." *The Harvard Crimson*. September 28, 1984.

20. Kochan, C. A., J. M. Budd. "The Persistence of Fraud in the Literature: The Darsee Case." *J. of American Society for Information Science*. 1992; 43(7): 488–493.

21. Medawar, P. "The Strange Case of the Spotted Mice and Other Classic Essays on Science." Oxford: Oxford University Press; 2006.

22. Hixson, J. *The Patchwork Mouse*. Anchor Press/ Doubleday: Garden City, New York; 1976. p. 5 et seq.

23. Medawar. op. cit. ch. 12.

24. Hixson, J. op. cit. p. 35 et seq.

25. Hixson, J. op. cit. p. 40 et seq.

26. Rasco, John. "Boyer Lecture 3: Sins of the Flesh— Big Ideas." ABC Radio National (Australian broadcasting corporation). October 17, 2018.

27. Cheng, Maria. Associated Press. "Stem Cells Used in Transplanting Women's Trachea." *The Times-Tribune*. November 19, 2008.

28. Williams, Juliet, and Alicia Chang. "Woman Can Speak Again after Voice Box Transplant." *Santa Maria Times* (Santa Maria, California). January 23, 2011.

29. France-Presse, Agence. "Groundbreaking Windpipe Operation Inspires Two More." *The Province* (Vancouver, British Columbia, Canada). November 24, 2011.

30. Walker, Andrea K. "Synthetic Windpipe Saved Md. Man's. Life Sets New Milestone." *The Baltimore Sun*. January 14, 2012.

31. Fountain, Henry. "Doctors Working to Rebuild Organs from Patient's Cells." *Austin American-Statesman*. September 16, 2012.

32. Alexander, B. "The Celebrity Surgeon Who Used Love, Money, and the Pope to Scam an ABC News Producer." *Vanity Fair*. January 5, 2016.

33. Rasko, J., and C. Power. "Dr Con Man: The Rise and Fall of a Celebrity Scientist Who Fooled Almost Everyone." *The Guardian*. September 1, 2017.

34. Andrews, Travis M. "Medical Scandal Jolts Nobel Panel." *The Philadelphia Inquirer*. September 8, 2016.

35. Claesson-Welsh, Lena. "Tracheobronchial Transplantation: The Swedish Academy of Sciences' Concerns." *The Lancet*. March 5, 2016.

36. Editorial. "Paolo Macchiarini Is Not Guilty of Scientific Misconduct." *The Lancet*. September 5, 2015.

37. Macchiarini, P. "Tracheobronchial Transplantation." *The Lancet*. January 23, 2016.

38. Horton, R. Editorial. "Offline: Paolo Macchiarini— Science in Conflict." *The Lancet*. February 20, 2016.

39. "'The Final Verdict:' *Lancet* Retracts Two Papers by Macchiarini." *Retraction Watch*. July 6, 2018.

40. Keefe, P. "The Family that Built an Empire of Pain." *The New Yorker* (internet). 2017 (cited May 7, 2019). Available from https:// www.newyorker.com/magazine/2017/10/30/ the-family-that-built-an-empire-of-pain.

41. Stewart, C. "Opioids Epidemic: The Prophets of Pain." *The Australian* (internet). 2019 (cited May 7, 2019). Available from https://www.theaustralian.com. au/inquirer/opioids-epidemic-the-prophets-of-pain/ news-story/28a4d249545f405e1a871901e1e84cb6.

42. Stewart, C. "Opioids Epidemic: The Prophets of Pain." *The Australian* (internet). 2019 (cited May 7, 2019). Available from https://www.theaustralian.com. au/inquirer/opioids-epidemic-the-prophets-of-pain/ news-story/28a4d249545f405e1a871901e1e84cb6.

43. Chappell, B. "Sackler Family's Donation to British Museum Is Quashed over Opioid Fallout." NPR Newscast. 2019.

44. Temple, J. *American Pain*. 1st ed. Guilford, Connecticut: Rowman & Littlefield; 2016.

45. Staff. "Doctor Sentenced on Illegal Distribution of Oxycontin." *Los Angeles Times* (internet). 2019 (cited May 7, 2019). Available from https://www.latimes.com/archives/la-xpm-2002-jun-21-na-oxycontin21-story.html.

46. Robertson, C. "Thirty-One Doctors, 32 Million Pills: Sweeping Opioid Case Revealed." *The Australian*. 2019.

47. Hakim, D., W. Rashbaum, R. Rabin. "The Giants at the Heart of the Opioid Crisis." *The New York Times*. 2019. *Sydney Morning Herald*. May 29, 2019.

48. "What Is Peer Review?" Elsevier.com (internet). 2019 (cited May 28, 2019). Available from https://www.elsevier.com/reviewers/what-is-peer-review.

49. Phillips, M. "Peer Review." *The Lancet*. 2000; 355(9204): 660.

50. Lock and Wells. op. cit. p. 11 et seq.

51. Bolsin, S., R. Pal, P. Wilmshurst, M. Pena. "Whistleblowing and Patient Safety: The Patient's or the Profession's Interests at Stake?" *Journal of the Royal Society of Medicine*. 2011; 104(7): 278–282.

52. Faunce, T., S. Bolsin, W. Chan. "Supporting Whistleblowers in Academic Medicine: Training and Respecting the Courage of Professional Conscience." *Journal of Medical Ethics*. 2004; 30(1): 40–43.

53. Freckelton, I. *Scholarly Misconduct*. 1st ed. Oxford: Oxford University Press; 2016. pp. 484 et seq. 53. Dyer, C. "Bristol Inquiry." *BMJ*. 2001; 323(7306): 181.

54. Dunn, P. "The Wisheart Affair: Paediatric Cardiological Services in Bristol, 1990–5." *BMJ*. 1998; 317(7166): 1,144–1,145.

55. Wisheart, J., J. Dhasmana. "The Bristol Affair: Lessons to Be Learned." *The Annals of Thoracic Surgery*. 2001; 71(4): 1,403–1,404.

56. Bolsin, S., J. Stewart. "The Wisheart Affair: Responses to Dunn. The Bristol Cardiac Disaster Editor's Response to Stephen Bolsin a Patient's Perspective." *BMJ.* 1998; 317(7172): 1,579–1,582.

57. Dyer, C. "Bristol Doctors Found Guilty of Serious Professional Misconduct." *BMJ.* 1998; 316(7149): 1,924–1,924.

58. Bolsin, S. "Professional Misconduct: The Bristol Case." *Medical Journal of Australia.* 1998; 169(7): 369–372.

59. Ramsay, S. "UK 'Bristol Case' Doctors Found Guilty of Misconduct." *The Lancet.* 1998; 351(9120): 1,935.

60. Vick, L. "Bristol Children's Heart Scandal: 20 Years on from the GMC Hearing." Enable Law. Oct. 17, 2017. Available from https://www.enablelaw.com/news/latest-news/bristol-childrens-heart-scandal-20-years-gmc-hearings/.

61. Hilts, P. J. "Crucial Research Data in Report Biologist Signed Are Held Fake: Nobelist to Ask Retraction on Paper He Defended." *The New York Times.* March 21, 1991: A1, B10.

62. Poehlman, E. T. "Effects of Endurance Training on Total Fat Oxidation in Elderly Persons." *Physiol.* 1985. Retracted.

63. Faunce, T., S. Bolsin. "Three Australian Whistleblowing Sagas: Lessons for Internal and External Regulation." *Medical Journal of Australia.* 2004; 181(1): 44–47.

64. Sudbø, J., J. J. Lee, S. M. Lippman, J. Mork, S. Sagen, N. Flatner, A. Ristimäki, A. Sudbø, L. Mao, X. Zhou, W. Kidal, J. F. Evensen, A. Reith, A. J. Dannenberg. "Non-Steroidal Anti-Inflammatory Drugs and the Risk of Oral Cancer: A Nested Case-Control Study." *The Lancet.* Oct. 15–21, 2005; 366(9494): 1,359–66. Retracted.

65. Krumholz, H., et al. "What Have We Learnt from Vioxx?" *BMJ.* 2007: 334,120.

66. Medow, J. "Bad Medicine." *The Sydney Morning Herald*. May 12, 2011.
67. Yamey, G. "Protecting Whistleblowers." *BMJ*. 2000; 320(7227): 70–71.
68. Thomas, H. "Don't Scare Whistleblowers into Silence." *The Australian*. October 21, 2019.
69. Fedele, R. "Blowing the Whistle." *Australian Nursing and Midwifery Journal*. May 22, 2019; 26: p. 14.

Suggested Further Reading

Walton, M. *The Trouble with Medicine*. St. Leonards, NSW: Allen & Unwin; 1998.

Freckelton, I. *Scholarly Misconduct*. 1st ed. Oxford: Oxford University Press; 2016.

Medawar, P. *The Strange Case of the Spotted Mice and Other Classic Essays on Science*. Oxford: Oxford University Press; 2006.

Keefe, P. "Empire of Pain." *The New Yorker* (internet). 2017 (cited May 7, 2019). Available from https://www.newyorker.com/magazine/2017/10/30/the-family-that-built-an-empire-of-pain

Hixson J. *The Patchwork Mouse*. Anchor Press/Doubleday. Garden City, New York 1976.

INDEX

Rimland, Barnard, 155
Roewer, Norbert, 108, 119
Roh, Sung-Il, 102
Rouse, Andrew, 152, 167
rubella, 140, 144, 146
"The Runaway Doctor"
 (Bissinger), 232

S

Sackler family, 263, 369, 371,
 389
Sarker, Sudip, 357–59, 387
Sasai, Yoshiki, 87–89, 91, 93-
 96, 351, 360
 death, 93-94
Scioto County, 243–44, 247,
 249, 251, 262, 265-66, 268
Shafer, Stephen, 113-14, 117
sinuses, 223–24, 226-27,
 231-32
Sister Maria (nursing sister in
 Dr. Bailey's clinic), 281-82
Skinner, Jillian, 318–19, 322
Snuppy (first cloned dog),
 100–102
somatic cell nuclear transfer
 (SCNT), 100, 104
Specogna, Monica, 232–35
STAP cells, 90-91, 93, 96
stem cells
 types of, 88
Stone, Sergio, 20–22, 27-28,
 30, 38, 41

Strike Force Tarella, 318, 341
Sudbø, Jon, 379, 391
Summerlin, William, 362–66,
 381
Swan, Norman, 195, 382
Sydney Swans, 133–35, 137

T

Tepperman, Rob, 97–98
thalidomide, 173, 176-80,
 182-85, 194-95, 198–200,
 205-6, 247, 351
The Lancet, 20, 45, 47, 148-
 49, 151-54, 157-61, 164-69,
 179, 199-200, 368-69, 373,
 379, 389-91
theriogenology, 99
"The Runaway Doctor"
 (Bissinger), 232
thimerosal, 154-55, 157, 168
Thomas, Hedley, 52, 83, 85,
 382, 385
Tri-State Healthcare, 258,
 260–262
Tuinal, 277, 294
2,4,5-T, 189-90

U

University of California–
 Irvine (UCI), 21–22, 26,
 28–31, 33-36, 40-41, 46-49
 settling dozen lawsuits, 41

Z